Essentials of Radiologic Science

Robert A. Fosbinder, B.A., R.T.(R)

Radiography Program Director
University of New Mexico
Albuquerque, New Mexico

Charles A. Kelsey, Ph.D.

Professor of Radiology
Department of Radiology
University of New Mexico School of Medicine
Albuquerque, New Mexico

McGraw-Hill
MEDICAL PUBLISHING DIVISION

New York   Chicago   San Francisco   Lisbon   London   Madrid   Mexico City   Milan
New Delhi   San Juan   Seoul   Singapore   Sydney   Toronto

McGraw-Hill

A Division of The McGraw·Hill Companies

Essentials of Radiologic Science

1234567890   KGPKGP   0987654321

ISBN 0-07-136452-8

This book was set in Caledonia by Rainbow Graphics, LLC.
The editors were Sally Barhydt and Muza Navrozov.
The production supervisor was Richard Ruzycka.
The index was prepared by Alexandra Nickerson.
Quebecor World/Kingsport was printer and binder.

This book is printed on acid-free paper.

Library of Congress Cataloging-in-Publication Data
Fosbinder, Robert.
    Essentials of radiologic science/Robert A. Fosbinder, Charles A. Kelsey.
      p. ; cm.
    Includes bibliographical references and index.
    ISBN 0-07-136452-8
    1. Radiography, Medical. I. Kelsey, Charles A. II. Title.
    [DNLM: 1. Technology, Radiologic. 2. Radiation Protection. WN 160 F746e 2001]
RC78.F574 2001
616.07'57—dc21

                                                       2001030062

Essentials of Radiologic Science

Contents

Preface

The field of radiography has changed rapidly since the discovery of x-rays in 1897 by Wilhelm Conrad Roentgen. Technical advances in medical imaging allow visualization of the human body in ways that were unimagined just 25 years ago. Yet in spite of these great technical advances, the basic concepts of radiography and image formation remain the same as they were 100 years ago. An understanding of these fundamental principles of radiography is vital to adapting to future changes in radiology. Our combined experience of over 40 years of teaching radiography students has taught us that the students have varied academic backgrounds with different strengths and weaknesses, especially in mathematics and science. This text is the result of our classroom teaching experience. Our goal in developing this text was to produce an understandable textbook written clearly and concisely without extraneous material. In our experience, the material in this text has produced graduates who are able to pass the American Registry of Radiologic Technologists (ARRT) examination in the three content-specific areas of radiation protection, equipment operation, and maintenance and image production.

We have highlighted the important points of each section in italics for emphasis and reinforcement, and we have provided a summary of the material at the end of each chapter. The practice questions at the end of each chapter provide positive feedback for those who understand the concepts of the chapter and identify those areas in which the student is having trouble and needs more help from the instructor. The chapter questions are written in the ARRT multiple-choice format to allow the students to become familiar with taking tests in this format.

This is not a self-study book; it is a textbook designed to be used under the direction of an instructor. We hope that instructors find this book easy for their students to read and understand, and we know they will find it a useful addition to their courses. The book is divided into five units: basic physics, circuits and x-ray production, image formation, special imaging techniques, and radiation protection. These units can be divided to form the basis of individual required classes within an approved School of Radiologic technology. This material has also proved valuable to practicing radiographers preparing for credentialing by the ARRT in advanced-level examinations in mammography, computed tomography, magnetic resonance imaging, and quality assurance/management.

Acknowledgments

We would both like to thank our past and present students who served to refine and improve this textbook. We would also like to thank our chairman, Fred A. Mettler, Jr., M.D., for his support during the time it took to bring this textbook to publication.

Charles A. Kelsey thanks his wife, Judy, for all her loving support. Robert A. Fosbinder thanks his wife, Tracy, and his children, Ryan and Kyle, for all their loving support during the time spent away from them while developing this textbook.

Essentials of Radiologic Science

Unit I

Basic Physics

1

Atoms and Atomic Structure

OBJECTIVES

Upon completion of this chapter, the student will be able to

1. Describe the Bohr model of the atom and its components.
2. Define electron binding energy.
3. Describe the process of ionization.
4. Define atomic mass and atomic number.
5. Identify the types of ionizing radiation.

INTRODUCTION

Knowledge of atomic structure and how atoms interact is fundamental to an understanding of how x-rays are generated and used to produce diagnostic images. In this chapter, we cover the Bohr model of the atom, atomic structure, and the ionization of atoms.

ATOMIC STRUCTURE

Atoms are the fundamental building blocks of nature. They cannot be broken into smaller parts by chemical means. Elements are substances made up of atoms of only one type. Atoms of the same or different elements can combine to form molecules. The combination of two hydrogen atoms with one oxygen

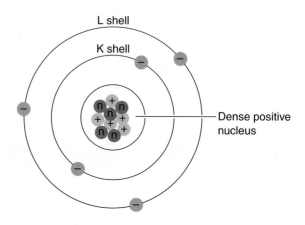

Figure 1.1 **The Bohr model of the atom.**

atom to form one water molecule is an example. Atoms are too small to see, even with the most powerful microscopes. Therefore, instead of describing the atom in terms of what we see, we use models to describe the atom. There have been many atomic models, beginning with those of the Greeks, who believed that there were four types of atoms: air, earth, fire, and water. Both Thomson and Dalton proposed models, but today the generally accepted atomic model is the Bohr model. The Bohr model describes the atom as a central dense, positive nucleus surrounded by electrons moving in shells or orbits similar to our solar system. Most of the space in an atom is empty. If the nucleus were the size of a pinhead, the diameter of the atom would be the length of a football field. The electrons are negative, and the nucleus is positive. Figure 1.1 illustrates the essential features of the Bohr model of the atom.

The nucleus contains nuclear particles called nucleons. **Nucleons** are either protons or neutrons. Protons have a single positive charge; neutrons have zero charge. Atoms are electrically neutral. The positive charges in the nucleus equal the negative electrons in their shells around the nucleus.

ELECTRON SHELLS

The electrons in an atom move around the nucleus in specific shells. The number of shells occupied in a particular atom depends on how many protons there are in the nucleus. There is a limit to how many electrons can occupy each shell. The shell closest to the nucleus is called the K shell and can hold no more than two electrons. If an atom has more than two protons within the nucleus, the additional electrons are located in shells that are farther from the nucleus. Atoms with more protons in the nucleus have more electrons in the surrounding shells. The shells are also identified by shell number—1, 2, 3, 4, and so on, in order of increasing distance from the nucleus. The order of

Table 1.1
Number of Electrons in Atomic Shells

Shell	Shell Number	Maximum Number That the Shell Can Hold
K	1	2
L	2	8
M	3	18
N	4	32
O	5	50
P	6	72
Q	7	98

the shell is important because the shell number indicates the maximum number of electrons the shell can hold.

The maximum number of electrons that can be contained in a shell is given by the equation

$$\text{Maximum number} = 2n^2$$

where n is the shell number. For shell number 3, also called the M shell, the maximum number of electrons that can occupy the shell is

$$\text{Maximum number} = 2 \times (3)^2$$
$$= 2 \times 9$$
$$= 18 \text{ electrons}$$

Table 1.1 presents the letter designations of the shells, the shell numbers, and the maximum number of electrons that can occupy each shell.

Figure 1.2 diagrams the shell structure for hydrogen, carbon, and sodium. Hydrogen has a single electron in its single shell. Carbon has two electrons in the K shell and four electrons in the L shell. Sodium has eleven electrons contained in three shells: two in the K shell, eight in the L shell, and one in the M shell.

Although the maximum number of electrons that a shell can hold is $2n^2$, there is another rule that may override this: The outer shell of an atom can never contain more than eight electrons.

ELECTRON SHELL BINDING ENERGY

Electron binding energy describes how tightly the electron is held in its shell. The negative electron is attracted to the positive nucleus by electrostatic

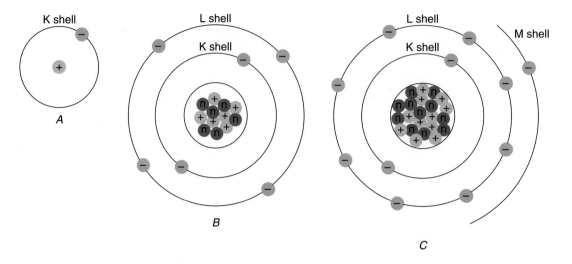

Figure 1.2 *A.* **Electronic shell structure for hydrogen (Z = 1).** *B.* **Electronic shell structure for carbon (Z = 6).** *C.* **Electronic shell structure for sodium (Z = 11).**

forces. Electrons in shells closer to the nucleus have a stronger attraction. The K shell always has the highest binding energy. The electron binding energy is the energy required to remove an electron from its shell. Small atoms with fewer protons in the nucleus have lower binding energies; larger atoms with more protons in the nucleus have higher binding energies. Electron binding energies can be as small as a few electron volts or as large as thousands of electron volts. An electron volt is a unit of energy.

IONIZATION

Ionization is the process of removing an electron from its shell. Radiation that has enough energy to remove an electron from its shell is known as ionizing radiation. The removed electron is called a **negative ion,** and the remaining positively charged atom is called a **positive ion.** Figure 1.3 shows the formation of a positive and a negative ion, also called an **ion pair.** The energy available to form the positive and negative ions must be sufficient to overcome the binding energy of the orbital electron or ionization will not occur.

Ionization always results in the formation of a positive ion and a negative ion. Ions can expose film, activate radiation detectors, and produce biologic effects.

The Bohr model of the atom consists of a dense central core containing positive protons and neutral neutrons surrounded by negative electrons

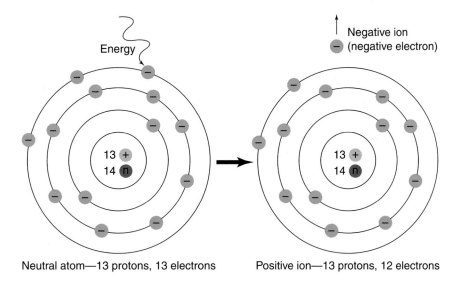

Figure 1.3 **Formation of an ion pair as an electron is removed from the atom.**

in orbits or shells. The maximum number of electrons that can occupy a shell is 2n², except that the outer shell can hold no more than eight electrons. Ionization is the removal of an electron from its shell. Electrons in shells closer to the nucleus have a higher binding energy, and so more energy is required to remove them from their orbits.

ATOMIC MASS

Because the masses of protons and neutrons are so small, the atomic mass unit (**AMU**) is used instead of the kilogram to describe the mass of an atom. The proton and neutron each weigh almost exactly 1 AMU. The electron is about 2000 times lighter. Table 1.2 gives the atomic mass, in kilograms and in AMUs, and the charge of the electron, the proton, and the neutron.

Table 1.2
Characteristics of Atomic Particles

Particle	Atomic Mass		Charge
	Kilograms	AMU	
Electron	9.1×10^{-31}	0.00055	−1
Proton	1.6726×10^{-27}	1.00728	+1
Neutron	1.6749×10^{-27}	1.00867	0

The **atomic mass** number is the mass of the atom in AMUs. It is the sum of the number of protons and the number of neutrons in the nucleus. The mass of the orbital electrons in an atom is so small that their contribution to the atomic mass is usually ignored. The atomic mass number is symbolized by A. It is written above and to the left of the chemical symbol. An element Y with atomic mass A is written ^{A}Y.

ATOMIC NUMBER

The **atomic number** is equal to the number of protons in the nucleus. The atomic number is symbolized by Z. An element Y with an atomic number Z and an atomic mass A would be written ^Z_AY, where Y is the chemical symbol for the element. The symbol for carbon with six protons and six neutrons is $^{12}_6$C. The atomic number Z is always smaller than the atomic mass number A, except for hydrogen, where A and Z are equal. Table 1.3 gives the chemical symbol, atomic mass in AMU, atomic number, and K-shell binding energies of some elements of interest in radiology. Larger atoms with higher atomic numbers and larger atomic mass numbers have higher binding energies.

PERIODIC TABLE

The periodic table of the elements lists the elements in ascending order of atomic number. Figure 1.4 presents a portion of the periodic table. The periodic table is arranged so that elements with similar chemical characteristics lie underneath one another. For example, fluorine, chlorine, bromine, and iodine all have similar chemical properties. That is, when they combine with hydrogen, they form acids; when they combine with sodium, they form crystals.

Table 1.3
Some Elements of Interest in Radiology

Element	Symbol	Atomic Mass (AMU)	Atomic Number	K-Shell Binding Energy (keV)
Hydrogen	$^1_1$H	1	1	0.01
Carbon	$^{12}_6$C	12	6	0.3
Oxygen	$^{16}_8$O	16	8	0.5
Aluminum	$^{27}_{13}$Al	27	13	1.6
Calcium	$^{40}_{20}$Ca	40	20	4.0
Iodine	$^{130}_{53}$I	130	53	33.2
Barium	$^{137}_{56}$Ba	137	56	37.4
Tungsten	$^{185}_{74}$W	185	74	69.6
Lead	$^{209}_{82}$Pb	209	82	88.0

1 H																	2 He
3 Li	4 Be											5 B	6 C	7 N	8 O	9 F	10 Ne
11 Na	12 Mg											13 Al	14 SI	15 P	16 S	17 Cl	18 A
19 K	20 Ca	21 Sc	22 Ti	23 V	24 Cr	25 Mn	26 Fe	27 Co	28 Ni	29 Cu	30 Zn	31 Ga	32 Ge	33 As	34 Se	35 Br	36 Kr
37 Rb	38 Sr	39 Y	40 Zr	41 Nb	42 Mo	43 Tc	44 Ru	45 Rh	46 Pa	47 Ag	48 Cd	49 In	50 Sn	51 Sb	52 Te	53 I	54 Xe
55 Cs	56 Ba	*	72 Hf	73 Ta	74 W	75 Re	76 Os	77 Ir	78 Pt	79 Au	80 Hg	81 Tl	82 Pb	83 Bi	84 Po	85 At	86 Rn
87 Fr	88 Ra	*															

* Rare-earth elements go here.

Figure 1.4 A portion of the periodic table of the elements.

The periodic table gets its name from the fact that the chemical properties of the elements are repeated periodically. The simplest element is hydrogen, with an atomic number of 1. The next heavier element is helium, a light inert gas with an atomic number of 2 and an atomic mass of 4. The first row of the periodic table is unusual because it contains only two elements. The first element in the second row is lithium. Lithium has an atomic number of 3 and has one electron in the L shell. This lone electron in the outer shell makes lithium chemically reactive.

If the atomic number is increased by one, the number of electrons in the outer shells also increases by one. There are eight elements in each row because the outer shell can contain no more than eight electrons. Elements lying beneath one another in the periodic table have the same number of electrons in their outer shell. Their chemical characteristics are similar because the chemical characteristics are determined by the number of electrons in the outer shell. The first elements in the next three rows of the periodic table are sodium, potassium, and rubidium. Each of these elements has a single electron in the outer shell and has chemical characteristics similar to those of lithium. Each row in the periodic table ends with an inert nonreactive gas. These gases are inert because their outer electron shell is filled with eight electrons and thus has no need to combine with other atoms.

Figure 1.5 shows the information contained in each cell of the periodic table. In the periodic table, the atomic number is located above the chemical symbol and the atomic weight is listed below the symbol. The atomic weight shown in the periodic table is an average of the masses of the different isotopes and is usually not a whole number. For example, the chemical symbol for calcium is Ca. Its atomic number is 20, and its atomic weight is 40.08 AMU.

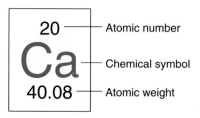

Figure 1.5 Information contained in a cell of the periodic table.

ISOTOPES

Atoms of the same element whose nuclei contain the same number of protons but a different number of neutrons are called isotopes. The **isotopes** of an element all have the same chemical characteristics because they all have the same number of outer-shell electrons. Table 1.4 shows some of the different isotopes of calcium.

Some isotopes do not occur in nature and must be artificially produced. Their natural abundance is zero.

ATOMIC WEIGHT

The **atomic weight** is an average of the atomic masses of all the isotopes of an element multiplied by the naturally occurring percentage of each.

Table 1.4

Different Isotopes of Calcium

Symbol	Number of Neutrons	Number of Protons	Natural Abundance
$^{39}_{20}$Ca	19	20	0.0
$^{40}_{20}$Ca	20	20	96.9%
$^{41}_{20}$Ca	21	20	0.0
$^{42}_{20}$Ca	22	20	0.6%
$^{43}_{20}$Ca	23	20	0.15%
$^{44}_{20}$Ca	24	20	2.1%
$^{45}_{20}$Ca	25	20	0.0

RADIOISOTOPES

Most isotopes are stable, but some are unstable and spontaneously transform into a different element. Unstable isotopes are termed **radioisotopes** or radioactive isotopes. Their nuclei have an excess number of protons or neutrons. Radioactivity is the spontaneous transformation of one element into another element, accompanied by the release of electromagnetic or particulate radiation. The atomic number of radioactive nuclei changes during the nuclear transformation. The transformation of radioactive nuclei into a different element is also termed **radioactive decay.**

Atomic mass is measured in atomic mass units (AMUs). The proton and the neutron each have a mass of 1 AMU. The number of nucleons in the nucleus is the sum of the number of protons and neutrons. The atomic mass of an atom is equal to the number of nucleons in the atomic nucleus. The atomic number is the number of positive charges in the nucleus, which is equal to the number of protons in the nucleus. Atoms that have the same number of protons but different numbers of neutrons in their nuclei are called isotopes. Isotopes of the same element have the same chemical characteristics but different atomic masses. Radioactive isotopes are unstable. They spontaneously transform into a different element and emit ionizing radiation during the transformation. The average of all naturally occurring isotopes of an element is its atomic weight. The periodic table arranges the elements in order of increasing atomic number. Elements located in the same column of the periodic table have similar chemical characteristics.

HALF-LIFE

The half-life of a radioisotope is the time required to transform half the atoms of the original element into the final element. The half-life depends on the radioisotope. For example, ^{39}Ca has a half-life of 0.8 second(s), the half-life of ^{41}Ca is 8×10^4 years, and the half-life of ^{45}Ca is 165 days. The amount of radioactivity remaining after a time T is shown in Table 1.5. mBq and a millicurie are units of radioactivity.

IONIZING RADIATION

A radioisotope can release different forms of ionizing radiation, which can be either electromagnetic or particulate radiation. X-rays and gamma rays are

Table 1.5
^{39}Ca Radioactivity Remaining after Time T

Time (s)	Number of Half-lives	Percent of Initial Radioactivity Remaining after Time T
0	0	100
0.8	1	50
1.6	2	25
2.4	3	12.5
3.2	4	6.25
4.0	5	3.13

forms of electromagnetic radiation. Alpha particles and beta particles are forms of particulate radiation. Ionizing radiation produces ion pairs when it passes through substances such as air or tissue.

Most radioisotopes emit gamma rays. Gamma rays and x-rays are both forms of electromagnetic radiation and differ only in their source or origin. Gamma rays are produced in the nucleus. X-rays are produced through interactions in atomic shells.

Alpha Particles

An alpha particle is a form of particulate radiation that consists of two protons and two neutrons. It has an atomic mass of 4 and an atomic number of 2. It is identical to the nucleus of a helium atom. An alpha particle is very large compared to other types of radiation but is not very penetrating. Alpha particles have no applications in diagnostic radiology.

Beta Particles

A beta particle is an electron. It has a single negative charge and a mass of about 1/2000 AMU. A beta particle is more penetrating than an alpha particle but less penetrating than a gamma ray or an x-ray. Beta particles are encountered in nuclear medicine applications.

Alpha particles, beta particles, gamma rays, and x-rays are forms of ionizing radiation. Ionizing radiation has enough energy to remove an orbital electron from its shell, producing a positive ion and a negative electron. Alpha particles have a very short range; they penetrate less than a millimeter into tissue. Beta particles penetrate several millimeters into tissue. X-rays and gamma rays penetrate many centimeters of tissue.

SUMMARY

The Bohr model of the atom consists of a dense positive nucleus surrounded by electrons in shells. The nucleus contains nucleons, which are either protons or neutrons. The proton has a positive charge and an atomic mass of 1 AMU. The neutron has zero charge and an atomic mass of 1 AMU. The atomic number Z is equal to the number of protons in the nucleus. The atomic mass A is equal to the sum of the number of neutrons and protons in the nucleus. The electron has a negative charge and a mass of almost zero. Electrons in an atom move only in specific orbits. Each orbit or shell has its own binding energy. The binding energy is the energy required to remove an electron from the shell. The shells closer to the nucleus have higher binding energies. Ionization occurs when an electron is removed from an atom. This results in an ion pair made up of one positive and one negative ion. Ionizing radiation consists of electromagnetic and particulate radiation with enough energy to ionize atoms. X-rays and gamma rays are forms of electromagnetic radiation. Alpha and beta particles are forms of particulate radiation.

Elements with similar electron shell structures have similar chemical properties. Isotopes are elements with the same atomic number but different atomic masses. Isotopes have the same chemical properties. The atomic weight of an element is the average of the atomic masses of naturally occurring isotopes. When elements are arranged in order of increasing atomic number, they form the periodic table of the elements. The chemical characteristics of the elements are repeated periodically, and elements that lie in the same column of the periodic table have similar chemical properties. Radioisotopes undergo spontaneous transformation. The atomic number and atomic weight of a radioisotope can change during radioactive transformation or decay. The half-life of a radioisotope is the time required for half the material to transform. Radioisotopes can emit electromagnetic radiation, beta particles, or alpha particles.

QUESTIONS

1. The Bohr model of the atom consists of the following:
   a. A dense positive nucleus surrounded by a diffuse cloud of negative charge
   b. A dense positive nucleus surrounded by electrons in definite shells
   c. A dense negative nucleus surrounded by a diffuse cloud of positive charge
   d. A dense negative nucleus surrounded by protons in definite shells

2. The nucleus of an atom contains which of the following?
   1. Protons
   2. Neutrons
   3. Electrons
   4. Gamma rays
   a. 1
   b. 1 and 2
   c. 2 and 3
   d. 1, 2, and 3
3. Nucleons consist of which of the following?
   1. Protons
   2. Neutrons
   3. Electrons
   4. Gamma rays
   a. 1
   b. 1 and 2
   c. 2 and 3
   d. 1, 2, and 3
4. The electron shell closest to the nucleus is termed the _____ shell.
   a. K
   b. L
   c. M
   d. N
5. The electron shell second closest to the nucleus is termed the _____ shell.
   a. K
   b. L
   c. M
   d. N
6. The third electron shell from the nucleus is termed the _____ shell.
   a. K
   b. L
   c. M
   d. N
7. The maximum number of electrons that the K shell can contain is
   a. 2.
   b. 4.
   c. 8.
   d. 18.
8. The outermost shell can contain no more than _____ electrons.
   a. 2
   b. 4
   c. 8
   d. 18

9. Which electron shell in an atom has the highest binding energy?
   a. K
   b. L
   c. M
   d. N
10. The binding energy of the _____ shell in an atom is greater than that of the _____ shell.
    a. L; K
    b. L; M
    c. M; K
    d. N; L
11. The electron binding energy is
    a. the energy of attraction between electrons in the shells.
    b. the energy required to remove the nucleus from an atom.
    c. the energy required to remove an electron from the nucleus.
    d. the energy required to remove an electron from its shell.
12. When an electron is removed from an atom, the atom is said to be
    a. neutralized.
    b. ionized.
    c. electrified.
    d. radioactive.
13. An ion pair consists of
    a. two positive ions.
    b. two negative ions.
    c. a positive ion and a negative ion.
14. The element $^{11}_{5}B$ has _____ protons.
    a. 5
    b. 6
    c. 11
    d. 16
15. The element $^{11}_{5}B$ has an atomic mass of
    a. 5.
    b. 6.
    c. 11.
    d. 16.
16. The element $^{11}_{5}B$ has _____ neutrons in its nucleus.
    a. 5
    b. 6
    c. 11
    d. 16
17. The atomic mass number of an atom is
    a. the number of protons.
    b. the number of neutrons.
    c. the number of protons and electrons.
    d. the number of protons and neutrons.

18. The atomic number is
    a. the number of protons.
    b. the number of neutrons.
    c. the number of protons and electrons.
    d. the number of protons and neutrons.
19. The periodic table of the elements lists the elements in order of increasing
    a. atomic number.
    b. atomic weight.
    c. atomic neutrons.
    d. atomic ionization.
20. Isotopes are
    a. atoms with the same atomic mass but different atomic numbers.
    b. atoms with the same atomic number but different mass numbers.
    c. atoms with the same number of neutrons.
    d. atoms with the same radioactivity.
21. The half-life of a radioisotope is
    a. the time required for half the atoms to be converted to electrons.
    b. the time required for half the electron shells to be filled.
    c. the time required for half the original atoms to be transformed.
    d. the time required for half the atoms to become radioactive.
22. Electromagnetic radiation includes
    a. x-rays.
    b. beta particles.
    c. alpha particles.
    d. neutrons.
23. The most penetrating ionizing radiation is
    a. alpha particles.
    b. beta particles.
    c. gamma rays.
    d. neutrons.
24. The least penetrating ionizing radiation is
    a. alpha particles.
    b. beta particles.
    c. gamma rays.
    d. neutrons.
25. Ionizing radiation consists of
    a. particulate radiation and electromagnetic radiation.
    b. particulate radiation and ultrasound radiation.
    c. electromagnetic radiation and ultrasound radiation.
    d. particulate radiation, electromagnetic radiation, and ultrasound radiation.
26. Elements in the same column in the periodic table have similar _____ properties.
    a. physical
    b. chemical
    c. electrical
    d. nuclear

ANSWERS TO CHAPTER 1 QUESTIONS

1.	b	14.	a
2.	b	15.	c
3.	b	16.	b
4.	a	17.	d
5.	b	18.	a
6.	c	19.	a
7.	a	20.	b
8.	c	21.	c
9.	a	22.	a
10.	b	23.	c
11.	d	24.	a
12.	b	25.	a
13.	c	26.	b

2

Electricity and Magnetism

OBJECTIVES

Upon completion of this chapter the student will be able to

1. Identify the four types of electrical materials.
2. State the laws and units of electrostatics.
3. Describe the action of an electric field on a charge.
4. State the laws and units of magnetism.
5. Identify different types of magnetic materials.
6. Describe the action of a magnetic field on a magnet.

INTRODUCTION

Radiology is based on the laws of electricity and magnetism. An understanding of the underlying principles of electricity and magnetism aids in understanding radiologic equipment and image production. In this chapter, we identify different types of electrical materials and review the laws of electricity and magnetism.

TYPES OF ELECTRICAL MATERIALS

There are four types of electrical materials: conductors, insulators, semiconductors, and superconductors.

Conductors

Electrons can move freely through a **conductor.** Tap water containing impurities and most metals are good electrical conductors. Copper and silver are very good conductors. Electric current flows freely through a conductor.

Insulators

The electrons in an **insulator** are held tightly in place and are not free to move. Rubber, wood, glass, and many plastics are good insulators. Electric currents do not flow in insulators.

Semiconductors

Semiconductors can act as either conductors or insulators, depending on how they are made and their environment. Rectifiers in an x-ray circuit are made of a semiconducting material. They conduct electrons in one direction but not in the other direction. Some semiconductors conduct or insulate, depending on surrounding conditions. A photodiode is a semiconductor that is an insulator in the dark but becomes a conductor when exposed to light.

Superconductors

Superconductors are materials that conduct electrons with zero resistance when they are cooled to very low temperatures. Superconductors are used to produce the magnetic fields in magnetic resonance imaging (MRI) units. Table 2.1 summarizes the four types of electrical materials.

The four types of electrical materials are insulators, conductors, semiconductors, and superconductors. Electrons cannot move in insulators, can move in conductors, and move with no resistance in superconductors. Semiconductors can act as either insulators or conductors, depending on outside conditions.

Table 2.1
Characteristics of Electrical Materials

Type of Material	Characteristics	Examples
Conductor	Electrons move freely	Copper, silver
Insulator	Electrons are fixed; no current can flow	Wood, plastic, glass
Semiconductor	Can be either a conductor or an insulator, depending on conditions	Silicon, germanium
Superconductor	Zero resistance at low temperatures; current will flow continuously once started	Special metal alloys

ELECTROSTATIC LAWS

Electrostatics is the study of stationary electric charges. Electricity is charges in motion and will be covered in Chap. 3.

There are four laws of electrostatics:

1. Like charges repel and unlike charges attract.
2. The force between two charges depends on their strength and the distance between them.
3. Electric charges concentrate on the surface of a conductor.
4. Electric charges concentrate at regions of highest curvature.

These electrostatic laws describe how electric charges interact. They are used in x-ray equipment, including x-ray image intensifier tubes and image display systems.

COULOMB'S LAW

The law describing the force between two charges is known as **Coulomb's law.** It describes the force between charges q_1 and q_2 separated by a distance d. It is written as

$$F = k(q_1 q_2)/d^2$$

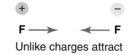

Unlike charges attract

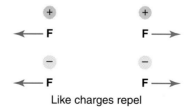

Like charges repel

Figure 2.1 Electrostatic laws of attraction and repulsion between charged objects.

where F is the force, k is a proportionality constant, and d is the distance between charges q_1 and q_2. Coulomb's law states that doubling the distance between two charges reduces the force by a factor of 4. Two charges of the same sign, either positive or negative, have a repulsive force between them. Two charges of opposite sign have an attractive force between them. The force between two charges increases as the strength of the charges increases, and increases as the distance between the charges decreases.

The basic charged particle is the electron. The unit of charge is the coulomb (C). One coulomb is much larger than the charge on an electron. There are 6.3×10^{18} electron charges in one coulomb. The charge of one electron is 1.6×10^{-19} C. Figure 2.1 illustrates the electrostatic laws of attraction and repulsion between charged particles.

DISTRIBUTION OF CHARGES

Charges remain in place on an insulator because they are not free to move. Charges accumulate on the surface of a conductor because they are free to move from the interior of the conductor, and they accumulate near regions of high curvature. Figure 2.2 shows how charges accumulate on the surface of a conductor and concentrate at regions of high curvature.

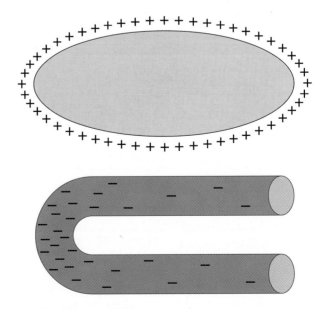

Figure 2.2 Charges accumulate on the surface of a conductor.

STATIC CHARGES

Static charges are stationary, nonmoving electric charges.

Everything in nature is electrically neutral; that is, all objects have the same number of positive and negative charges.

Negative and positive charges can be separated to produce a charged object. A positively charged object has an excess of positive charges; a negatively charged object has an excess of negative charges.

METHODS OF CHARGING

There are three methods of generating static electric charges:

1. Friction
2. Contact
3. Induction

Charging by Friction

Objects can be charged by rubbing them against a different material. Rubbing your shoes against a rug removes electrons from the rug and concentrates them on your body. Moist air is a good conductor and can carry off the excess charges. When the humidity is low, however, and there is less moisture in the air, the air becomes a poor conductor, and the charges will accumulate. On dry days, it is easy to build up a static charge. Walking across a rug on a dry day charges your body by friction. Approaching an uncharged object can produce a spark without your touching the object. The spark appears when the electric field breaks down the air. Lightning is the same process on a larger scale. Figure 2.3 illustrates charging by friction.

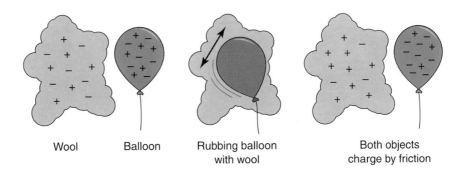

Wool   Balloon   Rubbing balloon with wool   Both objects charge by friction

Figure 2.3 Charging by friction.

When two dissimilar materials are rubbed against each other, electrons are removed from one material and accumulate on the other, resulting in two charged objects.

Charging by Contact

Charges flow from a charged conductor to an uncharged conductor during charging by contact. When a charged conductor touches an uncharged conductor, the excess charges are shared between the two conductors. Figure 2.4 illustrates charging by contact.

A charged conductor is brought near an uncharged conductor. As the two conductors approach each other, the charges in the uncharged conductor are attracted to the approaching opposite charges. When the two objects touch, the opposite charges cancel each other. This leaves the original charged conductor with less charge and the originally uncharged conductor with a charge.

Charging by Induction

Charging by induction uses a charged object to produce a second charged object without contact between the two objects. The three steps in charging by induction are as follows:

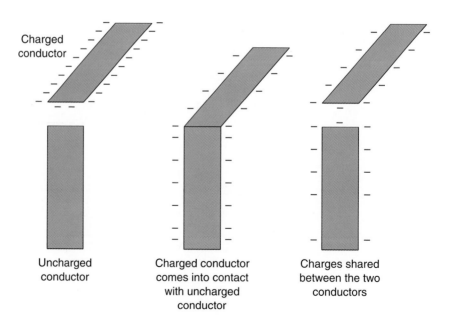

Figure 2.4 **Charging by contact.**

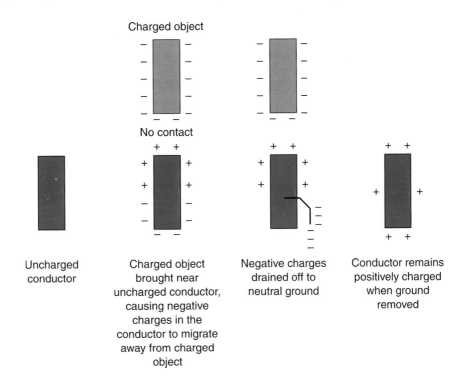

Figure 2.5 Charging by inductions.

1. A negative charge is brought near, but not in contact with, an uncharged conductor. This causes the charges in the conductor to be rearranged. The positive charges go to the end nearest the charged object, and the negative charges move to the other end.
2. The negative charge is drained off the uncharged conductor by connecting it to neutral ground, which can accept the extra charge. The earth is neutral ground. The positive charge is held in place by the nearby charged object.
3. The connection to ground is removed and the external charged object is removed. The object remains positively charged when the connection to ground is removed.

Figure 2.5 illustrates charging by induction. Induction is used in transformers and motors.

ELECTRIC FIELDS

An electric field describes the electrical force exerted on a charge. An electric field exists around all electric charges. The electric field is directed away from

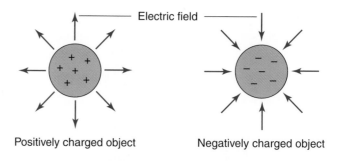

Figure 2.6 Electric field near a charged object.

positive charges and toward negative charges. When two charges are brought near each other, their fields interact. The resulting force of attraction or repulsion depends on the sign of the charges. There is no electric field around neutral objects, and an electric field does not exert a force on neutral objects. Figure 2.6 illustrates the electric field directions near positive and negative charged objects.

The laws of electrostatics describe how charges act on conductors and insulators. They are as follows:

1. *Like charges repel and unlike charges attract.*
2. *The force between two charges depends on their strength and the distance between them.*
3. *Electric charges concentrate on the surface of a conductor.*
4. *Electric charges concentrate at regions of highest curvature.*

The three methods of electrostatic charging are friction, contact, and induction. An electric field describes the force on an electric charge.

MAGNETISM

There are three types of magnetic materials:

1. Ferromagnetic materials, which react strongly in a magnetic field
2. Paramagnetic materials, which react weakly in a magnetic field
3. Nonmagnetic materials, which do not react in a magnetic field

Ferromagnetic materials are attracted to a magnet. These materials, such as iron, cobalt, and nickel, are made up of small groups of atoms called **domains.** These domains act like tiny magnets inside the material. When a ferromagnetic material is placed in a strong magnetic field, some of the domains

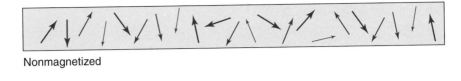

Nonmagnetized

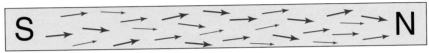

Magnetized—domains aligned in one direction

Figure 2.7 **Magnetization of magnetic materials by lining up the domains.**

are aligned. After the strong magnetic field is removed, the domains remain aligned, forming a permanent magnet. Figure 2.7 illustrates how ferromagnetic materials are magnetized by aligning the domains inside the material. Heating a magnet can destroy its magnetism because heat rearranges the domains into a random orientation, resulting in a loss of permanent magnetism.

Paramagnetic materials react weakly to magnetic fields. Aluminum and water are examples of paramagnetic materials.

Nonmagnetic materials do not react with magnetic fields. Wood, glass, rubber, and plastics are examples of nonmagnetic materials.

MAGNETIC FIELDS

A magnetic field describes the magnetic force exerted on a magnet. All magnets are surrounded by a magnetic field. A magnet placed in a magnetic field experiences a force. This magnetic force will align the magnet along the magnetic field. Every magnet has a north and a south pole. The magnetic field is directed away from the north pole and toward the south pole. Breaking a magnet in half produces two smaller magnets, each with a north and a south pole. Figure 2.8 illustrates how a magnet that is broken in half will produce two smaller magnets, each with its own north and south poles.

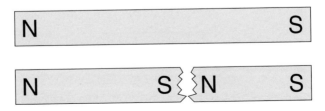

Figure 2.8 **Breaking a magnet produces two smaller magnets.**

LAWS OF MAGNETISM

There are three laws of magnetism:

1. Like poles repel; unlike poles attract.
2. Every magnet has a north and a south pole.
3. The magnetic force between magnets decreases as the square of the distance between them.

The first law of magnetism is shown in Fig. 2.9.

The north pole of a compass points toward the Earth's south magnetic pole, which lies under the ice in northern Canada. Figure 2.10 illustrates how the north pole of a compass points toward the south pole under the ice cap.

The end of the compass marked N is a north magnetic pole.

UNITS OF MAGNETISM

The units of magnetism are the **gauss** (G) and the **tesla** (T). One tesla is equal to 10,000 gauss. The earth's magnetic field is about 1 G or 10^{-4} T. A refrigerator magnet is about 1000 G or 0.1 T. Magnetic resonance imaging units typically have magnetic fields of 0.1 to 1.5 T. MRI imaging is discussed in Chap. 19.

The three types of magnetic materials are ferromagnetic, paramagnetic, and nonmagnetic materials. Ferromagnetic materials can be magnetized by aligning their internal domains with an external magnetic field. Magnetic materials are attracted to a magnet. Paramagnetic materials are weakly attracted to a magnet. Nonmagnetic materials are not attracted to a magnet. The three laws of magnetism

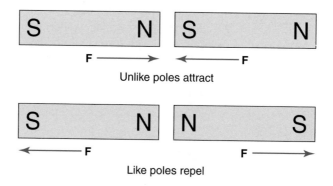

Figure 2.9 **Laws of magnetic attraction and repulsion.**

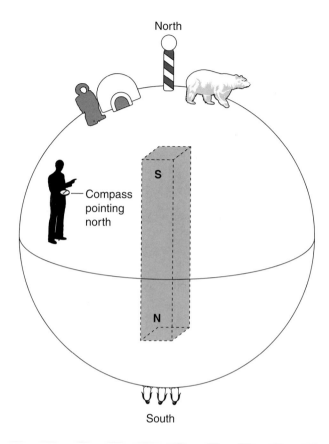

North

S

Compass
pointing
north

N

South

Figure 2.10 Earth's magnetic field.

are as follows: (1) Like poles repel, unlike poles attract; (2) every magnet has a north and a south pole; and (3) the magnetic force between magnets decreases with the square of the distance. All magnets are surrounded by a magnetic field.

SUMMARY

The four types of electrical materials are conductors, insulators, semiconductors, and superconductors. Electrons can move freely through an electrical conductor. Most metals are good conductors. Insulators limit the movement of electrons through the material. Rubber, wood, and plastic are good insulators. Semiconductors are materials that can act as conductors or insulators, depending on the surrounding conditions. Superconductors are materials that conduct electrons with no resistance at very low temperatures.

The three methods of generating static electric charges are friction, contact, and induction. The laws of electrostatics state that like charges repel, unlike charges attract, and the force between charges increases with increasing charge strength and decreasing distance between them. These are known as Coulomb's laws. Charges collect on the surface of a conductor and concentrate at areas of high curvature. An electric field exists near all electric charges.

Magnetic fields exist near all magnets. Ferromagnetic materials, such as iron, react strongly to a magnetic field. The laws of magnetism state that all magnets have a north and a south pole. Like magnetic poles repel, unlike poles attract, and the force between poles decreases as the distance between them increases. The units of magnetism are the tesla (T) and the gauss (G). One tesla equals 10,000 gauss.

QUESTIONS

1. The four types of electrical material are
   a. conductors, inflectors, semiconductors, and superconductors.
   b. conductors, insulators, semiconductors, and superconductors.
   c. convectors, insulators, semiconductors, and supercollectors.
   d. conductors, informers, semicolliders, and superconvectors.
2. Which material is not a conductor?
   a. Copper penny
   b. Silver dollar
   c. Wooden stick
   d. Saltwater
3. Which of these materials is not an insulator?
   a. Copper wire
   b. Plastic spoon
   c. Rubber knife
   d. Wooden ruler
4. A superconductor must be _____ to maintain its superconductivity.
   a. heated
   b. cooled
   c. magnetized
   d. energized
5. A(n) _____ will conduct an electric current with no resistance.
   a. insulator
   b. semiconductor
   c. conductor
   d. superconductor

6. The three methods of generating static charges are
   a. fraction, induction, and heating.
   b. friction, induction, and contact.
   c. function, instruction, and superconduction.
   d. friction, induction, and capacitance.
7. The unit of electric charge is the
   a. electron.
   b. proton.
   c. volt.
   d. coulomb.
8. What is the basic charged particle?
   a. Electron
   b. Neutron
   c. Volt
   d. Coulomb
9. The force between two positive charges is
   a. attraction.
   b. repulsion.
   c. zero.
10. The force between a positive and a negative charge is
    a. attraction.
    b. repulsion.
    c. zero.
11. The force between two negative charges is
    a. attraction.
    b. repulsion.
    c. zero.
12. The force between two uncharged particles is
    a. attraction.
    b. repulsion.
    c. zero.
13. The electrostatic law states that
    a. a proton will repel a neutron.
    b. an electron will repel a proton.
    c. an electron will repel an electron.
    d. a neutron will repel a neutron.
14. _____ is a very good conductor.
    a. Rubber
    b. Copper
    c. Glass
    d. Wood
15. The units of magnetism are the
    a. grass and the tesla.
    b. gauss and the tesly.
    c. gruss and the tesly.
    d. gauss and the tesla.

16. Which of these materials is not ferromagnetic?
    a. Iron
    b. Wood
    c. Nickel
    d. Cobalt

17. Which of these materials is ferromagnetic?
    a. Wood
    b. Glass
    c. Cobalt
    d. Plastic spoon

18. A ferromagnetic material is
    a. weakly influenced by magnetic fields.
    b. strongly influenced by magnetic fields.
    c. not influenced by magnetic fields.

19. Two magnets with the same poles facing each other will
    a. be attracted.
    b. be repelled.
    c. experience a force times the distance.
    d. experience no force.

20. Which statement is not one of the laws of magnetism?
    a. Like poles repel.
    b. Unlike poles attract.
    c. Stronger magnets have larger poles.
    d. The force between magnets decreases with the square of the distance between them.

21. The Earth's magnetic pole lying under the ice north of Canada is a(n)
    a. north magnetic pole.
    b. south magnetic pole.
    c. ice pole.
    d. equatorial pole.

ANSWERS TO CHAPTER 2 QUESTIONS

1.	b		12.	c
2.	c		13.	c
3.	a		14.	b
4.	b		15.	d
5.	d		16.	b
6.	b		17.	c
7.	d		18.	b
8.	a		19.	b
9.	b		20.	c
10.	a		21.	b
11.	b			

3

Electric Currents

INTRODUCTION

Moving electrons make up an **electric current.** There are several different currents flowing in an x-ray circuit, and it is important to recognize these different currents and their purpose in the production of a diagnostic image. In this chapter, we define current, voltage, and electric power. We also discuss the difference between alternating and direct current, induction, and transformers.

ELECTRIC CURRENTS

An electric current is a flow of electrons. The **ampere** (A) is the unit of current and is equal to one coulomb per second. The **coulomb** is the unit of electric charge. The **milliampere** (mA) is a smaller unit of current; it is equal to

Table 3.1
Typical Currents in an X-ray Tube

Location	Current
X-ray filament	2–5 amperes
X-ray tube	50–800 milliamperes

1/1000 of an ampere (10^{-3} A). Different current values are used in different parts of x-ray circuits. Table 3.1 presents typical currents associated with an x-ray tube.

The filament of an x-ray tube is supplied with a high current, which heats the filament and causes electrons to be boiled off the filament. X-ray tubes are discussed more completely in Chap. 6.

DIRECTION OF CURRENT FLOW

When Ben Franklin was working with electricity, he speculated about whether positive or negative charges come out of the battery. Unfortunately, he guessed wrong. He thought that positive charges flow from the positive terminal (the anode) of a battery to the negative terminal (the cathode). What really happens is that negative charges (electrons) flow from the negative cathode to the positive anode. In practice, all drawings of electric circuits are based on Ben Franklin's theory. We assume that current is flowing from positive to negative, even though we know that electrons are actually flowing in the opposite direction. Figure 3.1 shows the direction of current and electron flow in a wire.

In an electric circuit, electrons flow in one direction, and positive current flows in the opposite direction.

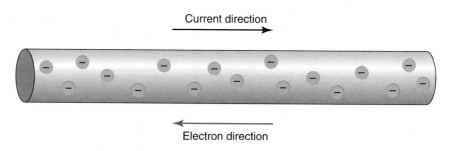

Figure 3.1 **The direction of current and electron flow in a wire.**

VOLTAGE

Voltage is the force or electrical pressure that produces electron movement and current flow. A voltage increase results in an increase in current, just as higher water pressure increases the amount of water flow. Voltage measures the electrical potential that causes electrons to flow in a conductor. The electrical potential is measured in volts (V) and is sometimes called the electromotive force, or **EMF.** Higher voltages give electrons higher energies. Voltages of 20,000 to 120,000 V are used in x-ray circuits to produce high-energy x-rays. One kilovolt (kV) is equal to 1000 (10^3) volts.

There does not have to be current flow for a voltage to exist, just as there can be water pressure in a pipe but no water flow if the valve is closed. Figure 3.2 illustrates how voltage is similar to water pressure in a hose. Higher water pressure causes more water to flow, and higher voltage produces more current flow.

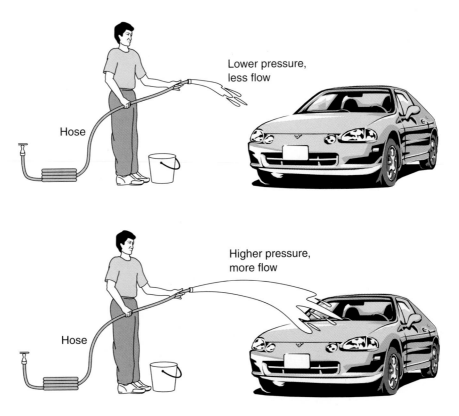

Lower pressure,
less flow

Hose

Higher pressure,
more flow

Hose

Figure 3.2 Voltage is like water pressure in a hose; higher voltage results in more current flow.

RESISTANCE

Resistance is the opposition to current flow. Resistance is measured in ohms (Ω). Higher resistance leads to less current flow. The resistance of a wire depends on its composition, length, and diameter. Copper and silver are superior electrical conductors because the electrons move very easily, resulting in less resistance. A larger-diameter wire has less resistance than a smaller-diameter wire because there is more area for current flow. Longer wires have more resistance. Resistance converts electric energy into heat when current flows through a wire.

RELATIONSHIP BETWEEN VOLTAGE, CURRENT, AND RESISTANCE

Voltage, current, and resistance are related by **Ohm's law.** This relation is given by

$$V = IR \qquad I = V/R \qquad R = V/I$$

where V = voltage, I = current, and R = resistance.

Ohm's law states that the voltage V is equal to the product of the current I flowing through a conductor and the resistance R of the conductor. Higher voltage and lower resistance result in higher current flow.

EXAMPLE 1:

Calculate the current in a circuit with a voltage of 9 V and a resistance of 2 Ω. From Ohm's law,

$$V = IR$$
$$9 = I \times 2$$
$$I = 9/2$$
$$I = 4.5 \text{ A}$$

If the current and voltage are known, the resistance can be calculated.

EXAMPLE 2:

What is the resistance of a circuit if the voltage is 100 V and the current is 5 A?

$$V = IR$$
$$100 = 5 \times R$$
$$R = 100/5$$
$$R = 20 \; \Omega$$

Figure 3.3 shows the circle of Ohm, which is an excellent way to remember the various combinations of Ohm's law. The figure shows that $V = IR$ or $I = V/R$ or $R = V/I$. Remember that V is always on top.

Current is the movement of electrons through a conductor. Current flows from positive to negative, and electrons flow from negative to positive. Current is measured in amperes. Resistance is the opposition to current flow. Resistance has units of ohms. Voltage is the pressure that forces the electrons to flow through a conductor. Voltage is measured in volts. Ohm's law states the relationship between voltage, current, and resistance.

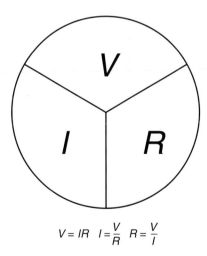

$$V = IR \quad I = \frac{V}{R} \quad R = \frac{V}{I}$$

Figure 3.3 The circle of Ohm.

DIRECT AND ALTERNATING CURRENTS

In **direct current (DC)** circuits, electrons flow only in one direction. **Alternating current (AC)** flows half of the time in one direction, and the other half of the time in the other direction. One AC cycle consists of one-half positive current flow and one-half negative current flow. Figure 3.4 shows how alternating current changes direction with time. Direct current has a constant direction.

In the United States, standard AC electric current has a frequency of 60 cycles per second. The duration of the positive half cycle is 1/120 second (s). The duration of the negative half cycle is also 1/120 s. One cycle per second is also known as one hertz (Hz).

ELECTRIC POWER

Power P is the rate of energy use. **Power** describes the amount of work done, or the amount of energy used per second. Electric power P is current I times voltage V. This is true for both AC and DC circuits. Electric power is measured in watts (W). One watt is produced by one ampere of current flowing with an electrical pressure of one volt. The relationship between power, current, voltage, and resistance is

$$P = VI \qquad P = I^2R \qquad P = V^2/R$$

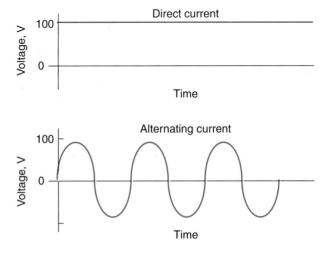

Figure 3.4 **Alternating and direct current.**

Direct current moves in only one direction; alternating current moves back and forth in the circuit. Electric power is the rate of energy use and is calculated by multiplying the voltage by the current. Power is measured in watts.

ELECTROMAGNETISM

A current flowing in a conductor creates a magnetic field around the conductor. Figure 3.5 shows the magnetic field around a current-carrying conductor. The accompanying magnetic field is a fundamental property of electric currents. The strength of the magnetic field increases with an increase in the current.

If the conductor is coiled in a circle, the magnetic fields from different parts of the coil add together and increase the magnetic field in the center of the coil. This is how an electromagnet works. Increasing the current or the number of turns in the coil produces a stronger magnetic field in the center of the coil. Adding a ferromagnetic material such as iron in the center of the coil also increases the magnetic field strength by concentrating the field through the center of the iron. Figure 3.6 shows how the magnetic field in the center of a coil is increased by adding turns to the coil and adding ferromagnetic material to the center of the coil. Transformers have iron cores to increase their efficiency.

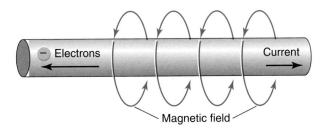

Figure 3.5 A magnetic field is always present around a wire that carries a current.

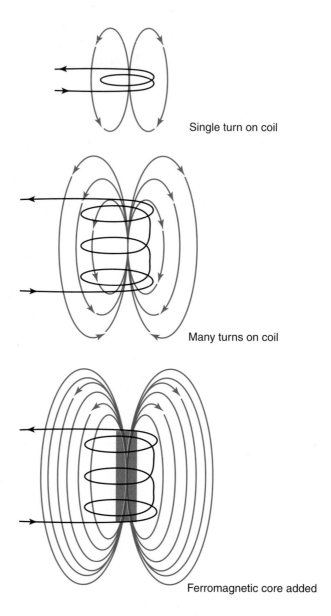

Single turn on coil

Many turns on coil

Ferromagnetic core added

Figure 3.6 A coil of wire produces a magnetic field in the center of the coil. More turns on the coil produce a stronger magnetic field. Adding a ferromagnetic core produces an even stronger magnetic field.

The relationship between current and changing magnetic fields is called **electromagnetic induction** and is the basis of transformer operation. A changing magnetic field produces an electric field. This electric field will cause electrons to flow in a conductor. Electromagnetic induction is the production of a current in a conductor by a changing magnetic field near the conductor. The magnetic field *must* be changing. A steady magnetic field does not induce an electric current.

CURRENT INDUCTION

A changing magnetic field will induce an electric current in a conductor. This principle is known as mutual induction. An electric current can be induced in a conductor in three ways.

One way is to move a magnet near a conductor. As the magnet approaches the conductor, the magnetic field around the conductor increases. As the magnet moves away from the conductor, the magnetic field decreases. The *change* in the magnetic field as the magnet approaches and recedes induces a current to flow in the conductor.

A second way to induce a current is by moving a conductor near a stationary magnet. In this case, the magnetic field is static and the conductor moves. The relative motion between the magnet and the conductor is the same regardless of which moves and which is stationary. In either case, a current is induced to flow in the conductor.

A third way of inducing a current is to hold the conductor stationary and generate the magnetic field with an AC electromagnet. The magnetic field from the electromagnet increases and decreases as the current through the magnet coils changes. This changing magnetic field induces a current to flow in the conductor. Alternating current flows in a conducting coil will produce a changing magnetic field in the center of the coil. A current will be induced to flow in a second nearby conducting coil.

In every case, the change in the magnetic field induces the current. The amount of induced current depends on the strength of the magnetic field and how fast it is changing. Direct currents do not have changing magnetic fields and do not induce currents. Figure 3.7 demonstrates the three ways in which current can be induced in a conductor.

Moving a magnetic field near a stationary conductor changes the strength of the magnetic field at the conductor and induces a current in the conductor. Moving a conductor through a stationary magnetic field also induces a current in the conductor. Changing the magnetic field strength near a conductor induces a current in the conductor. Alternating current in an electromagnet produces a changing magnetic field. This changing magnetic field will induce an alternating current to flow in a secondary coil of wire located in the magnetic field. This is the principle of transformer operation.

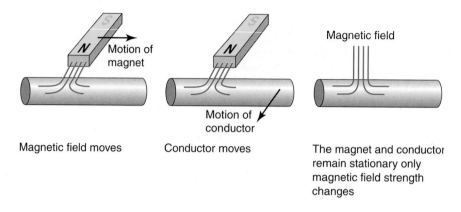

Magnetic field

Motion of
magnet

Motion of
conductor

Magnetic field moves   Conductor moves   The magnet and conductor
                                                         remain stationary only
                                                         magnetic field strength
                                                         changes

Figure 3.7 **The three ways in which current can be induced.**

TRANSFORMERS

Transformers are used to change low voltages into higher voltages or vice versa in an AC circuit. Transformers operate on the principle of mutual induction. Transformers can operate only with alternating current, not with direct current. A changing current is necessary in order to produce a changing magnetic field. Figure 3.8 illustrates the components of a transformer. An alternating current supplied to the primary coil changes the magnetic field around the coil. The changing magnetic field from the primary coil, or input, induces a current in the secondary coil, or output. The input voltage and current on the primary coil differ from the output voltage and current on the secondary coil.

The secondary coil of a transformer is linked to the primary coil by an iron core to improve its efficiency.

The voltage in the secondary coil of a transformer is related to the voltage in the primary coil by the transformer law:

$$V_{secondary} = V_{primary}(N_{secondary}/N_{primary})$$

where $N_{secondary}$ is the number of turns of wire in the secondary coil and $N_{primary}$ is the number of turns of wire in the primary coil. The turns ratio, $N_{secondary}/N_{primary}$, is the ratio of the number of turns in the secondary to the number of turns in the primary.

If there are more windings in the secondary coil than in the primary coil, the transformer is called a **step-up transformer.** A **step-down transformer** has more turns in the primary coil than in the secondary coil. This relationship states that the voltage in the secondary coil changes when either the primary voltage or the turns ratio changes.

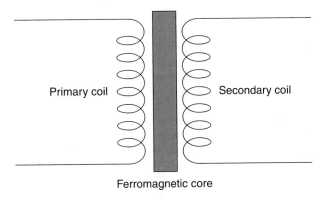

Figure 3.8 **The components of a transformer.**

EXAMPLE 4:

If the input voltage is 200 V, the number of turns in the secondary is 300,000, and the number of turns in the primary is 500, what is the secondary voltage?

$$V_{secondary} = ?$$
$$V_{primary} = 200$$
$$N_{primary} = 500$$
$$N_{secondary} = 300,000$$
$$V_{secondary} = 220 \times (300,000/500)$$
$$= 200 \times 600$$
$$= 120,000 \text{ V}$$

The output voltage in the secondary coil depends on the turns ratio and on the primary voltage. The induced voltage and current in the transformer coils are inversely related: Higher voltages in the secondary coil are accompanied by lower currents in the secondary coil. This occurs because the power output of the transformer cannot exceed the power input. When the secondary voltage is higher than the primary voltage, the secondary current must be less than the primary current. If the secondary voltage is lower than the primary voltage, the secondary current is higher than the primary current.

There are three types of transformers used in x-ray circuits: autotransformers, step-up transformers, and step-down transformers. **Autotransformers** allow the selection of input voltages to step-up and step-down transformers. Step-up transformers are used to provide high voltage to the x-ray tube. Step-down transformers are used to provide high current to the x-ray tube filament. Both step-up and step-down transformers have a fixed number of primary and secondary windings on their coils and a fixed turns ratio. If the turns ratio is constant, the only way to change the output of a transformer is to change the input voltage. Figure 3.9 shows a schematic of the three types of transformers used in x-ray circuits.

Autotransformers

The function of an autotransformer is to provide different voltages for input to the step-up and step-down transformers. The output of the autotransformer is connected to the primary coil of the step-up or step-down transformer.

An autotransformer has only one coil, which serves as both primary and secondary transformer windings. The output connections of an autotransformer are called **output taps.** In an x-ray circuit, the output of an autotransformer is used to change the voltage in the primary coils of the step-up and

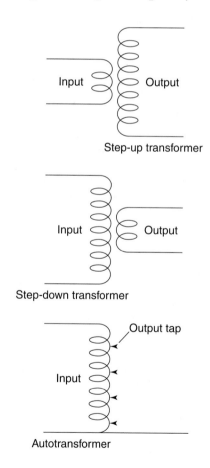

Step-up transformer

Step-down transformer

Autotransformer

Figure 3.9 **The three types of transformers used in x-ray circuits.**

step-down transformers. Different output voltages are obtained by selecting different autotransformer output taps. Changing the input voltage to the step-up or step-down transformer changes the output voltage.

As an example, if the input voltage of the autotransformer is 220 V and the output tap is selected for half the voltage, the input voltage to the primary coil of the step-up or step-down transformer is 110 V.

Step-up Transformers

A step-up transformer converts a lower AC voltage into a higher AC voltage and is also called the **high-voltage transformer.** Step-up transformers have more turns in the secondary coil than in the primary coil. The output voltage of a step-up transformer is higher than the input voltage, and the output current is always less than the input current. Step-up transformers are used to supply high voltages to the x-ray tube. Figure 3.10 shows the input and output voltages and currents from a step-up transformer.

Step-down Transformers

A step-down transformer produces an output voltage that is lower than the input voltage. The number of turns on the secondary coil of a step-down trans-

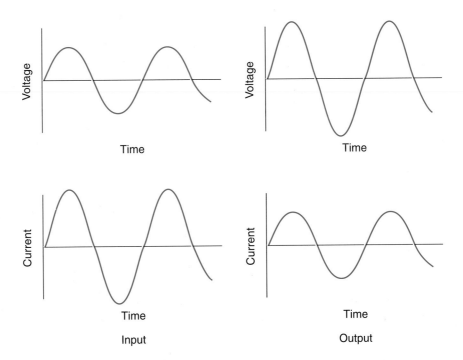

Figure 3.10 The input and output voltage and current waveforms from a step-up transformer.

former is less than the number of turns on the primary coil. The output current in the secondary coil of a step-down transformer is greater than the input current. Step-down transformers are used to supply high currents to the tube filament. Figure 3.11 shows the input and output voltages and currents from a step-down transformer.

A current flowing in a conductor forms a magnetic field around the conductor. An alternating current produces a changing magnetic field, which produces an electric field. This electric field can induce a current in a nearby conductor. This induction of current is the basis of all transformers. A step-up transformer has more windings in the secondary or output coil than in the primary or input coil. A step-down transformer has fewer turns in the secondary than in the primary. The input of either a step-up or a step-down transformer is connected to the single coil of an autotransformer to change the input voltage of the step-up or step-down transformer.

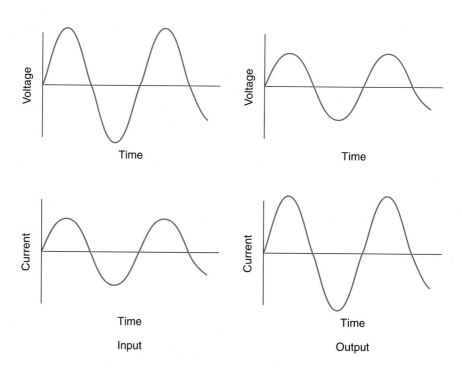

Figure 3.11 The input and output voltage and current waveforms from a step-down transformer.

ELECTRIC GENERATORS

An **electric generator** converts mechanical energy into electric energy. A current is induced in a conductor that is moved through a magnetic field across or perpendicular to the magnetic field lines. If the conductor moves parallel to the magnetic field, there is no current induced in the conductor. Figure 3.12 shows these two cases of a conductor moving through a magnetic field. The conductor must cut through the magnetic field lines in order to induce a current.

A wire bent into a coil can be rotated in a magnetic field. As the coil rotates in a magnetic field, the induced current rises to a maximum, drops to zero, then increases to a maximum in the opposite direction. No current is induced when the wire is moving parallel to the magnetic field. The induced current is an alternating current. Additional loops in the coil increase the voltage induced in the coil. Figure 3.13 shows how a coil rotating in a magnetic field produces an alternating current. In a generator, the mechanical energy of rotation is converted into electric energy.

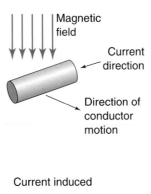

Current induced

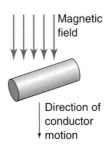

No current induced

Figure 3.12 Current is induced in a conductor moving perpendicular to a magnetic field. No current is induced in a conductor moving parallel to a magnetic field.

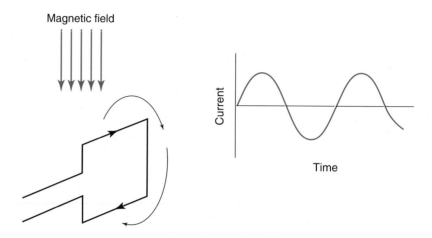

Figure 3.13 A rotating coil of wire produces an alternating current.

ELECTRIC MOTORS

A **motor** converts electric energy into mechanical energy. A current-carrying coil placed in an external magnetic field experiences a force. This is because current-carrying wires are surrounded by a magnetic field. The coil acts like a magnet. The external magnetic field and the magnetic field of the coil interact. Figure 3.14 illustrates the force on a current-carrying coil in a magnetic field.

The magnetic field forces the coil into alignment with the external magnetic field. The external magnetic field is produced by the stator. The rotating set of coils is called a **rotor.** The armature, which is part of the rotor, makes separate contacts with the individual coils. Alternating current flowing through the coils on the rotor produces continuous rotation because different coils are

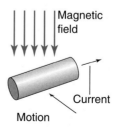

Figure 3.14 A current-carrying wire in a magnetic field experiences a force, which causes the wire to move. This is the principle on which the electric motor operates.

separately energized, so that they are always continuously forced toward alignment with the external magnetic field. Sliding brushes in contact with the armature provide current to the individual coils.

INDUCTION MOTORS

Induction motors also operate on the principle of mutual induction. Induction motors eliminate all electrical contacts with the rotor. In an x-ray tube, the rotating anode is driven by an induction motor. Both the motor rotor and the anode are sealed inside an evacuated glass envelope. The stators, located outside the glass tube, are electromagnets that produce changing magnetic fields by switching the current in the stator coils. The changing magnetic fields produced outside the glass envelope induce a current to flow in the coils of the rotor. The induced current in the rotor interacts with the changing external magnetic field, forcing the rotor to follow the external magnetic fields of the stator. The rotor and anode rotate because the external field is rotating. Figure 3.15 illustrates an induction motor in an x-ray tube.

An electric generator converts mechanical energy into electric energy by moving a conductor in a magnetic field. A motor converts electric energy into mechanical energy by placing a current-carrying wire in a magnetic field. The magnetic field forces the current-carrying wire to move.

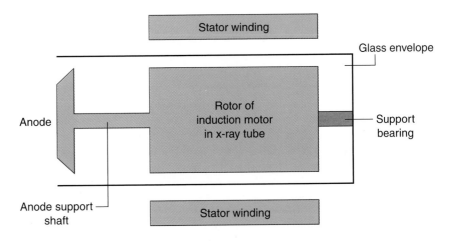

Figure 3.15 An induction motor induces current in the rotor and uses moving magnetic fields to produce motion of the rotor.

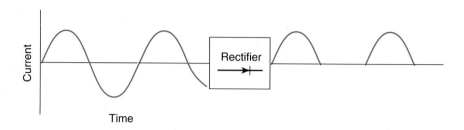

Figure 3.16 **A rectifier limits current flow to one direction only.**

RECTIFICATION OF ALTERNATING CURRENT TO DIRECT CURRENT

Many electronic circuits, including television tubes and x-ray tubes, operate on direct current. Electrons flow in only one direction in the x-ray tube, that is, from cathode to anode. These devices accelerate electrons toward the positive anode. If they were connected to an alternating current, the electron source would burn out when the AC voltage reversed. Therefore, these devices cannot operate on AC. It is necessary to convert AC to DC in the x-ray circuits. **Rectifiers** are semiconductors that allow current to flow in only one direction and convert AC into DC. Figure 3.16 illustrates the rectification of AC into DC.

Only positive current can flow through the rectifier. When negative current tries to flow back through the rectifier, it is blocked, and there is no current flow.

CAPACITORS

Capacitors are used to temporarily store electric charge. A capacitor consists of two conducting plates separated by an insulator. The two conducting plates are connected to the two terminals of a DC source. Positive charges flow to one plate; negative charges flow to the other plate. When the DC source is removed, the positive and negative charges on the plates remain attracted to each other, and the capacitor remains charged. If the capacitor is connected to a conductor such as a light bulb, a current will briefly flow from the positive to the negative plate of the capacitor until the positive and negative charges are balanced. The current flow from a capacitor usually takes only a fraction of a second. Capacitors are used to store electric energy in some portable x-ray units.

Alternating current can be changed into direct current using rectifiers. A rectifier circuit allows current to flow in only one direction. Electric energy can be temporarily stored in a capacitor.

SUMMARY

Electrons moving through a conductor make up an electric current. Current is the amount of electrons moving in a conductor per second and is measured in amperes or milliamperes. Current flows from the positive to the negative terminal in an electric circuit. Electrons flow from the negative to the positive terminal. Voltage is the electrical pressure or electromotive force applied to the electrons in the conductor and is measured in volts. Resistance, which is the opposition to current flow, is measured in ohms. Ohm's law, written $V = IR$, states the relationship between voltage, current, and resistance. Direct current flows only in one direction. One cycle of alternating current consists of current flow in one direction for half of the time and in the other direction for the other half of the time. One cycle per second is one hertz.

Power is the rate at which energy is used. The equation for electric power is $P = I^2R$ or $P = VI$. Power is measured in watts. Electrons moving through a conductor create a magnetic field around the conductor. A changing magnetic field induces a current in a conductor. This is known as mutual induction. Transformers change voltage and current into higher or lower values. The output of an autotransformer is used to change the input voltage to a step-up or step-down fixed winding transformer. A step-up transformer provides high voltage to the x-ray tube. A step-down transformer is used to supply current to the x-ray tube filament.

A generator converts mechanical energy into electric energy. A motor converts electric energy into mechanical energy. An induction motor is used to rotate the anode inside an x-ray tube. Rectifiers convert alternating current into direct current. Capacitors are devices that temporarily store electric charge.

QUESTIONS

1. Electric current is the flow of
   a. protons moving in a conductor.
   b. neutrons moving in a conductor.
   c. electrons moving in a conductor.
   d. atoms moving in a conductor.
2. The unit of electric current is the
   a. watt.
   b. ampere.
   c. volt.
   d. ohm.

3. The unit of electrical potential is the
   a. watt.
   b. ampere.
   c. volt.
   d. ohm.
4. The unit of electrical resistance is the
   a. watt.
   b. ampere.
   c. volt.
   d. ohm.
5. The unit of electric power is the
   a. watt.
   b. ampere.
   c. volt.
   d. ohm.
6. One milliampere is equal to _____ ampere(s).
   a. 1/1000
   b. 1/100
   c. 1/10
   d. 1000
7. Electrons move from
   a. positive to negative.
   b. negative to positive.
   c. neutral to positive.
   d. neutral to negative.
8. Conventional current flows from
   a. positive to negative.
   b. negative to positive.
   c. neutral to positive.
   d. neutral to negative.
9. Increasing the voltage in a circuit results in a(n)
   a. increase in current.
   b. increase in resistance.
   c. decrease in current.
   d. decrease in resistance.
10. As the diameter of a wire increases, the resistance
    of the wire
    a. increases.
    b. decreases.
    c. stays the same.
11. Ohm's law is
    a. $V = I/R.$
    b. $V = I \times R.$
    c. $V = I^2 \times R.$
    d. $V = R/I.$

12. In this figure,

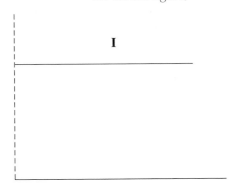
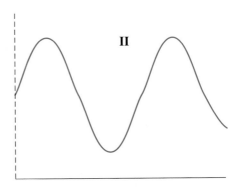

    a. I is AC, and II is DC.
    b. I is DC, and II is AC.
    c. I is AC, and II is AC.
    d. I is DC, and II is DC.

13. Electric power is calculated by the formula
    a. $P = IR$.
    b. $P = VI$.
    c. $P = VR$.
    d. $P = I/R$.

14. Which process is *not* a method of inducing a current?
    a. Moving a magnetic field next to a conductor
    b. Moving a conductor through a magnetic flux
    c. Holding a stationary magnetic field near a stationary conductor
    d. Changing a magnetic field near a conductor

15. A transformer converts
    a. low AC to high AC.
    b. low DC to high DC.
    c. low AC to high DC.
    d. low DC to high AC.

16. A transformer with a higher number of primary windings than secondary windings is a _____ transformer.
    a. step-up
    b. step-down

17. A transformer that produces an output voltage larger than the input voltage is a _____ transformer.
    a. step-up
    b. step-down

18. The current in the secondary coil of a step-up transformer is _____ the current in the primary coil.
    a. less than
    b. greater than
    c. the same as

19. A conducting wire moving in a magnetic field is a
    a. motor
    b. generator
    c. stator
    d. thermoliter
20. A current-carrying wire moving in a magnetic field is a
    a. motor.
    b. generator.
    c. stator.
    d. thermoliter.
21. Rectifiers are used to convert
    a. DC to AC.
    b. high voltage to low voltage.
    c. AC to DC.
    d. low voltage to high voltage.
22. An electronic device that is used to store an electric charge is called a
    a. motor.
    b. rectifier.
    c. transformer.
    d. capacitor.

ANSWERS TO CHAPTER 3 QUESTIONS

1.	c		12.	b
2.	b		13.	b
3.	c		14.	c
4.	d		15.	a
5.	a		16.	b
6.	a		17.	a
7.	b		18.	a
8.	a		19.	b
9.	a		20.	a
10.	b		21.	c
11.	b		22.	d

4

Electromagnetic Radiation

OBJECTIVES

Upon completion of this chapter, the student will be able to

1. Identify the different forms of electromagnetic radiation.
2. Define frequency, amplitude, wavelength, and intensity.
3. Describe the relationships between frequency, wavelength, velocity, and energy of electromagnetic radiation.
4. Describe the relation between radiation intensity and distance from the source.

INTRODUCTION

In this chapter, we discuss the different forms of electromagnetic radiation, the ways to describe x-rays and other forms of radiation, and how x-ray intensity changes with distance from the x-ray source. X-rays are an important part of the electromagnetic spectrum. This chapter discusses the characteristics of electromagnetic radiation.

ELECTROMAGNETIC RADIATION

Electromagnetic radiation is one of the many types of energy and may appear in the form of visible light, x-rays, infrared radiation, or radio waves. These vary in energy, frequency, and wavelength. The energy of the radiation is measured in electron volts (eV).

The entire band of electromagnetic energies is known as the electromagnetic spectrum. Figure 4.1 illustrates the different regions of the electromagnetic spectrum, from long-wavelength, low-energy radio waves to short-wavelength, high-energy gamma rays. Although Fig. 4.1 seems to indicate that there are sharp transitions between the types of radiation, there are no clear boundaries between the various regions in the electromagnetic spectrum.

Radio Waves

Radio waves are long-wavelength (1 to 10,000 m), low-energy radiation waves. Radio frequency (RF) radiation is used in magnetic resonance imaging.

Radar and Microwaves

Radar and microwaves have shorter wavelengths (10^{-1} to 10^{-4} m) and higher energy than radio waves and are used in ovens, in navigation, and in traffic control, where law enforcement officers monitor the speed of cars. In a microwave oven, the microwave energy forces the water molecules in food to vibrate rapidly, thus heating the food.

Infrared Radiation

Infrared radiation, or heat, has shorter wavelengths and higher energy than radar and microwaves (10^{-5} to 10^{-6} m). Infrared radiation can heat nearby objects. You can feel the heat from your toaster. The high-energy end of the infrared region is visible and can be seen in the red heating elements of your toaster.

Visible Light

Visible light selectively activates cells in the eye. It occupies a narrow band in the electromagnetic spectrum, with wavelengths between 10^{-6} and 10^{-7} m. The color red has the longest wavelength and lowest energy. The colors blue and violet have the highest energy and the shortest wavelengths in the visible spectrum.

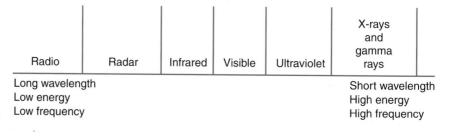

Figure 4.1 **The electromagnetic spectrum.**

Table 4.1
Regions of the Electromagnetic Spectrum and Their Characteristics

Spatial Region	Wavelength, m	Energy, eV	Frequency, Hz
Radio	$10^0–10^4$	$10^{-6}–10^{-10}$	$10^8–10^4$
Radar	$10^{-1}–10^{-4}$	$10^{-5}–10^{-2}$	$10^9–10^{12}$
Infrared	$10^{-5}–10^{-6}$	$10^{-1}–10^0$	$10^{13}–10^{14}$
Visible light	$10^{-6}–10^{-7}$	$10^0–10^1$	$10^{14}–10^{15}$
Ultraviolet	$10^{-7}–10^{-9}$	$10^1–10^3$	$10^{15}–10^{17}$
X-rays/gamma rays	$10^{-9}–10^{-16}$	$10^3–10^{10}$	$10^{17}–10^{24}$

Ultraviolet

Ultraviolet is the part of the spectrum just beyond the visible light region. Ultraviolet wavelengths range from 10^{-7} to 10^{-9} m. Ultraviolet light has enough energy to destroy bacteria and produce changes in the skin layers. Ultraviolet lights are used in biologic laboratories to destroy airborne bacteria. Ultraviolet light is believed to be responsible for the majority of sunburns and skin cancers.

X-rays and Gamma Rays

X-rays and gamma rays have very short wavelengths, between 10^{-9} and 10^{-16} m. They are high-frequency, high-energy radiation. Their energy is measured in thousands of electron volts (keV), and they are capable of ionization. Ionizing radiation such as x-rays and gamma rays has enough energy to remove an electron from its orbital shell.

The x-rays used in radiology come from interactions with electron orbits. Gamma rays come from nuclear transformations and are released from the nucleus of a radioactive atom. The only difference between x-rays and gamma rays is their origin. Some x-rays used in radiology have higher energy than some gamma rays. X-ray production is discussed in Chap. 7.

Table 4.1 lists the regions of the electromagnetic spectrum with their energies, wavelengths, and frequencies.

CHARACTERISTICS OF ELECTROMAGNETIC RADIATION

Electromagnetic radiation consists of vibrations in electric and magnetic fields. These vibrations have no charge and no mass and travel at the speed of light. Electromagnetic radiation moves in sinusoidal waves. These waves consist of electric and magnetic fields. Electromagnetic radiation is described in terms of the following characteristics:

> Velocity
> Frequency
> Period
> Wavelength
> Amplitude
> Energy
> Intensity

Velocity

All electromagnetic radiation in a vacuum travels at 3×10^8 meters per second (m/s) [186,000 miles per second (mi/s)]. Even though this is incredibly fast, light still requires a considerable amount of time to travel huge distances. For example, it takes 8 minutes (min) for light from the sun to reach the earth.

Sometimes electromagnetic radiation acts as a wave, and sometimes it acts as a particle. When it acts as a particle, this particle is called a **photon**. When electromagnetic radiation acts as a wave, it has a definite frequency, period, and wavelength. Whether it acts as a particle or as a wave, its velocity is the same.

Frequency

The **frequency** of a wave is the number of cycles per second. That is, the frequency is the number of peaks or valleys occurring each second. The unit of frequency is the hertz (Hz), which is one cycle per second. In the United States, electricity has a frequency of 60 Hz, that is, 60 cycles per second. A typical radio wave is 700,000 Hz (700 kHz). One thousand Hz is equal to one kilohertz (kHz). One megahertz (MHz) is equal to one million (10^6) hertz or cycles per second.

Period

The period of a wave is the time required for one complete cycle. A wave with a frequency of 2 cycles per second has a period of ½ second; that is, one complete wave cycle occurs each half second. Figure 4.2 illustrates the relationship between frequency and period in a sine wave.

Wavelength

The distance between adjacent peaks or adjacent valleys of a wave is the wavelength and is represented by the Greek letter lambda (λ). Wavelength is one of the important characteristics determining the properties of x-rays. Electromagnetic radiation with shorter wavelengths will have higher energy and frequencies and greater penetration. Wavelength is measured in meters, cen-

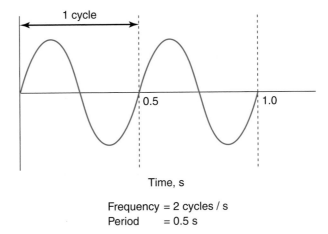

Figure 4.2 **The relationship between frequency and period.**

timeters, or millimeters. Figure 4.3 illustrates the relation between wavelength and frequency.

Electromagnetic wave velocity, frequency, and wavelength are related by

$$c = f\lambda \tag{4-1}$$

where c is the speed of light, f is the frequency, and lambda (λ) is the wavelength.

EXAMPLE 1:

Green light has a frequency of 6×10^{14} Hz. What is the wavelength of green light?

$$\lambda = c/f$$
$$\lambda = (3 \times 10^8)/(6 \times 10^{14})$$
$$= 5.0 \times 10^{-7} \text{ m}$$

As mentioned previously, the speed of light in air in a vacuum is 3×10^8 m/s. Frequency and wavelength are inversely proportional. If the frequency increases, the wavelength decreases. If the frequency decreases, the wavelength increases.

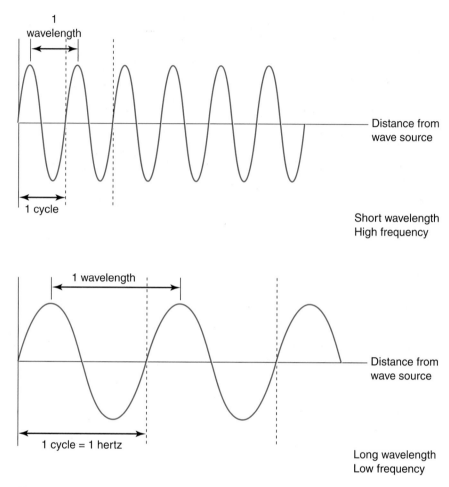

Figure 4.3 The relationship between wavelength and frequency.

Amplitude

The amplitude of a wave is the maximum height, or difference from zero (in either direction), of the peaks or valleys. Figure 4.4 compares the amplitudes of two electromagnetic waves as a function of time.

> *Electromagnetic energy comes in many forms. Radio and radar waves are low-energy forms of electromagnetic radiation; infrared and visible light are intermediate-energy forms of electromagnetic radiation; ultraviolet, x-rays, and gamma rays are higher-energy forms of electromagnetic radiation. X-rays and gamma rays often move as waves. A wave has a velocity, a frequency, a period, a wavelength, and an amplitude.*

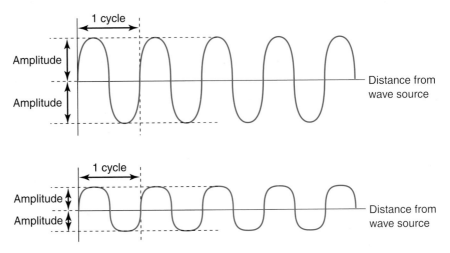

Figure 4.4 **Two waves of different amplitudes.**

ENERGY: ELECTROMAGNETIC RADIATION AS A PARTICLE

Electromagnetic radiation can act as a wave or a particle. When electromagnetic radiation acts as a particle, that particle is called a **photon**. The energy E of a photon is related to its frequency by

$$E = hf \tag{4-2}$$

or

$$E = hc/\lambda \tag{4-3}$$

where h is a conversion factor called **Planck's constant**, f is the frequency, c is the speed of light, and λ is the wavelength. The energy and frequency of a photon are directly proportional, but wavelength and energy are inversely proportional. The higher the energy, the shorter the wavelength and the higher the frequency. The value of Planck's constant is 4.2×10^{-15} eV $\cdot$ s.

EXAMPLE 2:

What is the energy of a green light photon whose frequency is 6×10^{14} Hz?

$$E = hf$$
$$= (4.2 \times 10^{-15}) \times (6 \times 10^{14})$$
$$= 2.5 \text{ eV}$$

RADIATION INTENSITY AND THE INVERSE SQUARE LAW

All electromagnetic radiation travels at the speed of light and diverges from the source at which it is emitted. Intensity is energy flow per cm² and is measured in watts per centimeter squared (W/cm²). The intensity of the radiation decreases with an increase in the distance from the source. This is because the x-ray energy flow is spread over a larger area. This relation is known as the inverse square law. It is called the **inverse square law** because the intensity is inversely proportional to the square of the distance. Figure 4.5 illustrates how the intensity decreases as the distance from the source increases.

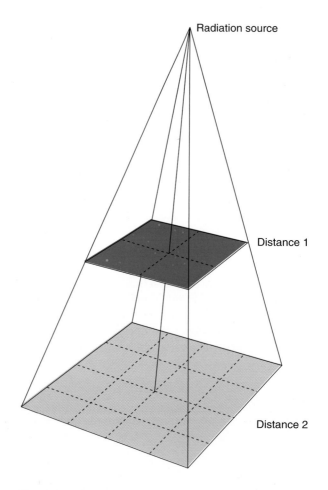

Figure 4.5 **The inverse square law relates the radiation intensity to the distance from the source.**

Mathematically, the inverse square law states that the intensity I_2 at a distance d_2 is related to the intensity I_1 at a distance d_1 by

$$I_2 = I_1(d_1/d_2)^2 \qquad\qquad (4\text{-}4)$$

Thus, the intensity is inversely related to the square of the distance. If the distance increases, the intensity decreases; if the distance decreases, the intensity increases.

If the distance from the x-ray source is doubled, the intensity decreases by a factor of 4. That is, the intensity at twice the distance is one-fourth the original value. If the distance from the x-ray source is halved, the intensity is four times greater. The exposure and exposure rate from an x-ray source also follow the inverse square law.

EXAMPLE 3:

What is the exposure rate 4 m from a source that has an exposure rate of 32 milliroentgens per hour (mR/h) at a distance of 1 m from the source?

If I_1 is the exposure rate at 1 m and I_2 is the exposure rate at 4 m, then

$$I_2 = I_1 \times (d_1/d_2)^2$$
$$I_2 = I_1[(1)^2/(4)^2]$$
$$= 32(1/16)$$
$$= 2 \text{ mR/h}$$

EXAMPLE 4:

The x-ray intensity is measured at 40 mR/h at 36 inches (in). What is the intensity at 72 in?

$$I_2 = I_1 \times (d_1/d_2)^2$$
$$(36)^2 = 1296$$
$$(72)^2 = 5184$$
$$(40 \times 1296)/5184 = 10 \text{ mR/h}$$

The energy of x-rays is directly proportional to the frequency and inversely proportional to the wavelength; as the energy of x-rays increases, the wavelength decreases. Higher-energy x-rays have shorter wavelengths. The inverse square law relates the intensity of the radiation from a source to the distance from the source. Doubling the distance to the source reduces the intensity to one-fourth the original value.

SUMMARY

The electromagnetic spectrum ranges from low-energy, low-frequency, long-wavelength radio waves to high-energy, high-frequency, short-wavelength gamma rays. Waves have an amplitude, frequency, period, and velocity. All electromagnetic radiation travels at the speed of light. Different forms of electromagnetic radiation have different frequencies, wavelengths, and energies.

Frequency is the number of wave cycles per second and is measured in hertz. One hertz is equal to one cycle per second. Wavelength is the distance between corresponding peaks or valleys of the wave. The period of a wave is the time for one wave cycle. The amplitude of a wave is the maximum extent or height of the wave (the distance of the wave from zero in either direction).

X-rays are a short-wavelength, high-frequency, high-energy form of electromagnetic radiation. X-rays have enough energy to ionize atoms and pass through many materials.

The inverse square law describes how the intensity of electromagnetic radiation changes with distance from the source. As the distance increases, the intensity of the electromagnetic radiation decreases. Doubling the distance decreases the intensity to one-fourth. Reducing the distance to half the original distance increases the intensity four times.

QUESTIONS

1. Which of the following is *not* a form of electromagnetic radiation?
   a. Microwaves
   b. Ultrasound
   c. Infrared
   d. X-rays
2. Ionizing radiation has enough energy to
   a. remove the nucleus from the atom.
   b. heat atoms to vaporization.
   c. reduce ionization to zero.
   d. remove electrons from the atom.

3. Select the order of increasing energy.
    1. X-rays
    2. Microwaves
    3. Visible light
    4. Radio
  a. 1, 2, 3, 4
  b. 4, 2, 3, 1
  c. 1, 2, 4, 3
  d. 4, 3, 2, 1
4. Light travels at a speed of
  a. 340 mi/s.
  b. 100,000 mi/s.
  c. 186,000 mi/s.
  d. 300,000 mi/s.
5. Because the speed of light is constant, an increase in frequency results in _____ in wavelength.
  a. an increase
  b. a decrease
  c. no change
6. For a constant speed of light c, an increase in wavelength results in _____ in frequency.
  a. an increase
  b. a decrease
  c. no change
7. The number of wave cycles per second for electromagnetic radiation is the
  a. wavelength.
  b. amplitude.
  c. frequency.
  d. intensity.
8. The distance between the same portions of adjacent waves is the
  a. wavelength.
  b. amplitude.
  c. frequency.
  d. intensity.
9. The variation between zero and the maximum height of the wave is the
  a. wavelength.
  b. amplitude.
  c. frequency.
  d. intensity.
10. Hertz is a measure of
  a. the number of cycles per millimeter.
  b. the number of cycles per second.
  c. energy per centimeter squared.
  d. intensity per millimeter.

11. One kilohertz is
    a. 1 cycle per second.
    b. 1000 cycles per second.
    c. 100,000 cycles per second.
    d. 1,000,000 cycles per second.
12. One megahertz is
    a. 1 cycle per second.
    b. 1000 cycles per second.
    c. 100,000 cycles per second.
    d. 1,000,000 cycles per second.
13. One hertz is
    a. 1 cycle per second.
    b. 1000 cycles per second.
    c. 100,000 cycles per second.
    d. 1,000,000 cycles per second.
14. X-rays and gamma rays differ in
    a. energy.
    b. origin.
    c. wavelength.
    d. speed.
15. The correct form of the inverse square law is
    a. $I_2 = I_1 \times (d_1/d_2)^2$.
    b. $I_2 = I_1 \times (d_2/d_1)$.
    c. $I_2 = I_1 \times (d_1/d_2)^2$.
    d. $I_2 = I_1 \times (d_2/d_1)^2$.
16. If the original exposure rate is 8 mR/h, moving from a distance of 4 m to a distance of 2 m results in a new exposure rate of _____ mR/h.
    a. 2
    b. 4
    c. 16
    d. 32
17. Doubling the distance from an x-ray source will
    a. increase the exposure rate by a factor of 2.
    b. increase the exposure rate by a factor of 4.
    c. decrease the exposure rate by a factor of 2.
    d. decrease the exposure rate by a factor of 4.
18. Reducing the distance to a radiation source to one-half the original distance will
    a. increase the exposure rate by a factor of 2.
    b. increase the exposure rate by a factor of 4.
    c. decrease the exposure rate by a factor of 2.
    d. decrease the exposure rate by a factor of 4.

ANSWERS TO CHAPTER 4 QUESTIONS

1.	b	10.	b
2.	d	11.	b
3.	b	12.	d
4.	c	13.	a
5.	b	14.	b
6.	b	15.	c
7.	c	16.	d
8.	a	17.	d
9.	b	18.	b

Unit II

Circuits and X-ray Production

5

X-ray Circuits

Upon completion of this chapter, the student will be able to

1. Identify the difference between alternating and direct current.
2. Identify single-phase, three-phase, and high-frequency waveforms.
3. Describe the relationship between current and voltage in the primary and secondary sides of step-up and step-down transformers.
4. Identify the components of a typical x-ray circuit and their purpose.
5. Define voltage ripple.

INTRODUCTION

X-ray circuits convert electric energy into x-ray energy. Knowledge of the components of an x-ray circuit will assist the technologist in detecting and correcting problems with the technical settings used to produce the x-ray image. X-ray circuits generate x-rays using transformers that convert low voltage [100 to 400 volts (V)] into high voltage (thousands of volts). X-ray circuits utilize transformers to change the voltage, rectifiers to convert alternating current into direct current, and autotransformers to select the milliamperes and kilovolts peak applied to the x-ray tube. X-ray circuits were previously referred to as x-ray generators. However, the term *generator* used in this context has nothing to do with the generators described in Chap. 3, which are used to generate electric currents.

DIRECT AND ALTERNATING CURRENT

Electric current describes the amount of electric charge moving through a conductor and is measured in amperes or milliamperes. The two types of electric current are direct current and alternating current. Direct current (DC) flows in only one direction. Batteries and rectifiers produce direct current. Direct current is used in TV sets, microwave ovens, and x-ray tubes. Figure 5.1A is a graph of direct current as a function of time. The current flows in one direction at all times. In an alternating current (AC) circuit, shown in Fig. 5.1B, the current flows in the positive direction half of the time and in the negative direction the other half of the time.

The negative part of the curve represents current flow in the opposite direction. Alternating current is used in most electrical appliances. It is more economical to distribute electric power with AC than with DC. In the United States, the current frequency is 60 hertz. The voltage is measured at the peak of the AC cycle. An AC voltage of 2000 V is referred to as 2 kVp, where kVp means kilovolts peak.

SINGLE-PHASE AND THREE-PHASE CIRCUITS

The alternating current shown in Fig. 5.1B is a single-phase current. By adding more circuit elements, it is possible to add two more phases to form a three-phase circuit. The major advantage of a three-phase circuit is that the current and voltage are more nearly constant, which results in more efficient x-ray production. Figure 5.2 illustrates the current flow as a function of time in a three-phase circuit.

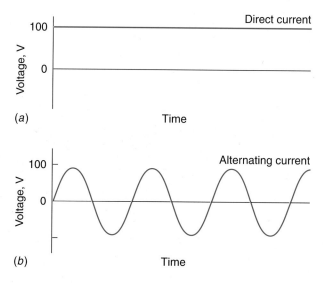

Figure 5.1 Direct current (a). Alternating current (b).

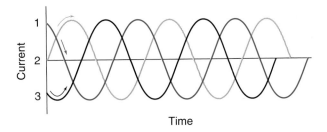

Figure 5.2 **Current from a three-phase circuit.**

HIGH-VOLTAGE CIRCUITS

High-voltage x-ray circuits contain transformers, kilovoltage (kVp) and milliampere (mA) selectors, rectifiers, and timing circuits. X-ray tubes operate only with direct current. In diagnostic radiology, the voltage across the x-ray tube can be set at values from 20,000 to 120,000 V or 20 to 120 kVp. This high voltage is required in order to produce diagnostic x-rays. A transformer is used to produce the high voltage. Transformers operate by mutual induction; they can work only with alternating current. A transformer converts an input voltage of a few hundred volts to an output voltage of many thousands of volts; rectifiers then convert the high-voltage AC to high-voltage DC. Finally, the high-voltage DC is applied to the x-ray tube and x-rays are produced.

Understanding the components of the x-ray circuit is important because changes in the circuit controls alter the x-ray image. Figure 5.3 shows a schematic diagram of a typical x-ray circuit.

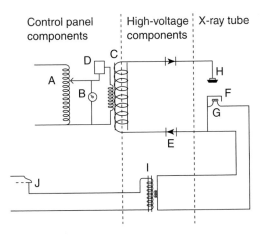

A. kVp selector
B. kVp meter
C. High-voltage transformer
D. Timer control
E. Rectifier
F. Cathode
G. Filament
H. Anode
I. Filament transformer
J. mA selector

Figure 5.3 **X-ray circuit.**

CONTROL PANEL COMPONENTS

The control panel components of the x-ray circuit appear on the left side of Fig. 5.3. The control panel components include the kVp, time and mA selectors, and the automatic exposure control circuit.

kVp and mA Selectors

The incoming electrical supply is connected to the autotransformer. The kVp and mA selectors are also connected to the autotransformer. The only way to change the output voltage of a transformer is to change its input voltage. The autotransformer is used to select the input voltage to either the step-up or the step-down transformer. The step-up or high-voltage transformer generates the high voltage used to produce the x-rays. The step-down or low-voltage transformer produces the mA tube current. Different autotransformers are used as the kVp and mA selectors.

Timing Circuits

Timing circuits shut off the high voltage to terminate the x-ray exposure after a selected exposure time. The timer opens a switch to cut off the high voltage from the x-ray tube and stop x-ray production. Exposure times are selected from the control panel to control the amount of x-rays produced. Short exposure times should be selected to minimize patient motion artifacts.

Automatic Exposure Control Circuits

An automatic exposure control (AEC) circuit measures the amount of radiation leaving the patient and turns off the x-ray beam when the correct amount of radiation has reached the detector. The AEC circuit is calibrated to produce the proper image density regardless of patient size. Figure 5.4 illustrates the operation of an automatic exposure control circuit.

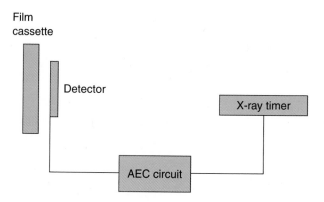

Figure 5.4 **Automatic exposure control (AEC) circuit.**

The purpose of the AEC unit is to provide the correct exposure regardless of patient size. At the control panel, the exposure mA and time can be selected independently, or the milliampere-time (mAs), which is the combination of milliamperes and time, can be selected, in which case the control circuits choose the highest mA and the shortest time allowed. The AEC detector is placed between the patient and the film cassette or image receptor.

In operation, the AEC circuit acts as the timer for the x-ray circuit. Rather than turning off the x-ray beam when a fixed time has been reached, the AEC unit turns off the x-ray beam when the proper amount of radiation has reached the image receptor. The AEC circuit still requires the technologist to set the mA and kVp correctly, although some units automatically select the highest mA allowable in order to reduce the exposure time and reduce the effects of patient motion.

Typical AEC systems have three rectangular-shaped detectors placed roughly at the corners of a triangle. In the past, automatic exposure control circuits were called phototimers because the detectors used were photomultiplying devices instead of ionization chambers. Figure 5.5 shows a picture of an image receptor holder with the position of the AEC detectors indicated.

The three detector cells can be selected to operate singly, in pairs, or all together, depending on the examination and patient orientation. A vast majority of examinations utilize the center detector. The detectors can be ionization chambers, scintillators, or solid-state detectors. Regardless of the type of detector used, the AEC unit keeps the x-ray beam on until enough x-rays have passed through the patient to provide proper exposure for the film or detector. The AEC unit must initially be calibrated for the film/screen combination used. If the film/screen combination is changed, the AEC unit must be recalibrated. Positioning is critical to allow the radiation to be detected through the part under examination.

AEC units have a provision for adjustments to give the technologist a way of modifying the overall density or blackness of the film. Each adjustment step produces about a 30 percent change in density.

Backup Timer

The backup timer terminates the exposure when the backup time is reached. It is necessary to set the backup timer in case something goes wrong. If the x-ray beam does not reach the AEC detectors, excess radiation could reach the patient and the tube could be damaged. This could happen if the x-ray beam and the detectors were not aligned. If the vertical Bucky AEC is selected and the x-ray beam is directed at the table, the x-ray beam will not turn off. The backup timer terminates the exposure before the tube limits are exceeded. Backup timers are usually set at 5 seconds (s).

The control panel portion of the x-ray circuit contains circuits to control the kVp, the mA, and the time. The kVp is changed by changing

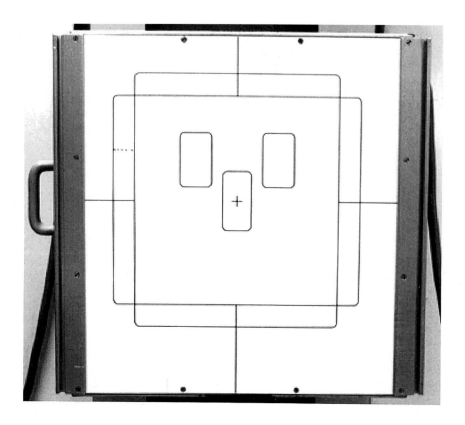

Figure 5.5 Photograph of image receptor (vertical Bucky) with the outline of the AEC cell locations indicated.

the input to the high-voltage step-up transformer, using an autotransformer. The mA is controlled by an autotransformer that changes the input to the step-down transformer. The timing circuit is used to select the exposure time. The automatic exposure control circuit measures the intensity of the x-rays leaving the patient and adjusts the exposure time to produce a proper-density image.

HIGH-VOLTAGE COMPONENTS

Components of the high-voltage circuit include the secondary windings of the step-up, high-voltage transformer, the secondary windings of the step-down transformer, and the rectifiers.

Transformers

A transformer consists of a pair of wire coils joined together around an iron core. This iron core provides coupling of the magnetic fields between the coils. X-ray transformers are usually placed inside a metal box about the size of a kitchen table or a desk. The box is filled with oil to provide electrical and thermal insulation to prevent electric shock and to cool the transformer. The current flowing through the coils produces heat in the transformer. A schematic representation of a transformer is shown in Fig. 5.6.

The voltage change between the primary or input side and the secondary or output side of the transformer depends on the ratio of the number of primary turns to the number of secondary turns.

A transformer with more turns on the secondary than on the primary is known as a **step-up transformer.** The output voltage on the secondary winding of a step-up transformer is greater than the input voltage on the primary winding. The output current on the secondary winding of a step-up transformer is less than the input current on the primary winding. The step-up transformer is used to produce high voltage or kilovoltage peak (kVp) between the cathode and anode of the x-ray tube.

Figure 5.7 shows a schematic of a step-up transformer with the current and voltage waveforms on the primary and secondary windings.

A transformer with fewer turns on the secondary than on the primary is a **step-down transformer**. In a step-down transformer, the output voltage on the secondary winding is less than the input voltage on the primary winding, and the output current on the secondary winding is greater than the input current on the primary winding. Figure 5.8 shows a schematic diagram of a step-

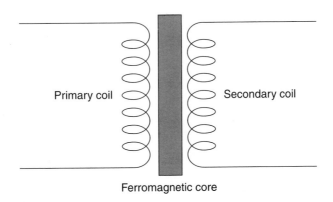

Primary coil

Secondary coil

Ferromagnetic core

Figure 5.6 Transformer with primary and secondary coils.

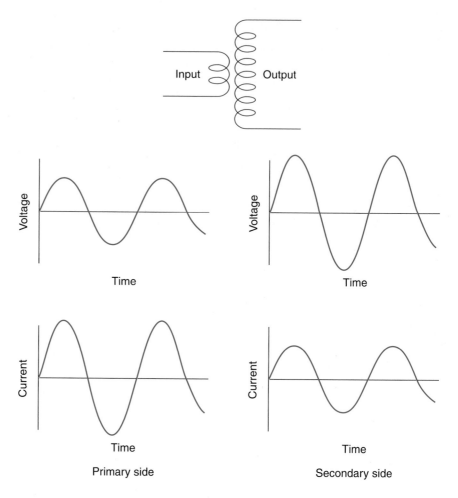

Figure 5.7 **Voltage and current on the primary and secondary sides of a step-up transformer.**

down transformer with the current and voltage waveforms on the primary and secondary windings. A step-down transformer is used in the filament circuit to produce high current to the filament to boil off the electrons that make up the tube current, or mA.

The ratio of the number of turns in the secondary to the number of turns in the primary of a transformer is called the **turns ratio.** The turns ratio determines the change in voltage from input to output. The input voltage is sometimes called the primary voltage because it is applied to the primary coil

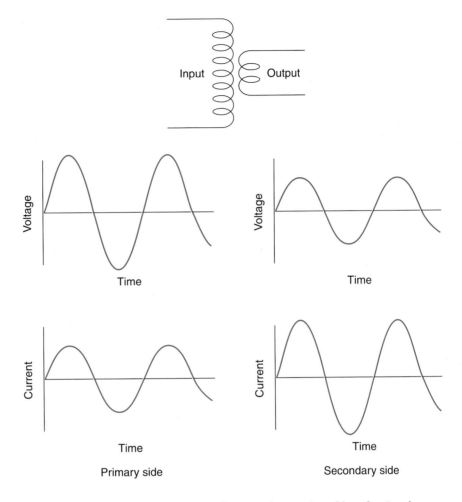

Figure 5.8 Voltage and current on the primary and secondary sides of a step-down transformer.

of the transformer. The output voltage is sometimes called the secondary voltage because it appears on the secondary coil of the transformer. Step-up transformers have a turns ratio greater than 1. Step-down transformers have a turns ratio less than 1.

Equation (5.1) gives the relationship between the primary voltage, the secondary voltage, the number of primary turns, and the number of secondary turns.

$$V_{secondary} = V_{primary} \left(N_{secondary}/N_{primary} \right) \tag{5.1}$$

EXAMPLE 1:

The number of windings on the primary coil of a transformer is 500, and the number of windings on the secondary coil is 400,000. What is the turns ratio?

SOLUTION:

$$\text{Turns ratio} = N_{secondary}/N_{primary}$$
$$= (400,000/500)$$
$$= 800$$

EXAMPLE 2:

If the input voltage on the primary winding of the transformer in Example 1 is 100 V, what is the output voltage on the secondary winding?

SOLUTION:

$$V_{secondary} = V_{primary}(\text{turns ratio})$$
$$= 100 \times 800$$
$$= 80,000 \text{ V}$$

Rectifiers

Rectifiers are solid-state devices that allow current to flow in only one direction. They are used to convert high-voltage AC from the secondary side of the step-up transformer to high-voltage DC, which is applied to the x-ray tube. Current flows from the positive terminal of the x-ray tube, which is called the anode, to the negative terminal of the x-ray tube, which is called the cathode. Although current is said to flow from positive to negative, in an x-ray tube electrons actually flow from the cathode to the anode. The construction and operation of x-ray tubes is discussed more completely in Chap. 6. Rectifiers are sometimes called diodes because they have two electrodes. Figure 5.9 illustrates the current flow through a typical rectifier in a single-phase circuit.

The output current shown in Fig. 5.9 is known as full-wave-rectified because both the positive and the negative parts of the single-phase input circuit are converted to positive current flowing in only one direction, or DC.

THREE-PHASE CIRCUITS

By the addition of two more circuits made up of transformers and rectifiers, 120° out of phase with each other and with the first circuit, the output voltage and current can be made more constant. The result, known as a three-phase

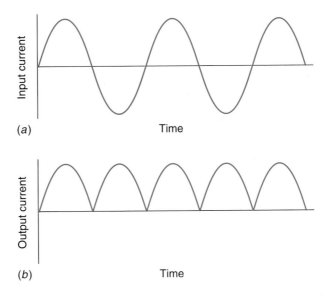

Figure 5.9 **Input current (*a*) and output current (*b*) from a single-phase full-wave-rectified circuit.**

circuit, provides more efficient x-ray production. Figure 5.10 shows the current from a full-wave-rectified three-phase, six-pulse circuit.

This circuit requires six rectifiers. By adding additional components, it is possible to produce three-phase, 12-pulse current. This provides a more constant voltage waveform. Increasing the number of pulses in the waveform by using 12-pulse 3-phase circuit increases the average voltage but does not increase the maximum voltage. Table 5.1 presents the number of rectifiers used in different forms of x-ray circuits.

HIGH-FREQUENCY CIRCUITS

Transformers operate more efficiently at higher frequencies because the coupling between the primary and secondary windings is more effective. A high-frequency transformer operating at 3000 Hz is much smaller and lighter than one designed to operate at 60 Hz.

High-frequency circuits first change the input frequency from 60 Hz to a higher frequency (500 to 3000 Hz) using a voltage inverter. The inverter converts the low-voltage AC to low-voltage DC using rectifiers, then switching the low-voltage DC on and off rapidly. This switching converts the low-voltage DC to low-voltage high-frequency AC. A transformer then increases the voltage (to 20,000 to 150,000 V), and a rectifier converts the AC into DC, which is

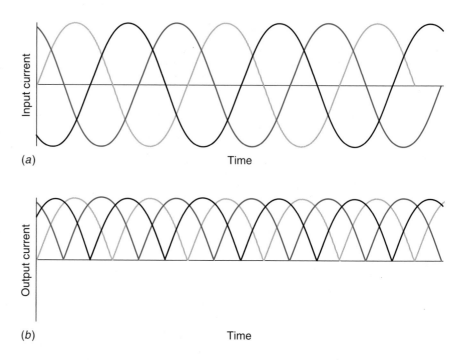

Figure 5.10 Input and output electrical waveforms from three-phase circuit: (a), unrectified; (b), rectified.

applied to the x-ray tube. Figure 5.11 illustrates the basic operation of the high-frequency x-ray circuit.

There are two main stages in the operation of a high-frequency x-ray circuit. The first stage converts 60-Hz 200-V AC to DC using rectifiers. The second stage rapidly switches the low-voltage DC on and off to produce high-frequency AC.

Although there are many different design details, all high-frequency circuits switch the low-voltage (200 V) DC rapidly on and off to produce high-frequency but still low-voltage AC. This is applied to the primary of a step-up transformer to produce a high-frequency high-voltage output. The secondary

Table 5.1
Number of Rectifiers in X-ray Circuits

Type of Circuit	Number of Rectifiers
Single-phase, full-wave	2 or 4
Three-phase, six-pulse	6
Three-phase, twelve-pulse	12

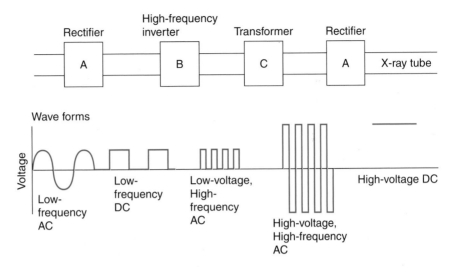

Figure 5.11 High-frequency inverter circuit used to convert low-voltage alternating current to high-voltage direct current.

voltage from the step-up transformer is then rectified to produce high-voltage DC, which is applied to the x-ray tube.

The advantages gained from the high-frequency circuit outweigh the cost and added complexity of the extra stages. The advantages of high-frequency circuits are smaller size, less weight, and improved x-ray production. Modern computed tomography (CT) scanners have high-frequency circuits mounted in the rotating gantry. High-frequency circuits with their lightweight transformers make spiral CT practical. Most x-ray units installed today have high-frequency circuits.

RIPPLE

Ripple measures the amount of variation between maximum and minimum voltage. Because most x-ray production occurs when the applied voltage is at maximum, the percent ripple provides a good indication of how much variation there is in the x-ray output. Lower-ripple circuits have more constant x-ray output and higher average voltage. Table 5.2 presents the average voltage and amount of ripple from different types of x-ray circuits.

The amount of ripple actually present at the x-ray tube depends on the length and type of x-ray cables and the details of the high-voltage circuit.

Three-phase high-frequency circuits produce higher average voltage, but single-phase and three-phase circuits have the same maximum voltage. At higher voltages, the x-ray production process is more efficient and the x-rays

Table 5.2
Average Voltage and Percent Ripple for Different Waveforms

Average Voltage	Max	Percent Ripple
Single-phase	0.71 V_{max}	100
Three-phase, six-pulse	0.95 V_{max}	13
Three-phase, twelve-pulse	0.99 V_{max}	3
High-frequency generator	1.00 V_{max}	1

are more penetrating, so three-phase and high-frequency circuits require fewer milliamperes or less time to obtain the same image density.

A step-up transformer is used to produce the high voltage applied to the x-ray tube. A step-down transformer is used to apply voltage to the filament and control the mA. Rectifiers convert AC to DC because they pass current in only one direction. High-frequency circuits use switches to convert 60-Hz AC to 3000 Hz. High-frequency circuits use smaller and lighter components. Ripple describes the variation of the DC high voltage applied to the x-ray tube. The backup timer prevents tube damage in case the automatic exposure unit fails to terminate the exposure.

SUMMARY

Direct current flows in only one direction. Alternating current flows in two opposite directions, half one way and half the other way. X-ray circuits convert low-voltage AC input to high-voltage DC, which is applied to the x-ray tube. The kVp selector is an autotransformer that changes the input to the step-up, or high-voltage, transformer. The mA selector is an autotransformer that changes the input to the step-down, or mA, transformer to control the filament current. The ratio of the number of turns on the secondary to the number of turns on the primary is called the turns ratio. A transformer with a turns ratio greater than 1 is a step-up transformer; the output voltage is greater than the input voltage. A transformer with a turns ratio less than 1 is a step-down transformer; the output voltage is less than the input voltage.

Ripple is a measure of the variation between the maximum and minimum voltage. Circuits with low ripple produce a more constant x-ray output. Three-phase and high-frequency x-ray circuits have less ripple and produce more constant output than single-phase x-ray circuits but do not change the maximum voltage.

21. An autotransformer functions as a(n)
    a. line-voltage compensator.
    b. kVp or mA selector.
    c. filament transformer.
    d. automatic exposure controller.
22. Ripple measures
    a. total tube voltage.
    b. variation between maximum and minimum mA.
    c. variation between maximum and minimum tube voltages.
    d. total mA.

ANSWERS TO CHAPTER 5 QUESTIONS

1.	a	12.	j
2.	d	13.	c
3.	a	14.	a
4.	e	15.	b
5.	h	16.	a
6.	b	17.	b
7.	i	18.	d
8.	i	19.	b
9.	c	20.	a
10.	g	21.	b
11.	f	22.	c

6

X-ray Tubes

OBJECTIVES

At the end of this chapter, the student will be able to

1. Identify and describe the components of a typical x-ray tube and their purpose.
2. Define thermionic emission.
3. Describe the line focus principle and the heel effect.
4. Define anode heat units.
5. Recognize allowed and forbidden tube heat loads.

INTRODUCTION

This chapter covers the components, operation, and limitations of x-ray tubes. The purpose of the x-ray tube is to produce an x-ray beam. The x-ray tube contains a negative electrode, the cathode, and a positive electrode, the anode.

X-RAY TUBE

The **filament** is heated to boil off the projectile electrons that make up the tube current. Projectile electrons are accelerated by high voltage from the negative cathode to the positive **anode,** where x-rays are produced. The energy of the projectile electrons is converted into heat and x-ray energy.

The filament is contained in the **cathode,** which is shaped like a cup to focus the projectile electrons onto the anode. The anode contains a focal spot that has an area of only a few square millimeters. The anode rotates in order to spread the heat from the projectile electrons over a larger area. The tube components are sealed inside an evacuated glass or metal envelope. The vacuum allows electrons to travel freely from the negative cathode to the positive anode.

TUBE HOUSING AND ENVELOPE

The glass or metal tube envelope is surrounded by oil, which provides electrical insulation and cooling for the tube. The x-ray tube and oil are contained in a metal housing. The housing protects against electric shock and absorbs **leakage radiation** emitted outside the x-ray beam. Regulations require that the leakage radiation through the tube housing be less than 100 milliroentgens per hour (mR/h) at 1 meter (m) from the tube. The x-rays that are emitted through the thin window of the envelope are called the **primary beam.** The thin window allows the maximum amount of x-rays to be transmitted, with very little absorption by the envelope. A fan is often used to transfer the heat from the housing to the room air by convection.

Figure 6-1 shows the components of a typical x-ray tube.

The metal housing that contains the cooling and insulating oil protects the x-ray tube from external damage. The housing also shields against leakage radiation, which must be reduced to less than 100 mR/h at 1 m.

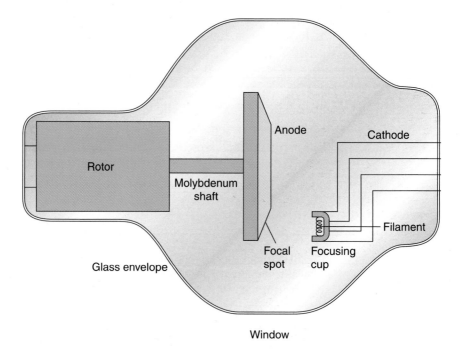

Figure 6.1 Components of x-ray tube.

CATHODE

The cathode is the negative electrode of the x-ray tube. It contains the filaments and focusing cup. Figure 6.2 shows a typical cathode, with two filaments located near the bottom of a focusing cup.

Focusing Cup

The filaments are contained within the focusing cup. The negative charge on the surface of the focusing cup forces the projectile electrons together into a narrow beam as they are accelerated to the anode. The anode region where the projectile electrons strike is called the **focal spot.** Figure 6.3 shows the focusing action of a typical cup-shaped cathode.

Filament

The purpose of the filament is to provide projectile electrons for acceleration to the positive anode. The filament, a coil of tungsten alloy wire, is heated to boil off electrons. The emission of electrons by heating of the filament is called **thermionic emission.** Changes in the filament current produce changes in the filament temperature. This causes a change in the number of projectile electrons boiled off the filament. An increase or decrease in the number of projectile electrons striking the focal spot changes the number of x-rays. The projectile electron current or tube current is termed the milliamperes (**mA**).

The size of the focal spot is determined by the size of the filament coil. X-ray tubes have two filaments, one large and one small. The large filament is used when high x-ray production is needed. The large filament produces a large focal spot, spreading the heat over a larger area, which allows higher tube

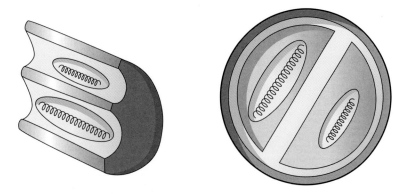

Figure 6.2 **Cup-shaped cathode with two filaments.**

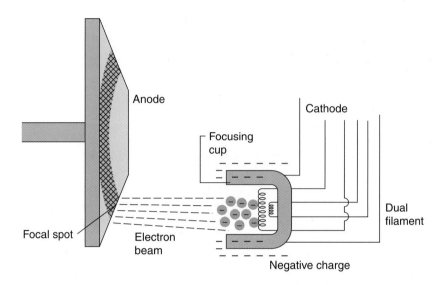

Figure 6.3 **Focusing action of the focusing cup.**

currents without damaging the anode. The small filament produces a small focal spot and is used when fine detail images are required. Lower tube currents should be used with small focal spots. Large filaments typically produce 1- to 3-millimeter (mm) focal spots; small filaments produce focal spots 1 mm or smaller. Focal spot size can be selected automatically by selecting larger or smaller mA stations or manually by selecting the focal spot size directly.

GRID-CONTROLLED TUBES

Grid-controlled tubes are designed to turn on and off quickly to produce very short exposure times. These tubes have extra electrical connections to apply a voltage that prevents the projectile electrons from leaving the cathode unless an activation voltage is applied. Grid-controlled tubes are used in cineradiography, digital subtraction radiography, and digital fluoroscopy when rapid multiple exposures are required.

TUBE AND FILAMENT CURRENT

There are two currents used in an x-ray tube, the filament current and the projectile electron current. The projectile electron or tube current is called the mA. Typical tube currents range from 50 to 800 milliamperes (mA). The mA

Table 6.1
Currents Used in X-ray Tubes

Filament current	2–5 amperes
Tube current	50–800 milliamperes

selector controls the amount of tube current by adjusting the filament current to change the filament temperature. Typical filament currents are 2 to 5 amperes (A), which is hundreds of times larger than tube currents. Filament currents are higher than tube currents because they must heat the filament so that thermionic emission can take place. Table 6.1 compares the magnitudes of the filament and tube currents.

The cathode is the negative terminal of the x-ray tube. The cathode structure contains the filaments and the focusing cup. Electrons are boiled off the filament by thermionic emission and then concentrated on the focal spot by the focusing cup. The anode, which is the positive electrode, contains the focal spot, or target, where the projectile electrons strike. Typical filament currents are several amperes, whereas typical tube currents are tens to hundreds of milliamperes.

ANODE

The positive anode contains the area where the projectile electrons stop. This area is called the focal spot. More than 99 percent of the electron energy is deposited in the anode as heat. Only about 1 percent of the projectile electron energy is converted to x-rays. Figure 6.4 illustrates the construction of a typical anode.

The focal spot on the anode can reach temperatures greater than 3000°C during an x-ray exposure. Most metals melt at these temperatures, and so the anode must be made of a material with a high melting point. Tungsten alloys that melt at 3400°C are commonly used in anode construction.

Anodes are disk-shaped structures 6 to 15 centimeters (cm) in diameter. The anodes in modern tubes are rotating anodes. They rotate to allow for better heat dispersion: When the anode rotates, the electrons strike a larger target area rather than a single spot. Anodes are made of a tungsten alloy chosen for its high atomic number and high melting point. The efficiency of x-ray production increases with the atomic number of the anode material. Materials with a higher atomic number produce more x-rays for the same tube current (mA).

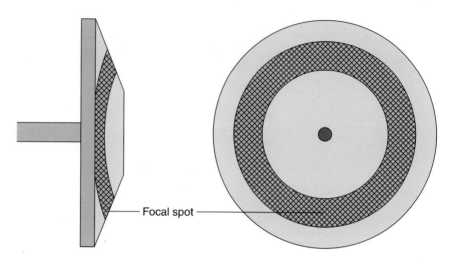

Focal spot

Figure 6.4 **Anode construction.**

Heat from the focal spot is carried to the rest of the anode by conduction. Anode heat is transferred from the anode to the walls of the tube housing by radiation. The housing walls are cooled by convection of room air, which may be increased by fans mounted on the housing.

Rotating Anode Tubes

The anode consists of a target, a shaft, and a rotor. Rotating anodes spread the heat from the electrons over a circular track rather than concentrating it in a single spot on the anode surface. The x-ray source remains fixed relative to the patient, but the heat is spread over a circular track as the anode rotates. Most anodes rotate at about 3600 revolutions per minute (rpm), but some high-speed tubes rotate at 10,000 rpm for greater heat dissipation. Changing the anode rotation speed changes the anode heat capacity but does not change the focal spot size.

The anode, shaft, and rotor are sealed inside an evacuated tube. Conventional motors using slip rings to provide electrical contact with the rotor are not used to drive the anode because the slip rings would destroy the vacuum inside the tube. Instead, an induction motor is used to rotate the anode. Electromagnets called **stators** are fixed on the outside of the glass envelope and activated by an electric current in a synchronized arrangement. Changes in the external magnetic field at the stators rotate the anode.

The shaft connecting the rotating anode to the rotor is made of molybdenum and is supported by bearings. Molybdenum is a strong metal with low heat conductivity. Its low thermal conductivity prevents the anode heat from reaching and damaging the rotor bearings. Bearing damage is a major cause of tube failure.

The anode is the positive terminal of the x-ray tube. It is constructed of a material that has high heat conductivity, a high melting point, and a high atomic number. Most anodes are made of tungsten alloys. Electrons from the cathode are concentrated by the focusing cup to strike the anode focal spot. X-ray tubes have a small focal spot for small detail imaging and a larger one for imaging thicker body parts, which requires higher tube currents. Typical x-ray tubes have 1- and 3-mm focal spots. More than 99 percent of the projectile energy deposited in the anode appears as heat. Diagnostic x-ray tubes have a rotating anode to spread the heat over the entire anode surface. Heat is transferred from the focal spot to the body of the anode by conduction. Heat is transferred from the anode to the tube housing by radiation. Heat is transferred from the tube housing to the room by convection.

LINE FOCUS PRINCIPLE

The line focus principle involves spreading the heat over a larger area while maintaining a smaller focal spot for sharper images. The sharpness of the final x-ray image is determined by the focal spot size. Smaller focal spots produce sharper images. The size of the focal spot as seen by the patient or the image receptor is known as the effective focal spot size and is smaller than the actual focal spot size because of the line focus principle. The surface of the anode is angled to spread the heat from the projectile electrons over a larger area. The angle between the anode surface and the x-ray beam, shown in Fig. 6.5, is called the **anode angle.** Figure 6.5 illustrates how reducing the anode angle reduces the effective focal spot size while maintaining the same area on the anode surface (actual focal spot). Radiographic tubes have anode angles from 12° to 17°. The smaller target angle results in a smaller effective focal spot size, better detailed images, and higher heat capacity. Spreading the heat over a larger area allows for increased mA values. This method produces sharper images because the effective focal spot is always smaller than the actual focal spot. The anode angle is set by the manufacturer during tube construction.

HEEL EFFECT

The heel effect produces an intensity variation between the cathode and anode sides of the x-ray tube. This causes a variation in density on the film. The heel effect exists because the x-rays are produced below the anode surface. The x-ray intensity is decreased toward the anode side of the tube because the x-rays emitted in that direction must pass through more anode material, or the heel of the anode.

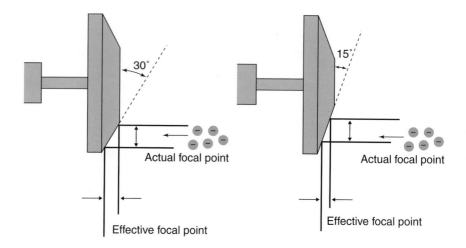

Figure 6.5 The line-focus principle uses an angled anode to spread the heat of the projectile electrons over a larger surface area.

Figure 6.6 shows how x-rays emitted toward the cathode side of the x-ray tube pass through less anode material than x-rays emitted toward the anode side of the field. The heel effect can produce intensity variations of more than 40 percent between the anode and cathode sides of the field. The heel effect is more noticeable with smaller anode angles, larger field sizes, and shorter source to image receptor distances (SIDs).

Smaller field sizes and larger SIDs reduce the heel effect. The heel effect is put to use in clinical situations to achieve a uniform density when there is a large variation in body part thickness across the x-ray field. The cathode side of the tube is placed over the thicker body part. An example of this would be imaging the thoracic spine in an anteroposterior projection. The cathode side would be placed over the lower thoracic spine with the anode at the upper thoracic area to produce a more uniform density over the entire thoracic spine.

OFF-FOCUS RADIATION

Off-focus radiation consists of x-rays produced at locations other than the focal spot. It occurs when projectile electrons strike other parts of the anode, away from the focal spot. Off-focus radiation causes radiographic images to appear unsharp, decreasing overall image quality. Most off-focus radiation is attenuated by the tube housing and the first stage collimator, which is located near the window of the glass envelope.

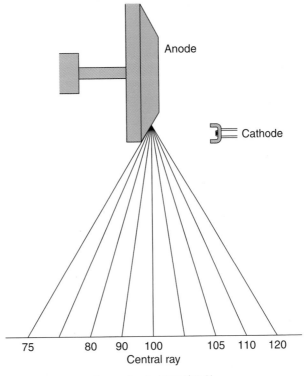

| 75 | 80 | 90 | 100 | 105 | 110 | 120 |

Central ray

Approximate intensity, %

Figure 6.6 **Heel effect.**

FOCAL SPOT BLOOMING

Negative projectile electrons repel one another while traveling from cathode to anode. Focal spot blooming refers to an increase in focal spot size with an increase in mA caused by this electrostatic repulsion. Focal spot blooming is important only with very high mA values and lower kilovoltage (kVp) settings.

The anode surface is tilted so that the effective focal spot as seen by the patient is smaller than the actual focal spot. The line focus principle allows the heat from the electron beam to be spread over a larger area while maintaining a small effective focal spot. Because most of the x-rays are produced below the surface of the anode, there are fewer x-rays on the anode side of the x-ray beam. This difference in intensity across the x-ray beam is known as the heel effect. Smaller anode angles spread the heat over larger areas and have greater heel effects.

HEAT UNITS

The heat deposited in the anode by the projectile electrons depends on the mA, kVp, and exposure time. Exposures with higher applied voltages, higher tube currents, and longer exposure times deposit more heat on the anode focal spot. The heat deposited in the anode is measured in heat units (HU). The number of heat units is obtained by

Single-phase	$HU = kVp \times mA \times seconds$
Three-phase, six-pulse	$HU = 1.35 \times kVp \times mA \times seconds$
Three-phase, twelve-pulse or high-frequency	$HU = 1.41 \times kVp \times mA \times seconds$

The 1.35 and 1.41 are factors used to adjust for the use of constant-potential, three-phase or high-frequency circuits. These circuits deposit more heat in the anode than a single-phase circuit for the same kVp and mA settings.

EXAMPLE 1:

What is the heat load in HU from a single-phase exposure with technical factors of 100 kVp, 200 mA, and 0.1 second (s)?

ANSWER:

$$HU = 100 \times 200 \times 0.1$$
$$= 2000 \text{ HU}$$

EXAMPLE 2:

What are the HU in Example 1 if the exposure is made using a high-frequency circuit?

ANSWER:

$$HU = 1.41 \times 100 \times 200 \times 0.1$$
$$= 2820 \text{ HU}$$

EXAMPLE 3:

The maximum heat load for an x-ray tube is 25,000 HU.
(A) What is the total heat load from three exposures?
(B) Will a series of three of these exposures in rapid succession, using a high-frequency circuit with technical factors of 120 kVp, 200 mA, and 0.15 s, exceed the heat limits of 25,000 HU for this tube?

ANSWER:

Calculate the heat units from three exposures.
Heat units from one exposure:

$$HU = 1.41 \times 120 \times 200 \times 0.15$$
$$= 5076 \text{ HU}$$

For three exposures, the total heat units is

$$HU_{total} = 3 \times 5076$$
$$= 15{,}228 \text{ HU}$$

(B) This series of exposures does not exceed the heat limits of the tube.

HEAT LIMIT CURVES

Heat limit or tube rating charts provide information about the amount of heat that can be safely deposited in the anode. Heat limit curves divide the technical factors of kVp, mA, and time into allowed and unallowed exposure regions. The region below and to the left of a heat limit curve is allowed; the region above and to the right of the curve is unallowed. Exposures in the allowed

EXAMPLE 4:

Is a small focal spot exposure of 100 kVp, 300 mA, and 0.1 s allowed? Use the curves of Fig. 6.7.

ANSWER:

To answer this question, locate the intersection of the 100-kVp and 0.1-s lines and ask whether the intersection point is above or below the 300-mA curve. In this case it is below and to the left of the curve, so this exposure is allowed.

EXAMPLE 5:

Is an exposure of 120 kVp, 400 mA, and 0.2 s on the small focal spot of the tube in Fig. 6.7 allowed?

ANSWER:

The intersection of 120 kVp and 0.2 s lies above and to the right of the 400-mA curve, so this exposure is not allowed.

Modern x-ray equipment has safety circuits to prevent the selection of a single unallowed exposure, but these circuits do not prevent multiple allowed exposures with no cooling between exposures. Even though a single exposure is allowed, repeat exposures using the same technique may exceed the total heat limit of the tube. It is essential to wait between multiple exposures to allow the anode to cool if each exposure is near the maximum heat capacity of the anode.

region will not harm the tube; exposures in the unallowed region could severely damage the tube. High-kVp, high-mA, long-time exposures are not allowed. Short-time, low-kVp, low-mA exposures are allowed. The heat limits are different for large and small focal spots because the large focal spot spreads the heat over a larger area on the anode surface. Figure 6.7 gives an example of a heat limit curve.

ANODE HEAT MONITORS

Some modern x-ray circuits are equipped with an anode heat monitor. This monitor displays the percent of maximum allowed heat that has been deposited in the anode. The monitor uses the mA, time, and kVp settings to calculate the heat units for each exposure. The anode cooling rate is included in the calculation.

TUBE LIFE AND WARM-UP PROCEDURES

An x-ray tube costs about the same as a new car. It is important to extend the life of the tube by properly warming up the tube before beginning clinical exposures. Tubes fail because of thermal factors. Excessive heat can cause filament failure, bearing damage, and anode cracks. Proper tube warm-up will extend tube life. Figure 6.8 shows an anode after a heat-induced crack split the anode into two pieces.

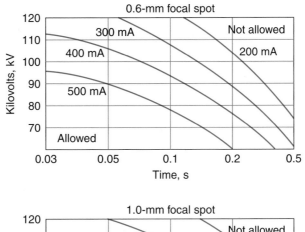

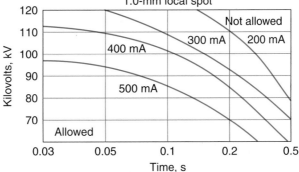

Figure 6.7 **Heat limit curves.**

Warm-up exposures eliminate anode cracking by spreading the heat over the entire target surface. A proper warm-up procedure uses at least a 1-s exposure so that the anode rotates many times during the exposure. A very short exposure on a cold anode concentrates the heat on a fraction of the anode surface. This can cause uneven thermal expansion of the anode and may crack the anode. A typical warm-up procedure would consist of two 70-kVp, 100-mA, 2-s exposures. Tube warm-up procedures should be performed whenever the x-ray tube has not been used for several hours.

While the x-ray unit is on, it remains in the standby mode, with a filament current of a few amperes keeping the filament warm and ready to be heated to its operating temperature. Just before the exposure is made, the anode begins rotating and the filament is heated to operating temperature by the boost current. This is called the prep stage of exposure. A safety circuit prevents exposure prior to the anode's reaching full rotation speed. The boost current raises the filament temperature to begin thermionic emission. The boost current is present while the exposure switch is activated. Maintaining the tube in the boost mode or prep stage after the x-ray exposure is completed can

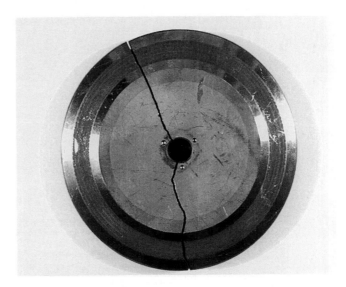

Figure 6.8 Anode after being split into two pieces by a heat-induced crack.

significantly shorten tube life by burning out the filament. The exposure switch should be released as soon as the exposure is completed. The standby mode does not shorten tube life.

Heat is the primary cause of tube failure. Heat increases rotor bearing wear. When tube bearings begin to fail, they emit a noticeable grinding noise after every exposure. Heat can also damage the anode surface.

The heat deposited in the anode is concentrated in the area of the focal spot. Heat units are calculated by multiplying the exposure time by the kVp and the exposure mA. Heat limit curves outline the allowed and unallowed exposure parameters. X-ray tubes must be properly warmed up before diagnostic exposures begin in order to prevent serious tube damage.

SUMMARY

The negative cathode of the x-ray tube contains the filament. Thermionic emission from the heated filament produces projectile electrons, which are accelerated to the positive anode. The anode is a disk-shaped structure constructed of a high atomic number alloy that has high thermal conductivity and a high melting point. The anode and cathode are contained in an evacuated glass or metal tube surrounded by oil inside a metal housing. The oil provides electrical insulation and cooling. The projectile electrons stop in the anode and produce x-rays. More than 99 percent of the electron energy is converted to heat in the anode; less than 1 percent is converted to x-rays. X-ray tubes utilize rotating anodes to distribute the heat around a circular track on the anode surface.

The line focus principle uses an angled anode to spread heat over a larger area (the actual focal spot) while still maintaining a smaller effective focal spot.

The heel effect causes different x-ray intensities at the cathode and anode ends of the tube, limiting the useful field size. The heel effect exists because some of the x-rays are produced below the anode surface. These x-rays are attenuated as they leave the anode. Thus, the intensity at the anode end is less than that at the cathode end of the field.

Heat units are the product of the kVp, the mA, and the exposure time. Heat units depend on the focal spot size and the type of x-ray circuit used. It is important to extend tube life by following proper warm-up procedures. Heat limit curves show the allowed and unallowed exposure regions for tubes. There are separate curves for the large and small focal spots.

QUESTIONS

1. Which component is not a part of the cathode structure?
   a. Filament
   b. Rotor
   c. Focusing cup
2. The heel effect
   a. exists because not all x-rays are produced at the surface of the anode.
   b. exists because x-rays produced inside the cathode are attenuated.
   c. depends on mA and kVp.
   d. is reduced by dual focal spots.
3. The principal means of heat transfer from the focal spot to the anode is
   a. conduction.
   b. convection.
   c. radiation.
   d. convention.
4. The line focus principle
   a. makes the focal spot appear larger than it really is.
   b. makes use of an angled cathode structure.
   c. produces x-ray lines.
   d. spreads the heat over a larger part of the anode.

5. The purpose of the cathode focusing cup is to
   a. alter the filament size.
   b. group the electrons for their passage to the anode.
   c. regulate anode rotation speed.
   d. increase the heat capacity of the tube.

If the maximum heat load of a tube in a single-phase circuit is 30,000 HU, which of the exposure series in Questions 6 to 10 is permitted on a cold tube? Answer A for allowed or B for not allowed.

6. _____ Five 100-kVp, 300-mA, 0.2-s exposures followed by one 100-kVp, 100-mA, 0.1-s exposure

7. _____ Five 120-kVp, 200-mA, 0.2-s exposures

8. _____ Five 80-kVp, 400-mA, 0.2-s exposures

9. _____ Six 75-kVp, 350-mA, 0.2-s exposures

10. _____ Five 80-kVp, 350-mA, 0.2-s exposures

11. A molybdenum shaft is used to connect the anode to the rotor because
    a. molybdenum is a poor heat conductor.
    b. molybdenum has a low bulk compressibility.
    c. molybdenum has a low moment of inertia.
    d. molybdenum has a 17.5-keV x-ray.

12. Many x-ray tubes have two filaments
    a. because the second filament can be used as a spare when the first burns out.
    b. to provide two focal spot sizes.
    c. to allow for cooling of the filament by alternating exposures.
    d. to improve tube cooling by sharing the heat between the two filaments.

13. The principal means of heat transfer from the anode to the housing is
    a. conduction.
    b. convection.
    c. radiation.
    d. convention.

14. The boost current in a filament
    a. maintains the filament at a standby temperature.
    b. is present while the x-ray machine is on.
    c. is used to improve the vacuum in the x-ray tube.
    d. raises the filament to its operating temperature.

In Questions 15 to 17, answer A for true or B for false.

15. _____ An increase in target angle will increase the heat capacity of the tube.

16. _____ An increase in focal spot size will increase the heat capacity of the tube.

17. _____ An increase in anode rotation speed will increase the heat capacity of the tube.

The number of heat units for a high-frequency exposure of 200 mA, 70 kVp, and 1 s is the maximum allowed. Are the exposures in Questions 18 to 22 also allowed? Answer A for yes or B for no.

18. _____ 100 mA, 70 kVp, 2 s
19. _____ 400 mA, 60 kVp, 1 s
20. _____ 100 mA, 110 kVp, 1 s
21. _____ 350 mA, 70 kVp, 2 s
22. _____ 200 mA, 80 kVp, 1 s
23. The transfer of heat by _____ is increased by mounting a fan on the tube housing.
    a. convection
    b. radiation
    c. conduction
    d. convention
24. Leakage radiation through the x-ray tube housing should be less than
    a. 10 mR/h at 1 foot
    b. 100 mR/h at 3 meters
    c. 100 mR/h at 1 meter
    d. 1000 mR/h at 1 meter

The effective focal spot will increase with which of the changes or conditions in Questions 25 to 27? Answer A for true or B for false.

25. _____ Very high mA
26. _____ Increasing the anode angle
27. _____ Increasing the anode rotation speed
28. Which of the following does not improve the heat capacity of the x-ray tube?
    a. A rotating anode
    b. A small target angle
    c. Larger focal spots
    d. Thermionic emission
29. What are the heat units for a high-frequency exposure taken at 120 kVp, 300 mA, and 0.6 s?
    a. 22,000
    b. 30,500
    c. 33,000
    d. 45,000
    e. 50,000
30. The principal means of heat transfer from the tube housing to the room is
    a. conduction.
    b. convection.
    c. radiation.
    d. convention.

31. The heel effect is more pronounced
    a. further from the focal spot.
    b. with a large focal spot.
    c. with a small cassette.
    d. with a small target angle.
32. The effective focal spot is determined by the target angle and the
    a. distance from the anode to the cathode.
    b. composition of the anode.
    c. diameter of the anode.
    d. filament size.
33. The major benefit of a small target angle is
    a. increased heat capacity.
    b. greater field coverage.
    c. a greater anode heel effect.
    d. more uniform radiographic density.
34. The focusing cup surrounds the
    a. anode.
    b. filament.
    c. rotor.
    d. stator.
35. A lateral skull tomogram requires 50 mA for 3 s at 75 kVp on a single-phase unit. How many heat units are generated by five exposures?
    a. 10,550
    b. 11,250
    c. 15,900
    d. 56,250
36. Electrons are emitted from the
    a. rotor.
    b. cathode.
    c. anode.
    d. stator.
37. X-rays are emitted from the
    a. rotor.
    b. cathode.
    c. anode.
    d. stator.
38. Thermionic emission
    a. is the emission of thermons.
    b. is the emission of electrons from the heated cathode.
    c. is the emission of electrons from the heated anode.
39. The tube current (mA) is changed by changing the
    a. filament current.
    b. anode voltage.
    c. focal spot size.
    d. time.

ANSWERS TO CHAPTER 6 QUESTIONS

1.	b		21.	b
2.	a		22.	b
3.	a		23.	a
4.	d		24.	c
5.	b		25.	a
6.	b		26.	a
7.	a		27.	b
8.	b		28.	d
9.	b		29.	b
10.	a		30.	b
11.	a		31.	d
12.	b		32.	d
13.	c		33.	a
14.	d		34.	b
15.	b		35.	d
16.	a		36.	b
17.	a		37.	c
18.	a		38.	b
19.	b		39.	a
20.	a			

7

X-ray Production

OBJECTIVES

At the conclusion of this chapter, the student will be able to

1. Describe the bremsstrahlung x-ray production process.
2. Describe the characteristic x-ray production process.
3. Identify the information contained in an x-ray spectrum.
4. Identify the changes in x-ray beam quality and quantity resulting from changes in kVp, mA, filtration, x-ray circuit waveform, and anode material.

INTRODUCTION

In this chapter, we cover the two x-ray production processes that take place in the anode, bremsstrahlung and characteristic. These processes differ in the amount and energy distribution of the x-rays they produce, and these differences influence the appearance of the final image. This chapter describes the two x-ray production processes and the changes in the x-ray beam produced by changes in the kVp, mA, filtration, x-ray circuit waveform, and anode material.

X-RAY PRODUCTION

Projectile electrons produced by thermionic emission in the cathode are accelerated by the high voltage to the anode, where either bremsstrahlung or characteristic radiation is produced. The bremsstrahlung process produces more than 80 percent of diagnostic x-rays; the rest are characteristic x-rays.

The kinetic energy of the projectile electrons is converted into heat and x-ray energy. Most of the projectile electron energy is converted into heat energy; only about 1 percent is converted into x-rays.

BREMSSTRAHLUNG

Bremsstrahlung is the German word for "braking radiation." Bremsstrahlung is the radiation produced when projectile electrons are suddenly stopped or slowed down in the anode.

The bremsstrahlung process produces x-rays of many different energies because the projectile electrons are slowed down at different rates. Figure 7.1 illustrates how projectile electrons produce bremsstrahlung radiation of different energies.

Projectile electrons that pass very close to the nuclei of the anode atoms produce higher-energy x-rays than those that pass further away. As the projectile electrons pass through the target atoms, they slow down, with a loss of kinetic energy. This loss of energy is converted to x-ray energy.

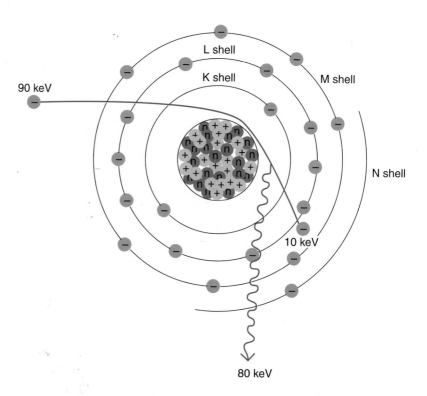

Figure 7.1 Production of bremsstrahlung radiation.

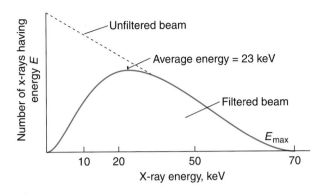

Figure 7.2 Continuous x-ray spectrum from the bremsstrahlung process.

X-RAY SPECTRA

A plot of the number of bremsstrahlung x-rays and their different x-ray energies is known as an x-ray spectrum. The x-ray spectrum in Fig. 7.2 shows that the bremsstrahlung process produces more low-energy x-rays than high-energy x-rays.

The maximum x-ray energy E_{max} produced by the bremsstrahlung process is equal to the energy of the projectile electrons. The bremsstrahlung process produces a continuous spectrum of x-ray energies; that is, there are no sharp peaks or valleys in the curve.

Figure 7.2 shows the number of x-rays with various energies in the x-ray beam emitted from the anode. Low-energy x-rays are filtered out or stopped before they reach the patient. The dotted line shows an unfiltered x-ray spectrum. All x-ray tubes have added filtration to absorb low-energy x-rays. These low-energy x-rays cannot penetrate through the patient and so will contribute no information to the x-ray image, but do contribute to the patient dose. The average energy of the x-ray beam depends on many factors. The majority of x-rays produced have an average x-ray energy of approximately one-third of the maximum energy E_{max}.

keV AND kVp

There are two energies associated with x-ray production. One is the energy of the individual x-rays; the other is the energy of the projectile electrons, which is determined by the voltage applied to the x-ray tube.

The energy of the individual x-rays is measured in kiloelectron volts (**keV**). The voltage applied to the x-ray tube is known as kilovoltage peak (kVp) and is equal to the energy of the projectile electrons. **kVp** is equal to the maximum energy of the x-rays, called E_{max}. Figure 7.2 shows that an applied voltage of 70 kVp produces an x-ray spectrum with an E_{max} equal to 70 keV and an average x-ray energy of about 23 keV.

CHARACTERISTIC X-RAYS

Characteristic x-ray production occurs when an orbital electron fills a vacancy in the shell of a tungsten atom. When a projectile electron removes an orbital electron from an inner electron shell of a tungsten atom in the anode, a vacancy is created. An outer-shell electron fills the vacancy and creates a characteristic x-ray. The difference in energy between the binding energy of the vacant shell and that of the outer shell is the characteristic x-ray energy. The vacancy is usually filled by an electron in the next outer shell, but it is possible to have transitions to the vacancy from shells farther from the nucleus. In diagnostic x-ray tubes with tungsten alloy anodes, the most common transition is from the L shell to the vacant K shell. Only K-shell vacancies from high atomic number elements produce characteristic x-rays with high enough energy to be useful in diagnostic radiology. K characteristic x-rays produce a discrete spectrum, meaning that only x-rays with the characteristic energies are present.

Figure 7.3 illustrates the filling of a tungsten K-shell vacancy with an L-shell or M-shell electron. All characteristic x-rays resulting from L-to-K transitions in a tungsten anode have an energy of 58 keV. This is the predominant characteristic x-ray from tungsten. A less likely transition would be an M-shell electron filling the K-shell vacancy. M-to-K transitions produce 67-keV characteristic x-rays. Figure 7.4 shows the characteristic x-ray spectrum from a tungsten anode.

To produce K characteristic x-rays, the K-shell orbital electron must be removed. The electron binding energy of the K-shell tungsten atom is 69.53 keV. The projectile electron must have an energy of at least 69.53 keV to remove a K-shell electron from a tungsten atom and produce K characteristic radiation. K characteristic x-rays are produced only at 70 kVp or above; with diagnostic x-rays in the 110 to 120 kVp range, only about 15 percent of the x-ray beam consists of K characteristic x-rays. The energy of characteristic x-rays does not vary.

X-rays are emitted from the anode when the projectile electrons from the cathode strike the anode. Some projectile electrons ionize the anode atoms, producing characteristic radiation. Characteristic radiation has specific energies. Other projectile electrons are slowed down or stopped in the anode material, producing bremsstrahlung radiation. Bremsstrahlung radiation has a continuous spectrum of energies.

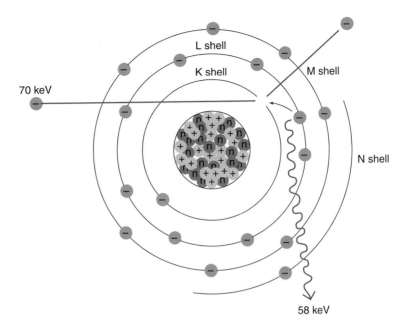

Figure 7.3 Production of characteristic radiation from a tungsten atom.

X-RAY BEAM QUALITY AND QUANTITY

X-ray beam quality describes the penetrating ability of the x-ray beam. It depends on the average x-ray energy of the x-ray beam, which is controlled by the kVp setting. X-ray beam quantity, or the amount of x-rays, is related to x-ray intensity. Intensity depends on the number and energy of x-rays in the beam. Beam quantity is controlled by the mA setting. Information about both

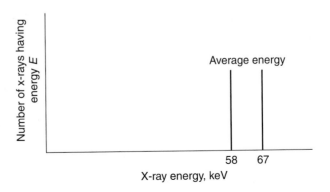

Figure 7.4 Discrete characteristic x-ray spectrum from a tungsten anode.

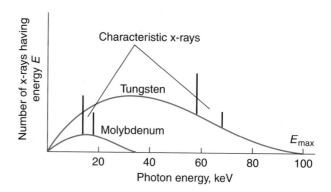

Figure 7.5 **X-ray production from tungsten and molybdenum anodes.**

beam quantity and beam quality is contained in the x-ray spectra curve. The intensity or quantity is represented by the area under the curve; the average energy is indicated by the peak of the curve.

X-RAY SPECTRA FROM DIFFERENT ANODE MATERIALS

Different anode materials produce different characteristic x-ray energies and different amounts of bremsstrahlung radiation. Tungsten alloy anodes are used in most diagnostic x-ray tubes, although tubes with molybdenum anodes are used in mammography. Figure 7.5 shows x-ray spectra produced from tungsten and molybdenum anodes. Tungsten has 58- and 67-keV characteristic x-ray energies, and molybdenum has 17- and 19-keV characteristic x-ray energies. Molybdenum anodes are used in mammography because their characteristic x-rays provide good contrast for breast imaging. The smooth curves represent the bremsstrahlung portions of the x-ray production curve; the discrete, sharp peaks represent the characteristic radiations from tungsten and molybdenum. The positions of the sharp peaks indicate the energy of the characteristic x-rays.

The four factors other than the anode material that can influence the x-ray spectra are shown in Table 7.1.

Table 7.1

Factors that Can Influence X-ray Spectra

1. kVp	The applied voltage controls the projectile electron energy, the intensity, the maximum energy, and the average energy of the x-ray beam. Changing the kVp does not change the energy of the characteristic x-rays.
2. mA	The mA controls the number of projectile electrons striking the anode and the intensity of the x-ray beam.
3. Beam filtration	Beam filtration influences the intensity and average energy of the x-ray beam.
4. Circuit waveform	The waveform influences the intensity and the average energy of the x-ray beam.

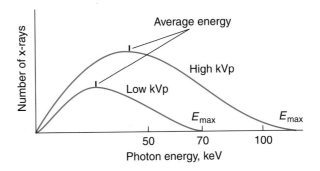

Figure 7.6 X-ray spectra resulting from exposures at 70 and 110 kVp. The average energy for each exposure is approximately one-third the maximum energy E$_{max}$.

KVP

Changes in the applied kVp change the average energy and the maximum energy of the x-ray beam. The quantity also changes with kVp because bremsstrahlung production increases with increasing projectile electron energy. Figure 7.6 shows the x-ray spectra resulting from exposures at 70 and 110 kVp. The x-ray intensity or area under the curve, the average energy, and the maximum energy E$_{max}$ all increase when the kVp is increased. The characteristic x-ray energy does not change with a change in kVp.

MA

Changes in mA change the quantity but not the energy of the x-ray beam. Changing the mA does not change either the average energy or the maximum x-ray beam energy. The number of characteristic x-rays increases with increasing mA, but the characteristic x-ray energy does not change. The quantity of the x-ray beam is directly proportional to the mA; doubling the mA doubles the quantity of the x-ray beam.

Figure 7.7 shows an x-ray spectra with a increase in x-ray quantity when the mA is increased from 100 to 200 mA.

FILTRATION

The purpose of filtration is to remove low-energy x-rays before they strike the patient. The filter is made of thin sheets of aluminum or some other metal attached to the output port of the tube housing. Adding filtration selectively

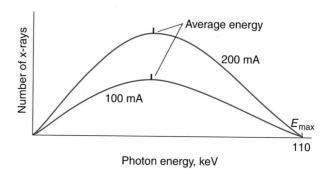

Figure 7.7 X-ray spectra from 100-mA and 200-mA exposures at 110 kVp.

removes more low-energy than high-energy x-rays. Thus, adding filtration increases the average x-ray energy and decreases the beam intensity. Filtration changes do not change either the maximum energy of the x-ray beam or the energy of the characteristic x-rays.

Figure 7.8 illustrates the change in the x-ray spectrum resulting from added filtration.

X-RAY CIRCUIT WAVEFORM

X-ray production depends on the type of x-ray circuit waveform. Different types of circuits are utilized for various types of x-ray equipment: single-phase, three-phase, and high-frequency circuits. Circuits that allow for more constant voltage result in higher intensity and higher average energies for the same mA and kVp settings. The maximum x-ray energy does not change with changes in waveform. Figure 7.9 illustrates the x-ray spectra from single-phase, three-phase, and high-frequency x-ray circuits.

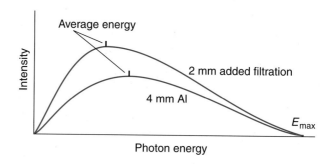

Figure 7.8 Changes in x-ray spectra resulting from addition of 2-mm Al filtration.

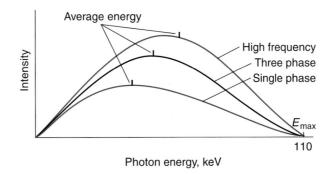

Figure 7.9 X-ray spectra from single-phase, three-phase, and high-frequency wave forms exposed at 110 kVp.

The x-ray output spectrum depends on the kVp, mA, filtration, anode material, and x-ray circuit waveform. The maximum energy of the x-ray beam can be changed only by changing the kVp. The characteristic x-ray energies can be changed only by changing the anode material. The intensity of the x-ray beam can be increased by increasing the kVp or mA, decreasing the filtration, or changing the x-ray circuit waveform to produce a more uniform kVp.

SUMMARY

X-rays are produced by either the bremsstrahlung process or the characteristic x-ray process. Bremsstrahlung x-rays are produced when the projectile electrons are slowed down or stopped in the anode. Over 80 percent of diagnostic x-rays are produced by the bremsstrahlung process. Characteristic x-rays are produced by transitions of orbital electrons that fill vacancies in atomic shells. The characteristic x-ray energy depends only on the anode material. An x-ray spectrum is a plot of x-ray intensity as a function of x-ray energy. The energy of individual x-rays is measured in keV. The kVp is the voltage applied to the x-ray tube. The kVp is equal to the maximum x-ray energy E_{max}. The average energy of the x-ray beam is one-third to one-half E_{max}. The x-ray spectrum depends on the kVp, mA, filtration, and x-ray circuit waveform. Beam quality is a measure of the penetrating ability or energy of the beam. Beam quantity measures the number of x-rays. Increasing the kVp increases the quantity, the average beam energy, and E_{max}. Increasing the mA increases the quantity but does not change the average energy or E_{max}. Increasing the filtration decreases the quantity and increases the average beam energy but does not change E_{max}. Changing from single to multiphase x-ray circuits increases the quantity and the average energy of the x-ray beam but does not change E_{max}.

QUESTIONS

1. The bremsstrahlung process produces x-rays when
   a. electrons are stopped in the cathode.
   b. a vacancy in an electron orbit is filled.
   c. a vacancy in the nucleus is filled.
   d. electrons are stopped in the anode.
2. Characteristic radiation is produced when
   a. electrons are stopped in the cathode.
   b. a vacancy in an electron orbit is filled.
   c. a vacancy in the nucleus is filled.
   d. electrons are stopped in the anode.
3. About _____ percent of the projectile electron energy is converted to x-ray energy.
   a. 1
   b. 10
   c. 25
   d. 99
4. X-ray tube filtration filters out
   a. low-energy electrons.
   b. high-energy electrons.
   c. low-energy x-rays.
   d. high-energy x-rays.
5. Interactions that produce x-rays in the anode include
   1. coherent
   2. Compton
   3. bremsstrahlung
   4. pair production
   5. characteristic
   a. 1, 3, and 5.
   b. 2 and 4.
   c. 3 and 5.
   d. 1, 2, 3, 4, and 5.
6. The voltage applied to the x-ray tube is the
   a. kVp.
   b. keV.

In Questions 7 to 12, match the different x-ray spectra with the corresponding technique change.

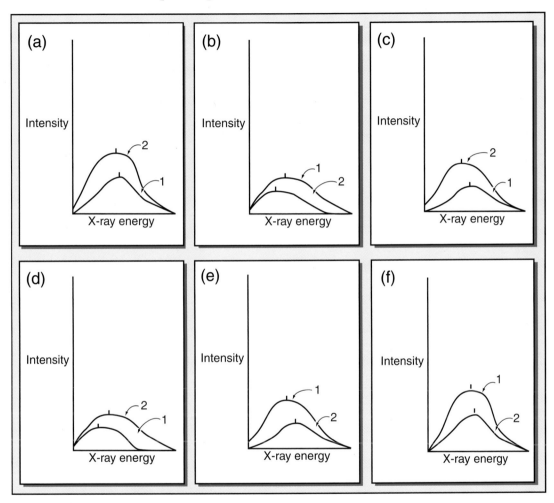

7. _____ mA increase
8. _____ mA decrease
9. _____ kVp increase
10. _____ kVp decrease
11. _____ Filtration increase
12. _____ Filtration decrease

13. Tungsten has the following binding energies:

Shell	K	L	M	N
Energy (keV)	69	11	2	1

Projectile electrons must have an energy of at least _____ keV to produce K characteristic x-rays from tungsten.
   a. 50
   b. 70
   c. 67
   d. 58

14. More than _____ percentage of an x-ray beam is made up of photons produced by the bremsstrahlung process.
   a. 1
   b. 10
   c. 80
   d. 99

15. The energy of the individual photons is known as the
   a. kVp.
   b. keV.

16. Bremsstrahlung produces a _____ energy spectrum.
   a. discrete
   b. continuous

17. Characteristic x-ray production produces a _____ energy spectrum.
   a. discrete
   b. continuous

18. Changing _____ will change the energy of the characteristic radiation.
      1. mA
      2. kVp
      3. filtration
      4. anode material
      5. waveform
   a. 1, 2, 3, 4, and 5
   b. 4
   c. 2
   d. 1, 2, 3, and 5

19. Changing _____ will change E_{max}.
      1. mA
      2. kVp
      3. filtration
      4. anode material
      5. waveform
   a. 1, 2, 3, 4, and 5
   b. 4
   c. 2
   d. 1, 2, 3, and 5

20. A technologist can control the quantity of x-rays striking the patient by adjusting the
    1. mA.
    2. kVp.
    3. rectification.
    4. anode material.
    a. 1
    b. 2
    c. 1 and 2
    d. 1, 2, and 4
    e. 1, 2, 3, and 4

21. The maximum kinetic energy of a projectile electron accelerated across an x-ray tube depends on the
    a. atomic number Z of the target.
    b. size of the focal spot.
    c. kilovoltage.
    d. type of rectification.

22. Beam quality is primarily determined by
    a. mA.
    b. kVp.
    c. focal spot size.
    d. target angle.

23. Beam quantity is primarily determined by
    a. mA.
    b. kVp.
    c. focal spot size.
    d. target angle.

Use the figure below for Questions 24 to 28.

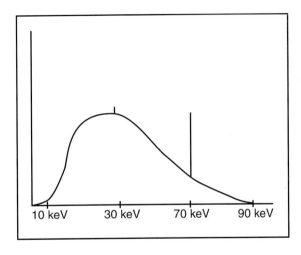

24. The average energy of this beam is
    a. 30 keV.
    b. 70 keV.
    c. 90 keV.
    d. 90 kVp.
25. The maximum energy of this beam is
    a. 30 keV.
    b. 70 keV.
    c. 90 keV.
    d. 90 kVp.
26. The energy of the characteristic x-rays is
    a. 30 keV.
    b. 70 keV.
    c. 90 keV.
    d. 90 kVp.
27. The applied voltage that produced this beam is
    a. 30 keV.
    b. 70 keV.
    c. 90 keV.
    d. 90 kVp.
28. The energy of the projectile electrons that produced this beam is
    a. 30 keV.
    b. 70 keV.
    c. 90 keV.
    d. 90 kVp.

ANSWERS TO CHAPTER 7 QUESTIONS

1.	d	15.	b
2.	b	16.	b
3.	a	17.	a
4.	c	18.	b
5.	c	19.	c
6.	a	20.	c
7.	a	21.	c
8.	f	22.	b
9.	d	23.	a
10.	b	24.	a
11.	e	25.	c
12.	c	26.	b
13.	b	27.	d
14.	c	28.	c

8

X-ray Interactions

At the completion of this chapter, the student will be able to

1. Distinguish between absorption, scattering, and transmission of x-rays.
2. Identify the factors that affect the amount of attenuation.
3. Define the half-value layer.
4. State five ways in which x-rays interact with matter.
5. Describe the two x-ray interactions important in image formation.

INTRODUCTION

X-rays entering a patient can be absorbed, scattered, or transmitted. These three processes are shown in Fig. 8.1.

When an x-ray is absorbed in a patient, all of the x-ray's energy is transferred into the patient's tissue. Scattering changes the x-ray's direction and reduces its energy. Scatter contributes to radiation fog and reduces image contrast. Transmitted x-rays pass through the patient without interaction. Most diagnostic x-rays are absorbed or scattered. Only about 1 percent of the incident x-rays are transmitted through the patient. Radiation leaving the patient is called exit radiation. Exit radiation consists of transmitted and scattered x-rays.

ATTENUATION

Attenuation is the removal of x-rays from the beam by either absorption or scattering. Attenuation occurs when there is a complete or partial loss of the x-ray energy in the patient. Figure 8.2 shows how both **absorption** and

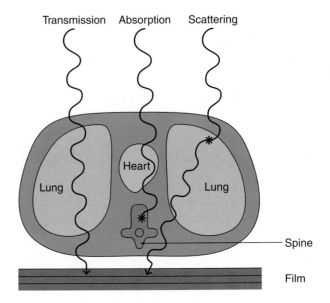

Figure 8.1 Absorption, scattering, and transmission of x-rays.

scattering contribute to attenuation. Absorption leads to complete energy loss. Scattering leads to partial energy loss.

The amount of attenuation depends on the

1. X-ray energy
2. Tissue thickness
3. Tissue density
4. Tissue material (atomic number)

These factors all influence the final radiographic image.

X-ray Energy

X-rays with higher energies (shorter wavelengths) have greater penetration and lower attenuation values. Changing the x-ray energy, the keV, by changing the kVp alters the penetration of the x-ray beam. Lower-energy x-rays have higher attenuation and lower penetration values.

Tissue Thickness

As the tissue thickness increases, more x-rays are attenuated, either by absorption or by scattering. More x-rays are attenuated by 22 centimeters (cm) of tissue than by 16 cm of tissue. Technical exposure factors (mAs and kVp) must be adjusted to compensate for different tissue thicknesses.

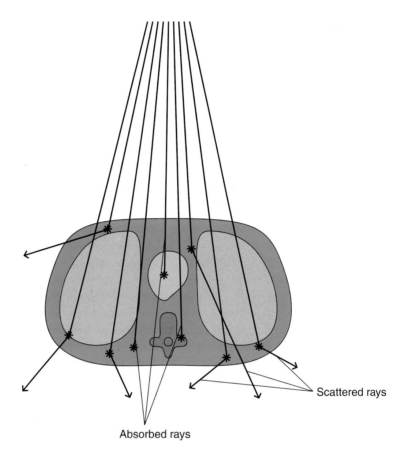

Figure 8.2 Both scattering and absorption contribute to the attenuation of x-rays.

Mass or Tissue Density

Mass density refers to how closely packed the atoms in a substance are. Density is measured in grams per cubic centimeter (g/cm³). X-ray attenuation is increased in dense tissue. In the body, air or gas has the lowest density. Muscle is more dense than fat. The attenuation of 1 cm of muscle is greater than that of 1 cm of fat. Bone is more dense than muscle; 1 cm of bone produces more attenuation than 1 cm of muscle or fat. Table 8.1 lists the densities of some body tissues and materials that are important in radiology.

Tissue Material (Atomic Number)

Materials with higher atomic numbers (Z) have higher attenuation values. Table 8.1 also gives the atomic number of some tissues and materials that are

Table 8.1
Attenuation Characteristics of Some Materials Important in Radiology

Material	Density (g/cm³)	Atomic Number
Air	0.0013	7.6
Lung	0.32	7.4
Fat	0.91	6.3
Muscle	1.0	7.4
Bone	1.9	13.8
Iodine	4.9	53
Barium	3.5	56
Lead	11.4	82

common in diagnostic radiology. Air, iodine, and barium are contrast materials that are often introduced into the body to improve image contrast. They are effective because their atomic numbers and/or densities are different from those of the surrounding body tissues. Substances that are highly attenuating are called **radiopaque.** Bone, barium, and iodine are examples of radiopaque substances. Substances that have low attenuation values are called **radiolucent**. Air and lung tissue are radiolucent. Lung is a combination of air spaces and tissue and has a density between that of air and of muscle.

HALF-VALUE LAYER

The half-value layer is defined as the amount of material required to reduce the x-ray intensity to half its original value. Twice the thickness of material does not produce twice the attenuation. At diagnostic x-ray energies, the half-value layer of soft tissue is about 4 cm. About 4 cm of tissue reduces the x-ray intensity to half its original value. The half-value layer describes the quality or penetration of the x-ray beam. More penetrating x-ray beams have greater half-value layers.

Figure 8.3 shows how two half-value layers reduce the intensity to one-quarter of its original value.

Attenuation is the reduction of the x-ray beam either by absorption or by scattering. The amount of attenuation depends on x-ray energy, tissue thickness, tissue density, and tissue material (atomic number). X-rays with higher energies have lower attenuation values. Thicker tissues have greater attenuation values. Tissues with higher densities or higher atomic numbers have higher attenuation values. The half-value layer is the amount of material required to reduce the intensity to half its original value.

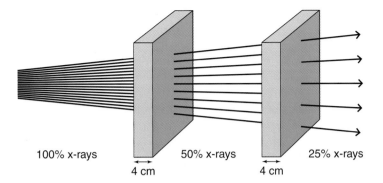

100% x-rays   50% x-rays   25% x-rays

4 cm   4 cm

Figure 8.3 Two half-value layers reduce the intensity to one-quarter of the original intensity.

TYPES OF X-RAY INTERACTIONS

The five x-ray interactions possible in tissue are

1. Coherent scattering
2. The photoelectric effect
3. Compton scattering
4. Pair production
5. Photodisintegration

These interactions take place between the incident x-rays and the target atoms in the tissue. Only photoelectric and Compton interactions are important in diagnostic radiology.

Coherent Scattering

Coherent scattering, sometimes called classical or Thompson scattering, occurs when the incident x-ray interacts with the entire target atom. Coherent scattering produces a change in x-ray direction with no change in x-ray energy. Coherent scattering, which is illustrated in Fig. 8.4, does not produce ionization. It occurs primarily at energies below 10 keV and is not important in diagnostic radiology. The other four interactions transfer some energy from the incident x-rays to tissue and do produce ionization.

The Photoelectric Effect

In a **photoelectric interaction,** the incident x-ray is completely absorbed by the atom. The x-ray energy is totally transferred to an inner-shell electron. The atom is ionized when this electron is ejected from the atom. The ejected electron is called a **photoelectron.** The photoelectron travels less than 1 millimeter

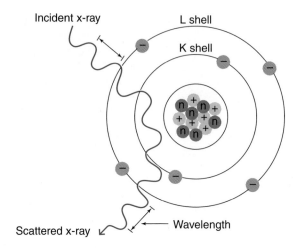

Figure 8.4 **Coherent scattering.**

(mm) in tissue. Filling the inner-shell vacancy, usually in the K shell, produces characteristic x-rays. Characteristic x-rays from tissue elements (carbon, nitrogen, and oxygen) have very low energies. They are called secondary radiation and act like scatter radiation. Most characteristic x-rays from tissue do not exit the patient because of their low energies. Figure 8.5 illustrates the photoelectric effect. The final result of the photoelectric effect is the complete absorption of the incident x-ray. There is no exit radiation after a photoelectric interaction. The photoelectric effect produces the lighter densities on the x-ray image.

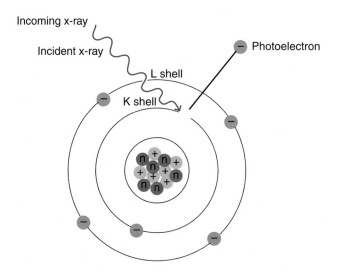

Figure 8.5 **Photoelectric interaction.**

Variation of the Photoelectric Effect with Atomic Number

The photoelectric effect increases with increasing atomic number Z. Atoms with higher atomic numbers absorb more x-rays. Bone absorbs more x-rays than soft tissue because bone has a higher atomic number than soft tissue; Fig. 8.6 shows that the photoelectric effect in bone is greater than that in soft tissue. The attenuation of bone is four times greater than the attenuation of soft tissue at an x-ray energy of 40 keV.

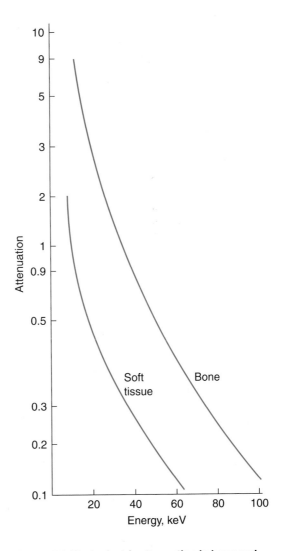

Figure 8.6 **Photoelectric attenuation in bone and soft tissue as a function of energy.**

Barium and iodine are used as contrast agents because of their high atomic number. This results in an increased photoelectric effect. Structures containing these radiopaque contrast agents appear lighter on the final radiographic image.

Variation of Photoelectric Effect with X-ray Energy

The photoelectric effect decreases as the x-ray energy increases. Figure 8.6 shows the photoelectric effect in bone and muscle as a function of energy. At higher kVp settings, there is less photoelectric effect in low atomic number structures such as soft tissue.

Compton Scattering

In Compton scattering, the incident x-ray is scattered by an outer-shell electron. The incident x-ray ionizes the atom by removing an outer-shell electron and continues on in a different direction. The energy of the incident x-ray is shared between the Compton scattered electron and the scattered x-ray. Figure 8.7 illustrates Compton scattering of an incident x-ray by an outer-shell electron. The Compton scattered x-ray has lower energy and longer wavelength than the incident x-ray.

Compton scattering is almost independent of changes in material (atomic number). The amount of Compton scattering decreases slightly with increasing x-ray energy. The amount of Compton scattering depends on the amount of tissue irradiated; larger field sizes produce more Compton scattering. Compton scattering reduces image contrast and is the major source of radiation received by the staff.

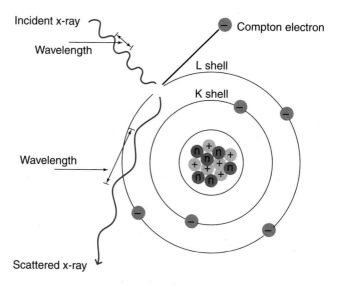

Figure 8.7 Compton scattering.

Only photoelectric and Compton interactions are important in diagnostic radiology. At low energies, the photoelectric effect is the dominant interaction; at higher energies, Compton scattering dominates. As the incident x-ray energy is increased, the relative amount of the photoelectric interaction decreases and the relative amount of Compton scattering increases. Figure 8.8 shows the relative importance of the photoelectric and Compton interactions as a function of x-ray energy.

At 26 keV (about 75 kVp), the number of Compton scattering and photoelectric interactions is equal in tissue.

Pair Production

The incident x-ray must have an energy of least 1.02 MeV for pair production to occur. In pair production, the incident high-energy x-ray is transformed into a positive and a negative electron pair when it passes near an atomic nucleus. The positive and negative electrons share the incident x-ray energy. Pair production does not occur at diagnostic radiology energies. Figure 8.9 illustrates pair production.

Photonuclear Disintegration

In photonuclear disintegration, the incident x-ray has enough energy (greater than 10 MeV) to break up the atomic nucleus. The nucleus splits into several fragments. Figure 8.10 illustrates photonuclear disintegration. Like pair production, photodisintegration requires extremely high energy x-rays and is not utilized in diagnostic radiology.

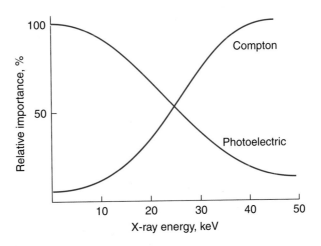

Figure 8.8 Relative importance of photoelectric and Compton interactions.

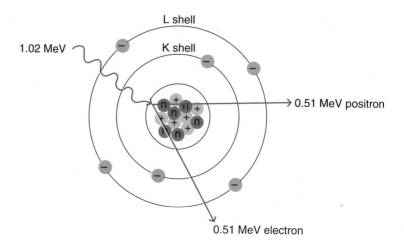

Figure 8.9 Pair production.

The five x-ray interactions possible in tissue are coherent scattering, the photoelectric effect, Compton scattering, pair production, and photodisintegration. Only the photoelectric effect and Compton scattering are important in the diagnostic energy range. The photoelectric effect is more important at lower energies; Compton scattering is more important at higher energies.

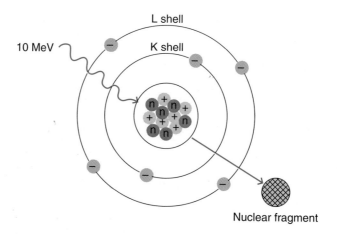

Figure 8.10 Photonuclear disintegration.

19. The HVL in tissue is about
    a. 2 cm.
    b. 1 cm.
    c. 2 cm.
    d. 4 cm.
20. The x-ray interaction that involves no loss of energy or ionization is
    a. coherent.
    b. photoelectric.
    c. Compton.
    d. pair production.
    e. photodisintegration.

ANSWERS TO CHAPTER 8 QUESTIONS

1.	b	11.	d
2.	a	12.	a
3.	a	13.	b
4.	a	14.	c
5.	b	15.	d
6.	a	16.	a
7.	a	17.	c
8.	b	18.	c
9.	b	19.	d
10.	c	20.	a

Unit III

Image Formation

9

Density and Contrast

OBJECTIVES

At the completion of this chapter, the student will be able to

1. Identify the factors that affect image density.
2. Describe the operation of an automatic exposure control (AEC) system.
3. Identify the factors that make up radiographic contrast.
4. Identify the factors that make up subject contrast.
5. Describe the difference between long-scale and short-scale contrast images.

INTRODUCTION

The appearance of an x-ray image used for a diagnosis depends on both the characteristics of the patient—that is, the x-ray interactions that occur in the different tissues of the patient—and the characteristics of the detector, usually film. These two factors—the subject contrast due to the patient and the film or detector contrast—combine to make up the overall or radiographic contrast. This chapter discusses the factors that influence radiographic contrast and image density and how the radiographer can alter the technical settings, such as kVp and mAs, to modify the image. The factors that influence film contrast are covered in Chap. 11.

OPTICAL DENSITY

Optical density or image density describes the degree of darkness or blackening of the x-ray image. Optical density is the logarithm of the ratio of the light intensity incident on the film to the light intensity transmitted through the film. Figure 9.1 illustrates the light intensity incident on and transmitted through the film.

The formula for the optical density (OD) is

$$OD = \log(I_i/I_t)$$

where I_i is the incident light intensity and I_t is the transmitted light intensity. In the example shown in Fig. 9.1, the incident light is 100 percent and only 1 percent of the light is transmitted through the film. The optical density of this film is equal to 2 because log 100 = 2.

Optical density is measured using an **optical densitometer.** This instrument is shown in Fig. 9.2.

Optical density is defined as a logarithm because the eye has a logarithmic response to changes in brightness, and so an image with twice the optical density will appear twice as dark.

Images in diagnostic radiology have ODs that range from 0.2 to 3.0, with most of the useful information in the 0.5 to 1.5 range. It is just possible to read a newspaper through a film with a density of 1.0.

The primary technical factors that influence the optical density on an image are milliampere-seconds (mAs) and source to image receptor distance (SID).

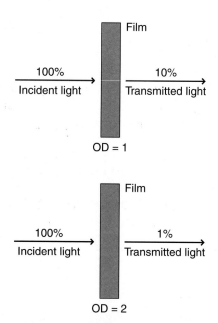

Figure 9.1 Optical density (OD) is the logarithm of the ratio of incident light intensity to transmitted light intensity. Films that transmit 10 percent and 1 percent of the incident light have optical densities of 1 and 2, respectively.

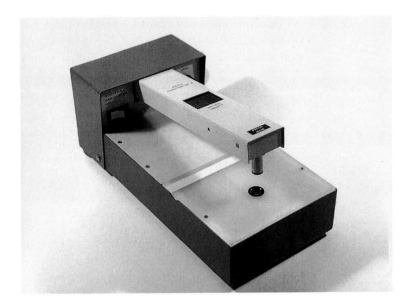

Figure 9.2 **An optical densitometer.**

mAs

The mAs is the product of mA and exposure time. The mA controls the number of x-rays in the beam or the quantity of x-rays. Larger mA values produce more x-rays. The exposure time controls the duration of the exposure. Longer exposure times result in the production of more x-rays. Larger mA values or longer exposure times produce darker, higher-density images. Doubling the mAs produces an image with greater optical density. Thicker body parts require higher mAs values to achieve the proper optical density. The mAs is the primary technical factor used to control image density.

SID

The intensity of the x-rays striking the film depends on the **SID.** The SID is the distance between the image receptor or film and the focal spot or x-ray source. Increasing the SID decreases the number of x-rays striking the film. This is an result of the inverse square law. Doubling the SID decreases the intensity to one-fourth of the original intensity. Reducing the SID to one-half the original value increases the intensity to four times the original intensity. Even though changes in the SID change the optical density of the film, the SID is usually not adjusted to change the optical density. The standard distances used in diagnostic imaging are 100 centimeters (cm) [40 inches (in.)] and 180 cm (72 in.). The mAs is used to change optical density at one of the standard SIDs.

The optical density describes the darkness of an image. Darker images have higher optical densities. The optical density of an image is influenced by the mAs and the SID. Lower mAs values and higher SID values produce images with lower optical densities.

AUTOMATIC EXPOSURE CONTROL

The automatic exposure control (AEC) adjusts the exposure time to produce acceptable image densities. The AEC measures the amount of exit radiation striking the film cassette and terminates the exposure when the proper number of x-rays have reached the film.

It is critically important that the kVp and mA be properly set because the AEC unit controls only the exposure time; the highest mA station compatible with tube limits should be chosen to ensure that the AEC utilizes the shortest exposure time to achieve the desired optical density while reducing motion unsharpness.

AEC Detectors

Ion chambers, scintillation detectors, or solid-state detectors are used as AEC detectors. Regardless of the type of detector used, there are usually three detectors located in a triangular configuration. Figure 9.3*A* shows the typical locations for the detectors. The two outer detectors are located on either side of the central detector.

The technologist is responsible for properly selecting the detectors and positioning the patient or the body part over the active detectors. The type of examination determines which detectors should be selected. For example, the posteroanterior chest examination employs either the two outer detectors or the right-sided detector to ensure proper density of the lung field rather than the spine, whereas the lateral chest examination uses only the central detector. Most examinations utilize the central detector when the central ray is centered through the part.

Figure 9.3*B* illustrates a typical control panel showing how various combinations of detectors can be selected. Careful positioning and selection of the proper combination of detectors are essential in producing a satisfactory radiograph with the AEC unit. With an AEC circuit in operation, changing the mA setting will not change the image density, because the AEC circuit will adjust the exposure time to obtain the same image density. Changing the kVp will change the image contrast but not the image density when an AEC circuit is operating.

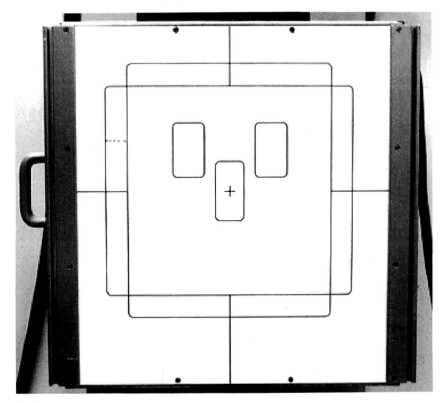

A

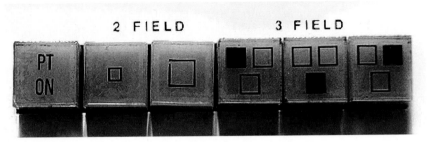

B

Figure 9.3 *A.* The location of AEC detectors on a vertical Bucky. *B.* Control panel showing locations of three AEC detector cells that can be selected.

BACKUP TIMER

The backup timer is designed to prevent catastrophic tube damage by terminating the exposure after a maximum time if the AEC fails. A backup timer is always set in case something goes wrong with the AEC circuit. A typical backup timer setting is 5000 milliseconds (ms). This means that the backup timer shuts off the x-ray beam after a 5-second (s) exposure. This might happen, for example, if a technologist neglected to empty a patient's pockets and there was a radiopaque object in one pocket that shielded the detector. Another common situation in which the backup timer is essential is when the wall Bucky remains selected and the x-ray tube is directed toward the table Bucky. Without the backup timer, the exposure would continue until the tube failed.

DENSITY CONTROLS

The AEC density controls of −2, −1, N, +1, and +2 permit adjustment of the image density to suit the preferences of individual radiologists. N is the normal setting. Each incremental step changes the image density by about 30 percent. A properly calibrated AEC unit should not require adjustment of the density controls to produce an acceptable radiograph. Changing the mA or kVp selectors on an x-ray unit with a properly functioning AEC will not change the image density. The AEC circuit changes the exposure time to maintain the same density following changes in mA, kVp, or distance.

The AEC adjusts the exposure time to produce acceptable image densities. Positioning the patient over the proper AEC detector is critical to the production of diagnostic images. Changing the kVp or mA control does not change the image density when the AEC is operating. The largest mA should be chosen in order to obtain the shortest exposure times and least patient motion artifacts.

CONTRAST

Contrast is the difference in density between two areas on the image. Radiographic contrast is made up of subject contrast and film contrast. Film contrast is the difference in optical density between different areas on the film. Film contrast is discussed in Chap. 11. Subject contrast describes the different amounts of exit radiation through different parts of the body. kVp is the primary controlling factor for radiographic contrast. Changing the mA, the exposure time, or the SID does not affect radiographic contrast. Figure 9.4 illustrates how bone, soft tissue, and lung have different amounts of exit radiation and different subject contrast.

Subject contrast depends on differential absorption of the x-ray beam. Differential absorption occurs because different areas of the body have different transmission and attenuation effects on the x-ray beam. Structures in the body that highly attenuate x-rays, such as bone, are called **radiopaque** structures. Those that only partially attenuate x-rays and allow a majority of them to be transmitted, such as lung, are called **radiolucent.** There are many factors that affect differential absorption and subject contrast: the thickness of the tissue, the atomic number and type of the tissue, the density of the tissue, the kVp setting, contrast media, and scatter radiation. Table 9.1 lists the factors that influence subject contrast.

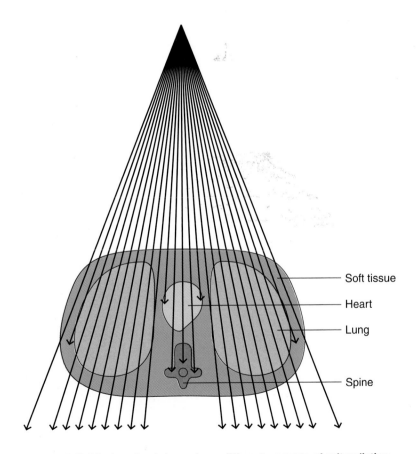

Soft tissue

Heart

Lung

Spine

Figure 9.4 Subject contrast depends on different amounts of exit radiation in adjacent areas, which is called *differential absorption*. Subject contrast describes how different areas of a patient attenuate x-rays differently.

Table 9.1
Factors that Influence Subject Contrast

1. Tissue thickness
2. Tissue type and atomic number
3. Tissue density
4. kVp or x-ray beam energy
5. Contrast agents
6. Scatter radiation

Tissue Thickness

Thicker parts of the body attenuate more x-rays. An increase of 4 cm in soft tissue thickness decreases the exit radiation by about a factor of 2. Two parts of the body with different tissue thicknesses will produce a difference in subject contrast. The two tissues will appear as two different densities on the radiograph. Figure 9.5 shows how an increase in tissue thickness decreases the number of x-rays leaving the body.

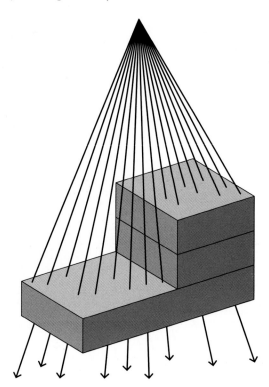

Figure 9.5 An increase in tissue thickness decreases the number of x-rays leaving the body.

Tissue Type and Atomic Number

Tissues with higher atomic numbers have greater attenuation values than tissues with lower atomic numbers. Bone, soft tissue, and fat all have different attenuation values. Bone has greater attenuation because bone has a higher atomic number than fat or soft tissue. Bone will appear as a lighter density than soft tissue on the radiograph, demonstrating a large difference in subject contrast.

Tissue Density

The density of the body part in grams per cubic centimeter (g/cm^3) affects the amount of attenuation. Fat has lower density than soft tissue, so 1 cm of soft tissue attenuates more than an equal thickness of fat. Bone is more dense and has a higher atomic number than soft tissue, so 1 cm of bone has more attenuation than 1 cm of soft tissue. Table 9.2 presents the density and atomic number of some materials encountered in radiology.

X-ray Energy

The kVp controls the energy of the x-ray beam. Higher-energy x-rays have less differential absorption because they are more penetrating. Higher-energy x-rays also produce more Compton scattering than lower-energy x-rays because Compton scattering predominates at higher x-ray energies. This combination of less differential absorption and more scattering results in less subject contrast at higher energies. Subject contrast depends on the average energy of the x-ray beam. Increasing the average energy of the x-ray beam by increasing the kVp or the beam filtration lowers the subject contrast. Lower kVp results in x-rays with less energy and more differential absorption, resulting in higher subject contrast. Mammography utilizes a low kVp to increase the subject

Table 9.2
Densities and Atomic Numbers of Some Materials Encountered in Radiology

Material	Density	Atomic Number
Air	0.13	7.6
Lung	0.32	7.4
Fat	0.91	6.3
Soft tissue	1.0	7.4
Bone	1.9	13.8
Iodine	4.9	53
Barium	3.5	56

contrast of the breast tissue. Figure 9.6 illustrates the change in subject contrast when the average energy of the beam is changed by changing the kVp.

Contrast Agent

Adding higher atomic number **contrast agent** to vessels or organs in the body increases the differential absorption and results in body structures' becoming

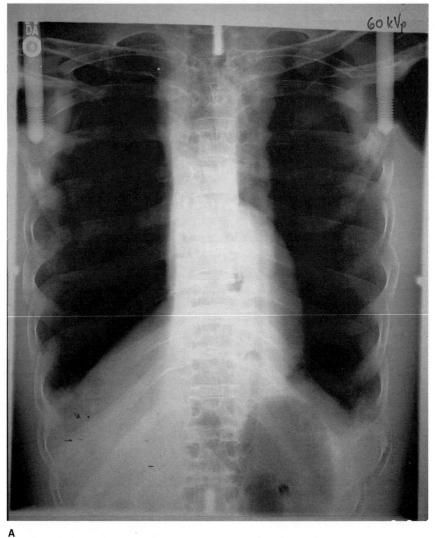

A

Figure 9.6 **Change in subject contrast produced by a change in average x-ray beam energy, demonstrated by radiographs of a posteroanterior chest phantom at 60 (A) and 120 (B) kVp.**

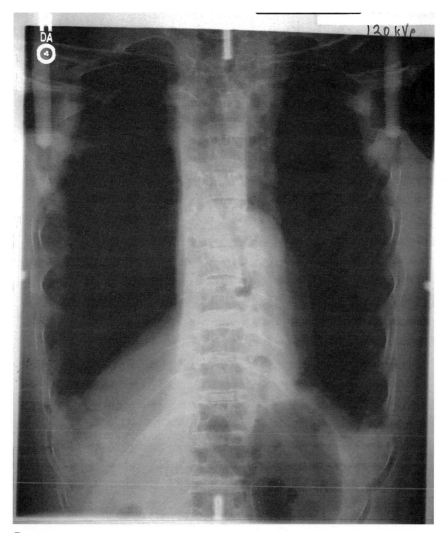

B

Figure 9.6 *(Continued)*

more visible. Iodine and barium are commonly used as contrast agents because they have high atomic numbers and high densities. Introducing barium into the intestines and introducing iodine into the kidneys are examples of the use of contrast agents in radiology. The increased attenuation makes the structures containing the contrast agent appear lighter than the surrounding tissues. Air is also used as a contrast agent. Air also increases differential absorption because it's lower density increases transmission through the air-filled structures.

Scatter

Scatter is radiation that has undergone one or more Compton interactions in the body. The presence of scatter reduces radiographic contrast. Grids are devices used to absorb and reduce the scatter before it reaches the film. The influence of scatter and the techniques used to remove scatter are discussed in Chap. 14.

Long-Scale and Short-Scale Contrast Images

The number of densities from black to white on a radiographic image is an indication of the range of the scale of contrast. The terms *long-scale* and *short-scale* describe the number of different densities between black and white on the image. A **long-scale contrast image** has many steps between black and white and is a low-contrast image. A **short-scale contrast image** has fewer steps between black and white and is a high-contrast image. High-kVp procedures produce long-scale contrast images. Low-kVp examinations produce short-scale contrast

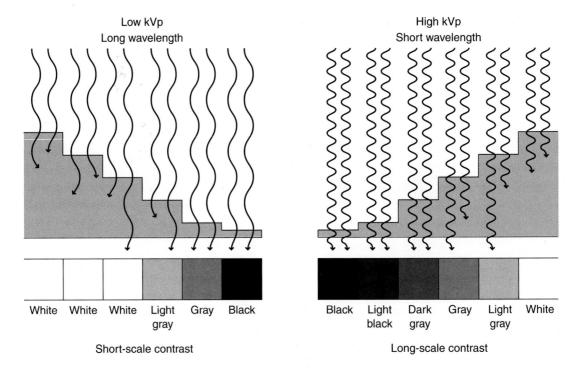

Figure 9.7 Production of short-scale and long-scale contrast images by x-ray beams of different energies. Step-wedge attenuator illustrates how high-kVp examinations produce long-scale contrast images.

images. The choice of mAs or SID will not affect radiographic contrast. Figure 9.7 shows a step wedge of graduated thickness to illustrate how higher-kVp examinations penetrate greater thicknesses and produce long-scale contrast images. Low-kVp examinations penetrate fewer thicknesses and have only a few steps between black and white, and so produce short-scale contrast images.

Contrast describes the difference in optical density between an object and the surrounding portions of the image. High-contrast objects have large density differences between their images and the surrounding tissues. Contrast material is often added to increase or decrease the attenuation of particular tissues in order to increase their contrast and make them more visible. Iodine, barium, and air are often used as contrast agents. Long-scale contrast images have many density differences between black and white and are low-contrast images. Short-scale contrast images have few density differences between black and white and are high-contrast images.

SUMMARY

Image density or optical density describes the degree of blackness of the radiographic image. Optical density is the logarithm of the ratio of the incident light intensity to the light intensity transmitted through a film. The most important technical factors influencing image density are mAs and distance. The mAs is the primary controlling factor for optical density. Increasing the mA or exposure time increases image density. Increasing the SID decreases image density. The purpose of an automatic exposure control circuit is to maintain the proper image density despite different patient thicknesses. The AEC detectors located between the patient and the image receptor terminate the exposure time when the proper density is achieved.

Contrast is the difference in optical densities between adjacent areas of the image. Radiographic contrast is a combination of subject and film contrast. Subject contrast arises from differences in exit radiation from different areas of the body. Film contrast is the difference in optical densities on the film. Subject contrast is influenced by thickness differences, tissue type, atomic number, tissue density, x-ray beam energy and kVp, contrast media, and scatter. The number of densities between black and white determines the contrast scale. A long-scale contrast image is a low-contrast image with many density differences between black and white. High-kVp examinations produce long-scale contrast images. A short-scale contrast image is a high-contrast image with fewer density differences between black and white. A low-kVp examination produces short-scale contrast images.

QUESTIONS

1. Radiographic contrast depends on
   a. tissue thickness.
   b. tissue density.
   c. kVp.
   d. all of the above.
2. If the optical density of the film is maintained the same, an image obtained with higher kVp is expected to have _____ contrast.
   a. higher
   b. lower
   c. the same
3. If the optical density of the film is maintained the same, an image obtained with higher mA and an appropriate reduction in time is expected to have _____ contrast.
   a. higher
   b. lower
   c. the same
4. Radiographic contrast consists of a combination of
   a. subject contrast and scattering.
   b. subject contrast and film contrast.
   c. film contrast and scattering.
   d. Compton and photoelectric scattering.
5. Subject contrast depends on
   a. tissue thickness.
   b. tissue density.
   c. x-ray beam energy.
   d. all of the above.
6. Radiographic contrast is
   a. the difference in densities between adjacent areas.
   b. the difference in attenuation between adjacent areas.
   c. the difference in scattering between adjacent areas.
   d. the difference in bremsstrahlung between adjacent areas.
7. Thicker body parts result in greater
   a. transmission.
   b. bremsstrahlung.
   c. attenuation.
   d. tissue density.
8. Materials with higher atomic numbers have lower
   a. transmission.
   b. bremsstrahlung.
   c. attenuation.
   d. tissue thickness.

9. Higher-energy x-ray beams have lower _____ than x-ray beams with lower energy.
   a. transmission
   b. bremsstrahlung
   c. attenuation
   d. tissue density
10. Tissues with greater density have greater
    a. transmission.
    b. bremsstrahlung.
    c. attenuation.
    d. tissue thickness.
11. Iodine and barium are used as contrast agents because they
    a. are liquids.
    b. have higher atomic numbers.
    c. are not flammable.
    d. are pure elements.
12. The presence of scatter
    a. improves contrast.
    b. degrades contrast.
    c. has no effect on contrast.
13. A long-scale contrast radiograph can be obtained by using
    a. higher kVp.
    b. lower kVp.
14. A short-scale contrast radiograph can be obtained by using
    a. higher kVp.
    b. lower kVp.
15. The most critical factor in obtaining diagnostic-quality images using an AEC circuit is the use of correct
    a. positioning.
    b. focal spot size.
    c. SID.
    d. backup time.
16. The contrast scale of an image can be measured by a(n)
    a. kVp meter.
    b. mA meter.
    c. ion chamber.
    d. step wedge.

17. List in order of increasing x-ray attenuation.
    1. Bone
    2. Fat
    3. Soft tissue
    4. Lung
    a. 1, 2, 3, 4
    b. 2, 4, 3, 1
    c. 4, 3, 2, 1
    d. 4, 2, 3, 1

18. Adjusting _____ on an x-ray circuit with an AEC will increase the image density.
    a. the kVp
    b. the mA
    c. the exposure time
    d. the AEC density control
    e. all of the above

19. Factors that affect the image density are
    a. mAs and distance.
    b. bremsstrahlung, photoelectric, and cathode.
    c. filament, single-phase, and electrical.
    d. fat, soft tissue, and pair production.

20. The primary factor that influences image density is the
    a. bremsstrahlung.
    b. filament.
    c. focal spot size.
    d. mAs.

21. The primary factor that influences image contrast is the
    a. kVp.
    b. distance.
    c. focal spot size.
    d. mAs.

22. When utilizing the AEC, changing the mA from 100 to 300 will result in
    a. more density.
    b. less contrast.
    c. a shorter exposure time.
    d. less distortion.

ANSWERS TO CHAPTER 9 QUESTIONS

1.	d		12.	b
2.	b		13.	a
3.	c		14.	b
4.	b		15.	a
5.	d		16.	d
6.	a		17.	d
7.	c		18.	d
8.	a		19.	a
9.	c		20.	d
10.	c		21.	a
11.	b		22.	c

10

Image Formation

OBJECTIVES

At the completion of this chapter, the student will be able to

1. Describe the factors that affect detail.
2. Describe the relationship between intensity, mAs, and SID.
3. Identify the exposure factors that affect the radiographic image.
4. Describe the various types of image distortion.
5. Describe the principles of magnification radiography.
6. Describe the principles of linear tomography.

INTRODUCTION

Conventional radiography forms a two-dimensional image from projections through a three-dimensional patient. This chapter covers the factors that influence the appearance of the radiographic image. There are many ways in which the x-ray images can be distorted, and it is important for the student to be able to recognize such distortions lest they result in missed or misleading diagnoses. The appearance of the final radiographic image is affected by the technical factors of milliamperes (mA), exposure time, kVp, distance, focal spot size, and the orientation of the x-ray beam with the patient. Proper selection of these factors by the technologist is an essential step in the production of diagnostic-quality radiographs. Magnification radiography is used to deliberately enlarge an object or area of interest but causes a distorted image. Tomography is an example of using motion to blur out portions of the image. This improves the visibility of structures at the location of interest.

MILLIAMPERES

Quantity of X-rays

The mA determines the number of x-rays produced and controls the optical density of the film. Changes in the mA control the number of projectile electrons flowing from the cathode to the anode in the x-ray tube, which results in changes in the quantity of x-rays produced. Doubling the mA doubles the number of x-rays. Milliampere selections on modern x-ray generators range from 25 to 1000 mA. Figure 10.1 shows the mA selector on a modern control panel.

Exposure Time

Exposure time also influences beam quantity. Exposure time can be expressed in milliseconds or as a decimal or a fraction of a second. Longer exposure times result in more x-rays striking the patient. Doubling the exposure time doubles the number of x-rays. The shortest or fastest exposure time should be selected in order to minimize patient motion artifacts.

Milliampere-Time (mAs)

Milliampere-time (mAs) is the combination of mA and time; it determines the optical density of the radiograph. mAs is obtained by multiplying mA times the exposure time. An increase in mA or in time results in an increase in x-ray quantity, which produces an increased optical density. To maintain the same optical density, the mA must be increased if the time is decreased.

> **EXAMPLE 1:**
>
> What is the mAs value of a 300-mA, 0.2-second (s) exposure?
>
> **ANSWER:**
>
> $$\begin{aligned} mAs &= mA \times time \\ &= 300 \times 0.2 \\ &= 60\ mAs \end{aligned}$$

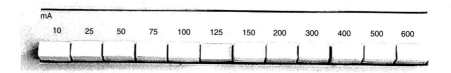

Figure 10.1 The mA selector panel on an operating console.

There are different combinations of mA and time that will give the same mAs value and the same image density. This is known as the **reciprocity law.** Larger mA values with a shorter time produce the same density as smaller mA values with a longer time and allow for less patient motion. Table 10.1 presents the relationship between the different methods of expressing mAs, with some typical mA values and exposure times.

If an image appears too light, the film is underexposed and the mAs must be increased to increase the image density. If an image appears too dark, the film is overexposed and the mAs must be reduced. When the image is underexposed or overexposed, the technologist needs to change the mAs by at least a factor of 2 to achieve a proper density. This would require the mAs to be doubled or halved. Slight changes in optical density will require at least a 50 percent change in mAs. Many modern x-ray circuits allow selection only of mAs values to eliminate the need for separate selection of mA and time values. Computer-based circuits reduce exposure times by selecting the highest mA value allowed for a specific mAs setting.

The quantity of x-rays reaching the image receptor is primarily controlled by the milliampere setting and the exposure time. The product of the time and the milliampere setting is known as the mAs. There are different

Table 10.1
Time and mA Combinations

Time			mAs from			
Milliseconds	Decimals	Fractions	25 mA	100 mA	300 mA	400 mA
10	0.01	1/100	0.25	1	3	4
25	0.025	1/40	0.625	2.5	7.5	10
50	0.050	1/20	1.25	5.0	15	20
100	0.1	1/10	2.5	10	30	40
200	0.2	1/5	5.0	20	60	80
250	0.25	1/4	6.25	25	75	100
333	0.33	1/3	7.5	33	99	132
500	0.50	1/2	12.5	50	150	200
1000	1.0	1	25	100	300	400

Milliseconds	Decimals	Fractions	mA		mAs
100	0.1	1/10	100	=	10
50	0.050	1/20	200	=	10
25	0.025	1/40	400	=	10

combinations of mA and time that should give the same optical density. This is known as the reciprocity law. The mAs must be changed by at least a factor of 2 for the change to be visible on the radiographic image.

KILOVOLTAGE

Quality of X-rays

Changes in the kVp alter the penetration or **quality** of the x-ray beam. Radiographic contrast depends on the quality of the x-ray beam. Increasing the kVp increases the amount of exit radiation through the patient and decreases differential absorption. High-energy x-rays are more penetrating and produce more scatter radiation.

The kVp setting is the primary controlling factor for radiographic contrast. Figure 10.2A, B, and C shows the image of an aluminum step wedge and a knee phantom taken at 50, 70, and 120 kVp. The high-kVp images have a long-scale contrast and smaller density differences between black and white. The mAs was adjusted to maintain the same central density. The number of density differences visible in the 50-kVp image is less than the number of density differences visible in the 120-kVp image. The 120-kVp image is a long-scale contrast, low-contrast image. The 50-kVp image is a short-scale contrast, high-contrast image.

DISTANCE

The Inverse Square Law

The distance between the x-ray source or focal spot and the image receptor influences the image density. This distance is called the source to image receptor distance **(SID).** An older term for this distance is the focal film distance **(FFD)** because the focal spot is the source of x-rays. Changes in SID do not change the quality of the beam or the radiographic contrast.

The x-ray intensity decreases with the square of the distance from the x-ray source. Doubling the distance decreases the x-ray intensity by a factor of 4. The x-rays are spread out over a larger area as the distance to the source increases. The variation of x-ray intensity as a function of distance is given by the inverse square law:

or
$$I_2 = I_1(D_1/D_2)^2$$
$$I_2/I_1 = (D_1/D_2)^2$$

where I_2 is the new intensity, I_1 is the old intensity, D_2 is the new distance, and D_1 is the old distance. This relation is known as the inverse square law because the new intensity is inversely related to the ratio of the distances squared.

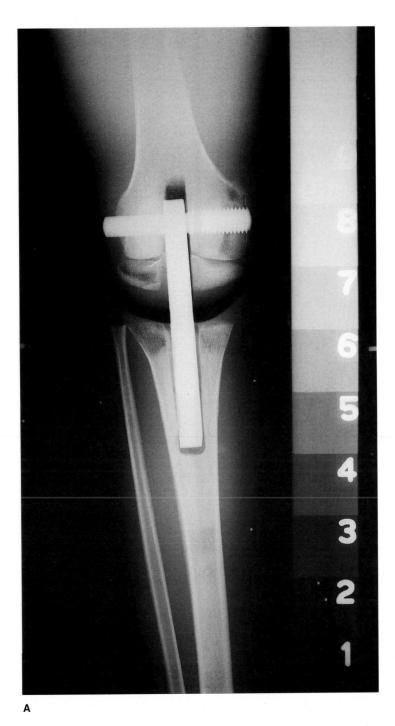

A

Figure 10.2 An aluminum step wedge and knee phantom with increases of 50 kVp (*A*), 70 kVp (*B*), and 120 kVp (*C*) show low kVp as short-scale contrast and high kVp as long-scale contrast. *(Continues)*

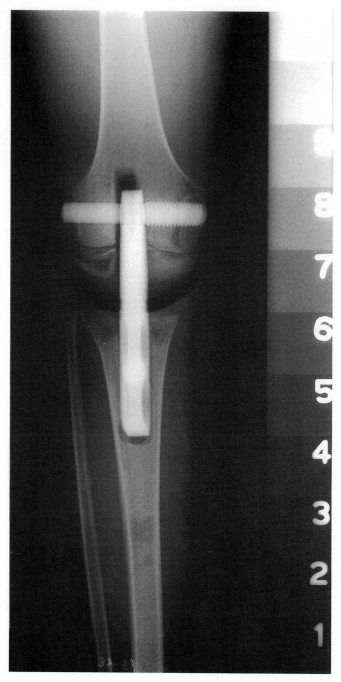

B

Figure 10.2 *(Continued)* 70 kVp.

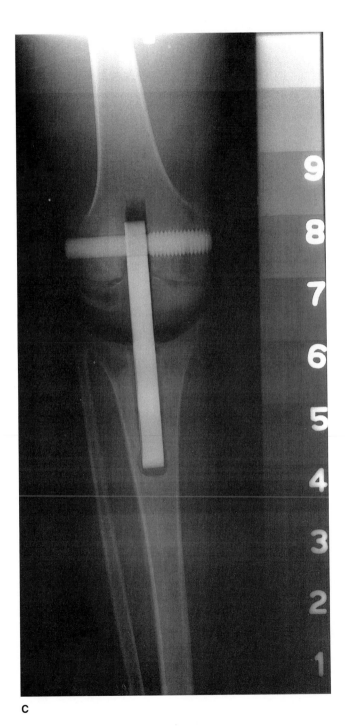

C

Figure 10.2 *(Continued)* 120 kVp.

An increase in distance results in a decrease in intensity. Other terms are also used to describe x-ray intensity when utilizing the inverse square law, such as x-ray exposure or x-ray output.

E X A M P L E   2 :

What is the intensity at 80 inches (in.) if the intensity at 40 in. was 60 milliroentgens (mR)?

$$I_1 = 60 \text{ mR}$$
$$D_1 = 40 \text{ in.}$$
$$D_2 = 80 \text{ in.}$$

A N S W E R :

$$I_2 = I_1(40/80)^2$$
$$I_2 = 60 \text{ mR} \times (1/2)^2$$
$$I_2 = 60 \times (1/4)$$
$$I_2 = 15 \text{ mR}$$

A decrease in the SID results in an increase in the number of x-rays striking the image receptor. The same principle is applied: When the distance is halved, the x-ray intensity will increase by 4 times. A decrease in SID results in more x-rays reaching the patient. Figure 10.3 illustrates the decrease in x-ray intensity as the distance to the source increases.

mAs and SID

Changes in SID will change the optical density unless the mAs is altered to compensate for the changes in distance. To maintain the same optical density, the mAs must be increased if the distance is increased. If the distance is decreased, the mAs must be decreased. In diagnostic radiology, the SID is standardized at either 40 in. [100 centimeters (cm)] or 72 in. (180 cm). The SID is not changed to compensate for changes in optical density; the mAs is the primary controlling factor for density.

If the distance is doubled, the mAs must be increased by a factor of 4 to compensate for the decrease in intensity caused by the greater distance.

To calculate the amount of mAs change required to compensate for changes in SID, the mAs-distance formula is used:

$$mAs_2 = mAs_1(d_2/d_1)^2$$

where mAs_2 is the new mAs, mAs_1 is the old mAs, d_2 is the new SID, and d_1 is the old SID.

The relationship between changes in mAs and distance is directly proportional, in contrast to the inverse square law relationship between intensity and

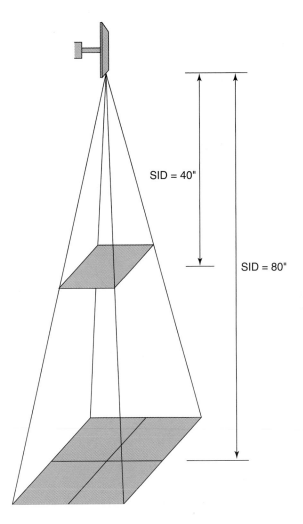

SID = 40"

SID = 80"

Figure 10.3 Increasing the distance from the x-ray source decreases the number of x-rays reaching the patient. This is an example of the inverse square law.

distance. In the mAs-distance relationship, the mAs must be increased to compensate for an increase in distance.

The mA and the exposure time control the quantity of the x-ray beam. mAs is equal to mA times time. The inverse square law relates the intensity of the beam to the distance from the source. Doubling the SID reduces the beam intensity by a factor of 4. Changes in the mAs can be used to compensate for changes in the SID.

EXAMPLE 3:

A lateral cervical spine projection examination in the emergency room was taken at 40 in., 70 kVp, and 10 mAs and produced an image with satisfactory density. A follow-up lateral is to be taken in a general x-ray room where a 72-in. SID is utilized. What new mAs should be selected for this new distance?

$$mAs_1 = 10$$
$$D_1 = 40 \text{ in.}$$
$$D_2 = 72 \text{ in.}$$

ANSWER:

The new mAs is given by

$$mAs_2 = mAs_1(72/40)^2$$
$$= 10 \times (1.80)^2$$
$$= 10 \times (3.2)$$
$$= 32 \text{ mAs}$$

KVP AND IMAGE DENSITY

A change in kVp will alter the image density because the penetration or quality of the x-rays will change. An increase in kVp results in an increase in exit radiation. When the x-ray quality is increased with higher kVp, because of the higher penetration of the beam, less x-ray quantity is needed to produce the same optical density. A 15 percent change in kVp is equivalent to changing the mAs by a factor of 2. This is called the **15 percent rule** for kVp. If the kVp is decreased from 100 kVp to 85 kVp, the mAs must be doubled to maintain the same image density. The same is true if the kVp is increased by 15 percent: The mAs should be decreased by a factor of 2.

Changes in kVp will change radiographic contrast when the 15 percent rule is utilized with the appropriate change in mAs. These changes will result in changes in the image contrast.

Table 10.2 presents ways in which density and contrast are altered by a change in technical factors.

The technologist must select different combinations of kVp and mAs to optimize image density and contrast. Higher mA settings should be chosen to minimize the exposure time and patient motion artifacts. It is often possible to obtain a further reduction in exposure time by increasing the kVp by 15 percent and reducing the mAs by one-half.

E X A M P L E 4 :

An intravenous contrast study of the urinary system obtained at 80 kVp and 10 mAs has acceptable density but lacks contrast. What mAs should be chosen if the new kVp is 15 percent less?

A N S W E R :

The kVp must be lowered to increase the contrast. A 15 percent decrease from 80 kVp results in a new voltage of 68 kVp. To maintain the same image density, the mAs must be doubled to compensate for the 15 percent decrease in kVp. The new mAs would be 20 mAs.

The calculation is

$$80 \text{ kVp} \times 0.15 = 12 \text{ kVp}$$
$$80 \text{ kVp} - 12 = 68 \text{ kVp}$$
$$\text{New mAs} = \text{old mAs} \times 2$$
$$10 \text{ mAs} \times 2 = 20 \text{ mAs}$$
The new kVp = 68 kVp; the new mAs = 20 mAs.

A 15 percent decrease in kVp requires a doubling of the mAs.

E X A M P L E 5 :

A technologist reduces the mAs by half to reduce motion artifacts. What new kVp should be selected to maintain the same density as is obtained from 60 kVp at 10 mAs?

A N S W E R :

$$\text{New mAs} = \tfrac{1}{2} \text{ old mAs}$$
$$\text{New mAs} = \tfrac{1}{2} \times 10$$
$$\text{New mAs} = 5 \text{ mAs}$$

The new kVp must be 15 percent higher than the old kVp. Therefore, the amount the kVp must be raised is 15 percent.

$$\text{Amount to raise the kVp} = 60 \text{ kVp} \times 0.15 = 9 \text{ kVp}$$
$$\text{New kVp} = 60 \text{ kVp} + 9 \text{ kVp} = 69 \text{ kVp}$$

New technical factors: 69 kVp at 5 mAs.

Table 10.2
How a Change in Technical Factors Affects Density and Contrast

Factor	Density Will	Contrast Will
mA increase	Increase	Be unchanged
mA decrease	Decrease	Be unchanged
Time increase	Increase	Be unchanged
Time decrease	Decrease	Be unchanged
kVp increase	Increase	Decrease
kVp decrease	Decrease	Increase
SID increase	Decrease	Be unchanged
SID decrease	Increase	Be unchanged
Focal spot increase	Be unchanged	Be unchanged
Focal spot decrease	Be unchanged	Be unchanged

VARIABLE-KVP TECHNIQUES

Before modern high-mA circuits became available, it was not possible, using short exposures, to produce images with acceptable density on heavy patients. Motion artifacts with longer exposures were unacceptable, so variable-kVp technique charts were developed. Technique charts were developed for a standard SID. The mAs was fixed, and the kVp was selected for a given patient thickness. The problem with the variable-kVp technique was that the radio- graphic contrast was different for different size patients. Today almost all exposures are made using fixed-kVp techniques. In fixed-kVp technique charts, the kVp selected is fixed for the various body parts being examined, and only the mAs is changed for changes in patient thickness. Proper radiographic contrast is achieved and the image density is maintained through changes in mAs.

Changes in the x-ray intensity caused by changes in the settings for the technical factors of mAs, SID, and kVp can be compensated for by corresponding changes in other technical settings. Fixed-kVp techniques change the mAs to obtain the correct image density. Variable-kVp techniques altered the kVp to obtain the correct image density.

IMAGE SHARPNESS

Detail, image sharpness, and spatial resolution are terms used to describe the sharpness of the image and how well the system images small features such as hairline fractures, edges, or borders of structures. Detail is defined as the smallest separation of two lines or edges that can be recognized as separate objects on the image. A system with 0.5-mm resolution can image two objects 0.5 mm apart as distinct objects. Objects closer than 0.5 mm imaged with this system are blurred together and cannot be recognized as separate objects.

Spatial resolution is measured in line pairs per millimeter (lp/mm). Imaging systems with better resolution can resolve more line pairs per millimeter.

Spatial resolution is measured using a high-contrast resolution phantom that has lead strips of different widths and separations. Figure 10.4 shows an x-ray of a resolution phantom taken with large and small focal spots. The image taken with the larger focal spot (Figure 10.4A)has poorer resolution and can image fewer line pairs per millimeter.

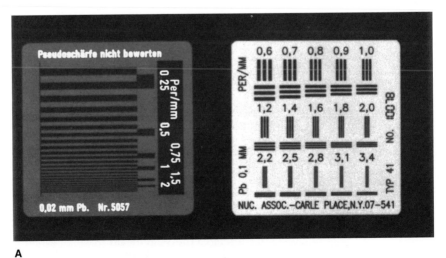

A

Figure 10.4 **Bar phantom images obtained with a large focal spot** *(A)* **and a small focal spot** *(B)*. **The image 10.4A taken with the large focal spot shows poorer resolution.** *(Continues)*

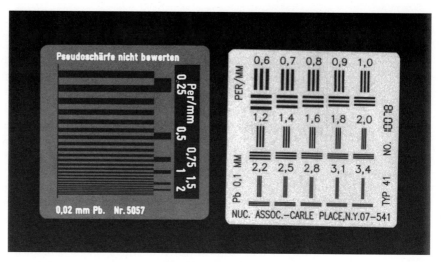

B

Figure 10.4 *(Continued)*.

FACTORS THAT AFFECT DETAIL AND GEOMETRIC UNSHARPNESS

The controlling factors that affect detail or sharpness are geometric factors. They include SID, focal spot size, object to image distance (**OID**), and source to object distance (**SOD**). The relationships between the factors that make up geometric unsharpness are summarized in Table 10.3. Figure 10.5 illustrates SID, OID, SOD, and focal spot size.

High-detail images are obtained with long SIDs, short OIDs, and small focal spots.

Focal Spot Blur

Focal spot blur degrades the detail of fine structures. X-rays diverging from different parts of the focal spot will blur the image of an edge. Larger focal spots produce greater blur.

The line focus principle makes use of an anode surface that is tilted or angled with respect to the x-ray beam. A small target angle produces an effective focal spot that is smaller than the actual focal spot. Because of the small anode angle, the effective focal spot is smaller on the anode side and larger on the cathode side. This results in less focal spot blur on the anode

Table 10.3
Effect of Technical Changes on Image Unsharpness

Factor	Image Unsharpness
SID decreases	Increases
SID increases	Decreases
Focal spot increases	Increases
mAs increases	Unchanged
OID increases	Increases
SOD increases	Decreases
kVp increases	Unchanged

side of the image and more blur on the cathode side. The amount of geometric unsharpness also depends on the SOD, the SID, and the OID. The relationships between focal spot size, SID, OID, and SOD are shown in Fig. 10.5*A, B,* and *C.*

Geometric unsharpness or focal spot blur was formerly called *penumbra.* Geometric unsharpness increases with a short SID, large effective focal spot, long OID, and short SOD.

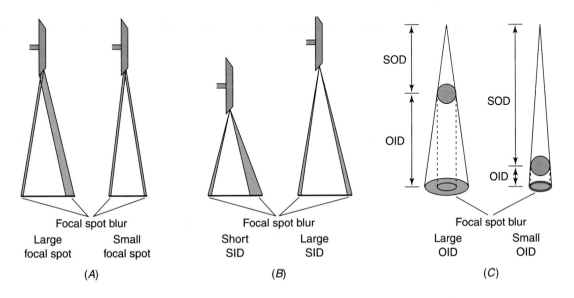

Figure 10.5 Geometric unsharpness depends on the focal spot size (*A*), SID (*B*), and SOD and OID (*C*).

Detail or spatial resolution describes how sharp the image is. Detail is determined by the focal spot size, SID, OID, and SOD. Geometric blur or penumbra is the blurring of the edges in the image of an object. A smaller focal spot, longer SID, shorter OID, and larger SOD produce better detail. Geometric unsharpness is greater on the cathode side of the image.

DISTORTION

Distortion is the misrepresentation of the size or shape of an object. Size distortion is called magnification. Shape distortion is called either elongation or foreshortening.

Size Distortion/Magnification

In magnification, the represented object appears larger on the final radiographic image. The primary controlling factor for magnification is the OID. The amount of geometric unsharpness is increased by magnification. As routine practice, magnification of a body part should be kept to a minimum to avoid masking other structures.

Magnification is the increase in the image size over the true object size, as shown in Fig. 10.6.

The amount of magnification of an object is given by the magnification factor, MF, which is the ratio of the image size I to the object size O:

$$MF = I/O$$

or

$$MF = SID/SOD$$

EXAMPLE 6:

What is the magnification factor of an image taken at 40 in. SID and 32 in. SOD?

ANSWER:

$$MF = 40/32$$
$$= 1.25$$

The magnification factor is 1.25, which means that the image will appear 25 percent larger than the object.

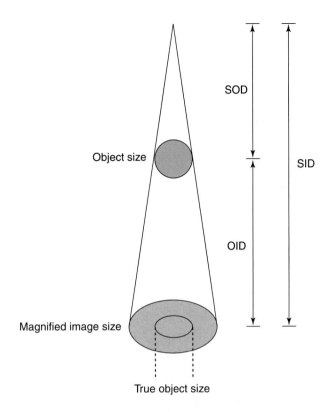

Figure 10.6 **Magnification is the ratio of image size to object size.**

EXAMPLE 7:

What is the size of an object radiographed at a 40-in. SID and a 10-in. OID if the image measures 2.4 in.?

ANSWER:

$$\text{Image} = 2.4 \text{ in.}$$
$$\text{SID} = 40 \text{ in.}$$
$$\text{OID} = 10 \text{ in.}$$
$$\text{SOD} = 40 - 10$$
$$= 30 \text{ in.}$$
$$\text{MF} = 40/30 = 1.33$$
$$\text{MF} = I/O$$
$$O = I/\text{MF}$$
$$O = 2.4/1.33 = 1.8 \text{ in.}$$

The actual size of the object is 1.8 in., and the magnification factor is 1.33.

where MF is the magnification factor, I is the image size, and O is the object size. The magnification factor is also determined by the ratio of the SID to the SOD. Images that are formed with small SOD values and short SID values have larger magnification factors. Remember, the SOD is the OID minus the SID. An object midway between the image plane and the source has a magnification factor of 2. A magnification of 1 means that the image is the same size as the object.

Shape Distortion

Shape distortion depends on the alignment of the x-ray tube, the body part, and the image receptor. The central ray is the line connecting the focal spot to the center of the image receptor. Figure 10.7 presents examples of foreshortening and elongation shape distortion resulting from changes in the alignment of the central ray. If the image is smaller than the object in one direction, the image is said to be foreshortened. If the image is longer than the object in one direction, it is said to be elongated. If the image is larger than the object in two directions, it is said to be magnified.

The alignment of the central ray is critical in reducing or eliminating shape distortion. The central ray must be perpendicular to the film cassette and the body part being examined to eliminate shape distortion. Proper alignment of the tube, the patient, and the film cassette is particularly important in portable examinations. There is no shape distortion along the central ray. Therefore,

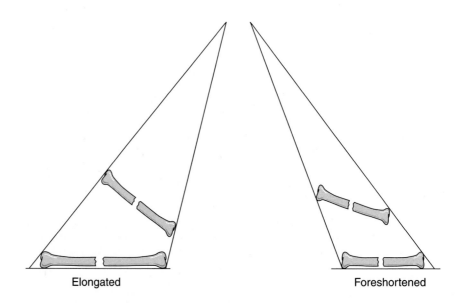

Elongated   Foreshortened

Figure 10.7 Depending on the relative positions of the object and the central ray, shape distortion can appear as either elongation or foreshortening.

the central ray should be centered on the body part of interest. Objects distant from the central ray will be distorted as a result of the divergent rays away from the central portion of the beam.

In some clinical situations, shape distortion is used to reduce the superposition of overlying structures. For example, the central ray can be angled in axial images; this will result in foreshortening or elongation of the structures overlying the ones of interest. Some such situations include imaging the skull, clavicle, and calcaneus.

Distortion is the misrepresentation of an objects size or shape. Magnification is a form of distortion that is used to enlarge the image of smaller objects. The magnification factor is the image size divided by the object size. Images that are formed with small SOD values and small SID values have larger magnification factors. Shape distortion can take the form of elongation or foreshortening. There is no shape distortion along the central ray. Proper alignment of the x-ray tube, patient, and film cassette is essential in eliminating shape distortion.

MOTION UNSHARPNESS

Motion unsharpness is distortion caused by movement of the patient during the x-ray exposure.

Patient motion is one of the major causes of repeated radiographs. Patient motion includes voluntary and involuntary movements. Involuntary movements include cardiac motion and peristaltic motion of the digestive tract. Voluntary movements include those motions that can be controlled by the patient, including breathing. Patient motion destroys fine detail in the image. Motion unsharpness can be reduced by using shorter exposure times or by immobilizing the part being imaged. Good communication skills can induce the patient to remain still and reduce voluntary motion. The shortest exposure times with higher mA values should be chosen to reduce unsharpness due to patient motion.

LINEAR TOMOGRAPHY

Linear tomography is a special technique used to improve the visualization of selected objects by burring out structures away from the objects of interest. Tomography has been partially replaced by magnetic resonance imaging and computed tomography. Figure 10.8 illustrates the principles of tomography. The x-ray tube and film cassette are moved in opposite directions during the exposure. The exposure time must be long enough to provide continuous exposure during the tomographic motion. Tomographic exposures

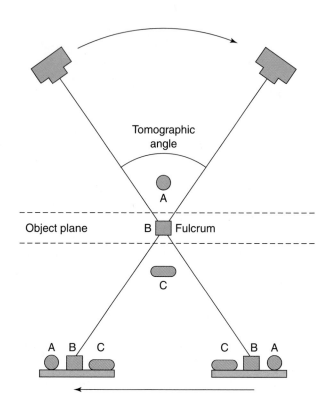

Figure 10.8 **Principles of linear tomography.**

employ longer exposure times with lower mA values. The x-ray tube and film cassette pivot at the fulcrum. The location of the fulcrum defines the object plane or focal plane. Structures above and below the object plane appear blurred in the tomographic images, whereas objects in the object plane are sharp.

The images of points *A* and *C* in Fig. 10.8 are spread over the entire image receptor, while the position of point *B* remains fixed on the image receptor throughout the tomographic motion. The thickness of the object plane or section is determined by the extent of the tube and image receptor motion. The thickness of the object plane is called the tomographic cut and is defined by the tomographic angle or amplitude. The tomographic angle determines the amount of tube and image receptor motion and is measured in degrees. Larger tomographic angles produce thinner tomographic cuts. Smaller tomographic angles produce thicker tomographic cuts. A tomographic angle of 50° produces a 1-mm-thick object plane; a tomographic angle of 10° produces a 6-mm-thick object plane.

The position of the object plane is defined by the location of the fulcrum. It is changed by changing this location to allow the body part being examined to lie within the object plane. This may be done by raising or lowering either the table or the fulcrum, and it is always done in increments of millimeters or centimeters. The tomographic motion in which the tube and film cassette move in a straight line is known as linear tomography. There are also more complicated motions, such as circular, elliptical, hypocyclodial, and trispiral, that are used to image smaller structures. The principal advantage of tomography is improved radiographic contrast as a result of the blurring of tissues outside of the object plane.

BONE MINERAL DENSITOMETRY

Bone mineral densitometry (**BMD**) measures the density of bone mineralization to assist the diagnosis of osteoporosis. BMD is different from a bone scan. A bone scan involves injection of a radioactive isotope into the patient. With BMD, a pencil beam of x-rays is scanned through the spongy or trabeculated portion of the bone; the patient's vertebrae, proximal femur, distal radials, and ulna are most commonly scanned and analyzed. BMD can detect bone mineral loss of a few percent, which may indicate the beginnings of osteoporosis. Some BMD units use two different x-ray energies to improve the analysis of the data.

Patient motion causes blurring. Shorter exposures reduce motion blurring. Linear tomography uses tube and film cassette motion to deliberately blur out tissue structures above and below the plane of the tomographic cut. Bone mineral densitometry measures the bone mineral content of the spine or other bones.

SUMMARY

X-ray quantity is determined by mAs, which is the product of milliamperes and time. Image density is primarily controlled by mAs. Image contrast is primarily controlled by kVp. High-kVp techniques produce images with long-scale contrast or low contrast. Low-kVp techniques produce images with short-scale contrast or high contrast. The inverse square law states that x-ray intensity varies inversely with the square of the SID. For example, the intensity decreases by a factor of 4 when the SID is doubled. Image density decreases as intensity decreases. To compensate for density changes produced by SID changes, the mAs must be changed. A 15 percent change in kVp is equivalent to changing the mAs by a factor of 2. Image sharpness or detail indicates how well small structures are recorded on the image. Detail depends on focal spot size, SID, OID, and patient motion. Sharp, high-detail images are obtained using small focal spots, large SIDs, short OIDs, and short exposure times. Distortion is the misrepresentation of the size or shape of an object. Magnification is size distortion and depends on SID and OID. Magnification increases geometric unsharpness. Shape distortion depends on the alignment of the central ray, the body part, and the image receptor. Shape distortion can appear as elongation or foreshortening. Tomographic motions selectively blur out overlying structures to improve the contrast of structures lying in the object plane. The thickness of the object plane is determined by the tomographic angle. Thin tomographic cuts or object planes are produced using large tomographic angles.

QUESTIONS

In Questions 1 to 3, match the technical changes with the effect produced on the image. (You need not use all the answers.)

1. _____ Increased kVp
2. _____ Decreased kVp
3. _____ Larger focal spot
   a. Greater unsharpness
   b. Less contrast, longer contrast scale
   c. Lower fog
   d. Shorter contrast scale, greater contrast
4. In a radiographic image, geometric unsharpness is decreased by increasing
   a. the size of the x-ray field.
   b. the size of the focal spot of the x-ray tube.
   c. the distance from the focal spot to the patient.
   d. the patient motion.
5. Which of the following would improve radiographic quality if patient motion is a problem?
   a. 0.6-mm focal spot, 100 mA, 0.25 s
   b. 0.6-mm focal spot, 200 mA, 0.125 s
   c. 0.6-mm focal spot, 300 mA, 0.083 s
   d. 1.2-mm focal spot, 500 mA, 0.050 s
6. An x-ray exposure of 85 kVp and 200 mAs produces a correct density but too much contrast. What mAs should be used if the kVp is raised to 100 kVp?
   a. 50
   b. 100
   c. 200
   d. 400

7. Radiographs are obtained utilizing 70 kVp and 10 mAs for proper density. The kVp is decreased by 15 percent. In order to obtain the same film density, the mAs must be
   a. 2.5.
   b. 5.
   c. 20.
   d. 40.
8. If the distance from the source is increased by a factor of 2, the mAs must be _____ to maintain the same image density.
   a. increased by a factor of 2
   b. decreased by a factor of 2
   c. increased by a factor of 4
   d. decreased by a factor of 4
9. If the distance from the source is increased from 36 in. to 72 in. SID, the exposure at 36 in. used 70 kVp and 10 mAs, what new mAs should be chosen to maintain the same image density?
   a. 2.5 mAs
   b. 5.0 mAs
   c. 20 mAs
   d. 40 mAs
10. If the distance from the source is decreased by a factor of 2, the mAs must be _____ to maintain the same image density.
    a. increased by a factor of 2
    b. decreased by a factor of 2
    c. increased by a factor of 4
    d. decreased by a factor of 4
11. The factor that alters image unsharpness is
    a. mAs.
    b. kVp.
    c. anode material.
    d. focal spot size.
12. The factor that alters x-ray beam quality is
    a. mAs.
    b. kVp.
    c. distance.
    d. focal spot size.
13. The factor that alters x-ray beam quantity is
    a. mAs.
    b. kVp.
    c. magnification.
    d. focal spot size.

14. An exposure at 40 in. SID, 200 mA, 2 s, 80 kVp is changed to 40 in. SID, 100 mA, 2 s. What kVp should be chosen to produce the same image density?
    a. 70 kVp
    b. 80 kVp
    c. 92 kVp
    d. 110 kV

15. The larger the tomographic angle, the
    a. thicker the cut or object plane.
    b. thinner the cut or object plane.
    c. faster the cut.
    d. larger the body part.

16. The advantage of tomography is improved
    a. density.
    b. radiographic contrast.
    c. detail.
    d. patient exposure.

17. The location of the object plane is determined by the
    a. focal spot size.
    b. tomographic angle.
    c. SID.
    d. fulcrum location.

18. A fixed-kVp technique changes the _____ to obtain proper image density.
    a. kVp
    b. mAs
    c. mAs and SID
    d. OID

19. A radiograph of the sella turcica was performed using an SID of 40 in. The sella turcica has a 10-in. OID. What is the magnification factor of the sella turcica?
    a. 0.25
    b. 0.75
    c. 1.33
    d. 4.0

20. The primary controlling factor for magnification is
    a. kVp.
    b. mAs.
    c. focal spot size.
    d. OID.

21. Changing the kVp from 60 to 70 kVp and decreasing the mAs by one-half results in
    a. a shorter scale of contrast.
    b. increased optical density.
    c. a longer scale of contrast.
    d. decreased optical density.

22. At 60 in., the x-ray intensity is 90 mR. What is the intensity at 36 in.?
    a. 32 mR
    b. 180 mR
    c. 250 mR
    d. 360 mR

ANSWERS TO CHAPTER 10 QUESTIONS

1.	b	12.	b
2.	d	13.	a
3.	a	14.	c
4.	c	15.	b
5.	d	16.	b
6.	b	17.	d
7.	c	18.	b
8.	c	19.	c
9.	d	20.	d
10.	d	21.	c
11.	d	22.	c

11

Radiographic Film

OBJECTIVES

At the completion of this chapter, the student will be able to

1. Identify the components of radiographic film.
2. Identify the stages of image formation.
3. Identify the important portions of the characteristic curve.
4. Identify the optical density, speed, contrast, and latitude of a radiographic film.

INTRODUCTION

In this chapter, we address the composition of x-ray film, the formation of the latent image, and the film characteristic curve. The film characteristic curve contains information on the speed, contrast, and latitude of a film. It is important for the student to understand the characteristics of x-ray film and how changes in the film characteristics can change the appearance of the x-ray image

FILM CONSTRUCTION

Radiographic film is produced in a variety of sizes. Table 11.1 lists the most commonly used sizes in both centimeters and inches.

Radiographic film is composed of a layer of emulsion applied to one or both sides of a transparent polyester plastic base. The emulsion is attached to the polyester base by a thin layer of transparent adhesive. The soft emulsion layer is covered by a supercoat of hard gelatin. The supercoat layer protects

Table 11.1
Commonly Used Sizes of X-ray Film

Size in centimeters	Size in inches
18 × 24	8 × 10
24 × 30	10 × 12
28 × 35	11 × 14
35 × 43	14 × 17

the emulsion during storage, loading, and handling. Figure 11.1 shows a cross section of a typical double-emulsion film.

Polyester Base

The polyester base provides support for the emulsion. It is constructed from polyester plastic about 0.2 millimeter (mm) thick. The base layer is strong, flexible, and transparent. It is usually tinted to reduce viewer eyestrain.

Emulsion Layer

The **emulsion layer** is made up of silver halide crystals uniformly distributed in a clear gelatin. The gelatin holds the silver halide crystals in place.

The silver halide crystals are made up of silver, bromine, and iodine atoms. All the atoms are in an ionic form. The silver ion is positive because it has one electron missing from its outer shell. The bromine and iodine ions are negative because they have an extra electron in their outer shells. The presence of bromine and iodine ions in the crystal results in a negative charge on the crystal surface. Impurities are added to the silver halide crystals to form a sensitivity speck. Changing the size and mixture of the silver halide crystals changes the response characteristics of the film. Films with larger crystals generally are

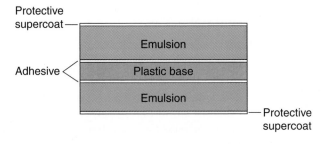

Figure 11.1 A radiographic film with emulsion layers on both sides of the supporting plastic base.

faster—that is, they are more sensitive to radiation and light—than films with smaller crystals.

The **Gurney Mott theory** indicates that x-rays and visible light cause ionization of the atoms in the crystal. Ionized crystals are said to be exposed. The free electrons from the ionization are attracted to the sensitivity speck. The collection of negative electrons at the sensitivity speck attracts positive silver ions to the sensitivity speck, where they are neutralized to form silver atoms. When silver atoms are collected at the sensitivity speck, the charge structure outside the crystal is altered and the exposed crystal becomes part of the latent image. The **latent image** is the distribution of exposed and unexposed crystals in the undeveloped film, caused by differential absorption in the patient. The latent image must be developed to become visible. Developing converts the silver ions in the exposed crystals to black metallic silver.

Figure 11.2 illustrates the migration of silver ions to the sensitivity speck, where they form silver atoms, altering the charge pattern of the silver halide crystal.

The silver halide crystals are designed to be sensitive to different wavelengths or colors of light. Conventional blue-sensitive film is sensitive to blue wavelengths of light. Green-sensitive, or orthochromatic, film is sensitive to green wavelengths of light. These films are matched to the spectrum of light emitted from the intensifying screens. The construction and application of intensifying screens is covered in Chap. 13.

Supercoat Layer

The outer or supercoat layer is made of a hard transparent gelatin that protects the film from damage during storage and handling. It softens during processing to allow the developing chemicals to reach the crystals in the emulsions.

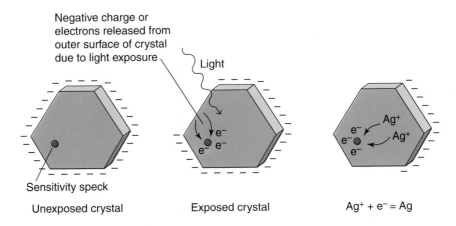

Figure 11.2 **The charge patterns surrounding silver halide crystals in the emulsion are changed after exposure.**

FILM PROCESSING

The pattern of silver halide crystals, exposed and unexposed, before developing is called the latent image. The film must be processed or developed to turn the latent image into a visible image. The processing chemicals convert the exposed silver halide crystals to black metallic silver. The unexposed crystals are then dissolved by the fixer, resulting in clear areas on the film.

Radiographic film is composed of an emulsion layer applied to a polyester base. A supercoat protects the film during storage and handling. The emulsion contains silver halide crystals, which can be changed by exposure to light. The Gurney Mott theory explains how light interacts with the crystals to produce a latent image. The latent image is the spatial distribution of exposed but undeveloped silver halide crystals.

SENSITOMETRY AND DENSITOMETRY

The sensitometer and densitometer are utilized in radiology department quality assurance programs. Sensitometry is the measurement of a film's response to different amounts of light. A **sensitometer** exposes the film to light through a series of progressively darker filters. The image formed by the sensitometer is a series of steps progressing from clear to black. This pattern is known as a step wedge pattern.

A **densitometer** measures the blackness of the film in units of **optical density.** Darker films have higher optical densities. Optical density is obtained by measuring the light transmission through a film with the densitometer, which consists of a light source and a light detector. The densitometer compares the intensity of the light passing through a point on the film to 100 percent light transmission. Figure 11.3A shows a photograph of a sensitometer and a densitometer, and Fig. 11.3B shows an example of a gray scale pattern produced by a sensitometer.

Optical density is defined as the logarithm of the ratio of the light intensity incident on the film to the light intensity transmitted through the film. In mathematical terms, optical density is defined as

$$OD = \log (I_i/I_t) \tag{11.1}$$

where I_i is the incident light intensity and I_t is the transmitted light intensity.

Optical density is useful because the human eye has a logarithmic response. If film A has an optical density one-half that of film B, then film A will appear twice as bright as film B.

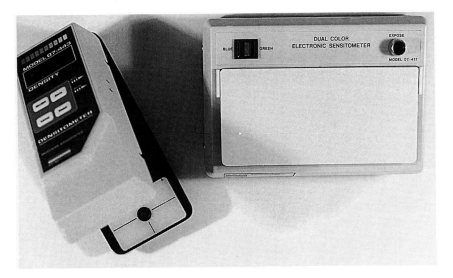

A

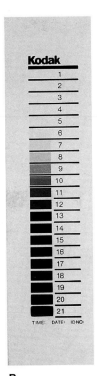

B

Figure 11.3 **Photograph of a densitometer and a sensitometer (*A*), and the gray scale image produced by the sensitometer (*B*).**

Table 11.2
Relation between Light Transmission and Optical Density

Percent Light Transmission	Optical Density	Image Appearance
100	0	White
10	1	Light gray
1	2	Dark gray
0.1	3	Black

Table 11.2 gives the optical densities of films with 100, 10, 1, and 0.1 percent transmission. Darker films have smaller transmission values and higher optical density values.

Figure 11.4 shows the transmission of light through a film that transmits 1 percent of the incident light and has an optical density of 2.

Most diagnostic films in radiology have optical densities in the range of 0.2 to 3.0. An optical density of 0.2 is just noticeable, and an optical density of 3.0 is very black.

EXAMPLE 1:

A film transmits 10 percent of the incident light. What is its optical density?

ANSWER:

$$I_i = 100\%$$
$$I_t = 10\%$$
$$I_i/I_t = 10$$
$$\log (10) = 1$$
$$\log (I_i/I_t) = 1$$

The optical density of this film equals 1.

CHARACTERISTIC CURVE

The three most important characteristics of a radiographic film are speed, contrast, and latitude. A plot of the optical density as a function of the logarithm of the exposure is called the **characteristic curve.** The characteristic curve shows the speed, contrast, and latitude of a particular film. Changing the

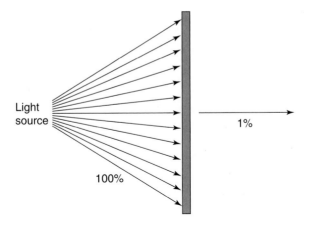

Figure 11.4 Transmission of light through a film and the meaning of optical density.

emulsion thickness or the size or distribution of the silver halide crystals changes the film characteristics. The characteristic curve is also known as the sensitometric or H&D curve. Figure 11.5 shows a typical characteristic curve. The four regions of the characteristic curve are the base plus fog, toe, straight-line, and shoulder regions.

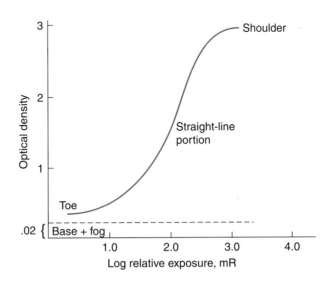

Figure 11.5 Typical characteristic curve showing the toe, straight-line region, and shoulder regions of the curve.

The base plus fog region describes the initial film density. Base plus fog arises from the tint of the polyester support base and exposure to background radiation, heat, and chemicals during storage. The optical density in the base plus fog region should be less than 0.2. In the toe region, only a few of the silver halide crystals have been exposed. The optical density in the toe region ranges from 0.2 to 0.5.

In the straight-line portion of the curve, there is a linear relationship between optical density and the logarithm of the relative exposure (log relative exposure). The straight-line portion of the characteristic curve is the range used in radiology. The optical density of the straight-line portion of the curve ranges from 0.5 to 2.5.

In the shoulder region of the curve, most of the silver halide crystals have been exposed, and any additional exposure does not produce much additional blackening. The optical density in the shoulder region is greater than 2.5.

Film Speed

Film speed describes the exposure required to produce an optical density of 1.0 above base fog. The terms *faster* and *slower* survive from the early days of photography, when portrait photos required sitting still for long periods of time. Using a faster film meant a shorter sitting time because the film required less exposure. A faster film requires less exposure and a lower mAs setting to produce the same optical density. Figure 11.6 shows the characteristic curves for two films with different speeds. Film A is the faster, and film B is the slower. Film A is faster than film B because it requires less exposure to achieve an optical density of 1 above the base plus fog level.

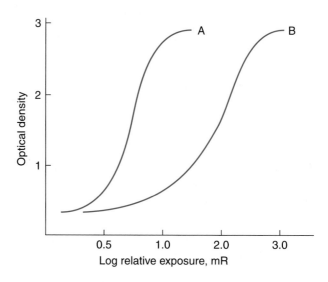

Figure 11.6 Characteristic curves of films having different speeds.

Film Contrast

Film contrast is the difference in optical density between two areas in the image. The contrast of a particular radiographic film is fixed by the manufacturer. Film contrast is described by the slope of the straight-line portion of the characteristic curve, which is also called the film gamma (Γ). Films with steeper straight-line portions have higher contrast. Films can be purchased with high, medium, or low contrast for different imaging applications.

Latitude

Latitude describes the range of exposures that produce an acceptable radiograph. Films can have wide or narrow latitude. Wide-latitude films have low contrast; narrow-latitude films have higher contrast. Wide-latitude films produce acceptable images over a greater range of technical factors. Conversely, a film with a narrow latitude requires the mAs and kVp to be set close to the optimal settings to produce an acceptable radiographic image. Figure 11.7 shows the characteristic curves of films with different latitudes.

Film A has a narrower latitude and higher contrast than film B. Films with narrow latitudes produce high-contrast images. Film B has a wider latitude and produces lower-contrast images. Generally, higher-speed films have higher contrast and narrower latitude; slower-speed films have lower contrast and wider latitude.

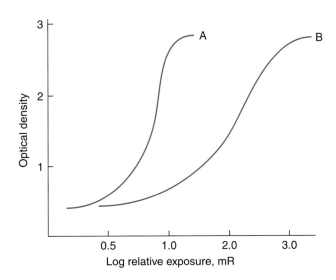

Figure 11.7 **Characteristic curves of films having different contrast and latitude values.**

Film speed describes how many x-rays are required to produce a proper density image. Faster films require fewer x-rays. The characteristic curve presents optical density plotted against the logarithm of the exposure. Film speed and film contrast can be identified from the characteristic curve. Film contrast is the difference between the optical density of an area and that of the surrounding areas.

SPECIALTY TYPES OF FILM

Specialty types of film used in radiology include mammographic, hard copy, duplication, and roll film. All specialty films are single-emulsion films. A single-emulsion film has emulsion on only one side of the polyester film base. Single-emulsion film is processed in the same manner as double-emulsion film. It provides better resolution than double-emulsion film because with double-emulsion film, the images from the two sides are not exactly superimposed unless they are viewed directly head on, whereas with single-emulsion film, the image is on only one side of the base, and so small objects and sharp edges are not blurred as much. In addition, there is a possibility that light from one intensifying screen will pass through the emulsion and film base to expose the opposite emulsion. Such "crossover" light is spread out and reduces the sharpness of the image.

It is possible to identify the emulsion side, even in the darkroom under safelights, because light reflection makes the emulsion side look dull and the base side appear shiny. The manufacturers place notches on one edge of single-emulsion film to aid in identification of the emulsion side in the dark. When the film is positioned with the notches at the upper right corner of the film, the emulsion is facing up. It is important to have the emulsion side of single-emulsion film facing the intensifying screen, which is the light source. If the film is facing backward, the image will be blurred because the light must pass through the base before reaching the emulsion.

Mammographic Film

Mammographic film is single-emulsion film with very fine crystals. Mammographic films are a compromise between the need for high sensitivity with low patient dose and very high spatial resolution. Mammographic films are designed to be used with a single high-resolution screen. The emulsion is always placed in contact with the intensifying screen.

Duplication Film

Duplication film is a specialty film that is used to produce copies of conventional radiographs. It is available in the same standard sizes as conventional film. Duplication film is a single-emulsion film that is designed to be sensitive to ultraviolet light from the duplicating machine. The duplicating film is placed in contact with the original film and exposed in the duplicator for a few seconds. No x-rays are used. The duplication film is then processed in the usual manner. Duplication film is designed so that clear areas on the original film produce clear areas on the duplicate film. It is sometimes called reversal film because its response to light is reversed from that of normal film. With normal film, longer exposures result in darker images; with duplication film, longer exposures produce lighter images.

Hard Copy, Laser Printer, or Multiformat Film

Hard copy film is used to provide a permanent record of an electronically displayed image. Digital images from computed tomography, ultrasound, nuclear medicine, or magnetic resonance imaging units are initially presented on monitors or as electronic "soft" displays, and only certain images are selected for the permanent hard copy record. Hard copies can be produced by a laser printer or a multiformat camera. The spatial resolution of the laser printer is superior to that of the multiformat camera. The number of images on one film, known as the image format, can be selected by the operator. Typical image formats are four, six, or twelve images on one film.

Roll Film

Roll film is used to record cine or spot film images. Cine film is movie film. It is used primarily for angiographic and cardiology examinations where moving vessels of the heart are imaged. Cine film comes in two widths, 16 mm and 35 mm, in 300-foot rolls. The 35-mm size is most commonly used. The images are less than 16 or 35 mm wide because the sprocket holes used to advance the film occupy about 35 percent of the width. A 16-mm film image is about 7×10 mm; a 35-mm image is 23×35 mm. Serial imaging is also done with 105-mm film. This film is used for recording images displayed on the image intensifier. Spot film images on 105-mm film are used in gastrointestinal studies, where the structures move more slowly. The difference between cine and spot film recording is the rate of image recording. Cine film is usually taken at 30 or 60 frames per second, whereas spot films are usually taken at less than 10 frames per second.

Specialty films, including mammographic, laser printer, and hard copy films, are single-emulsion films—the emulsion is coated on only one side of the polyester film base. Single-emulsion films have better spatial resolution than double-emulsion films.

FILM STORAGE AND HANDLING

Film is very sensitive to storage and handling conditions. Improper storage or handling can produce fog or artifacts. Fog is an increase in density over the entire film. **Artifacts** are unwanted local densities on the final image. Radiographic film is sensitive to light, temperature, humidity, radiation, and improper handling. Exposed but undeveloped film is much more sensitive to radiation than unexposed film.

Light

Radiographic film is designed to be sensitive to light from the intensifying screens. It is also sensitive to visible light and will fog if it is exposed to room lights. It must be handled and loaded in a darkroom. Darkrooms are equipped with safelights. Safelights are designed to filter out light that is energetic enough to expose the film. Blue-sensitive film is not sensitive to amber light, so an amber safelight filter is used with blue-sensitive film. Green-sensitive, or orthochromatic, film is sensitive to an ordinary amber safelight and therefore requires a special deep red safelight filter, such as a **GBX filter.**

Temperature and Humidity

Film should be stored in a cool, dry place with a temperature less than 70°F and with less than 60 percent relative humidity. Storage under heat conditions above 75°F will increase the fog and decrease image contrast. Storage under conditions of low humidity, less than about 40 percent, will increase static artifacts.

Radiation

Film must be shielded from radiation exposure. Even a few milliroentgens will produce a noticeable increase in fog. Exposure to scattered radiation in fluoroscopy rooms is a possible source of radiation fog.

Improper Handling of Film

Unexposed film is sensitive to shock, pressure, and improper handling. Dropping a box of unexposed film can cause artifacts on the edge or corner that strikes the floor. The sensitivity of film to pressure can be demonstrated by placing a piece of paper over an undeveloped film and writing on the paper. The pressure of the pen through the paper will alter the emulsion so that the writing will show after the film is developed. Film boxes should always be stored on end to avoid abrasion and pressure artifacts. Rough handling can cause crease densities to appear on the developed film. Rapid removal of unexposed film from the storage box can produce static artifacts.

Radiographic film is sensitive to light, radiation, temperature, and humidity. Film handling is critical to the production of diagnostic-quality images. The undeveloped film must be stored on end in a cool, dry place to avoid film artifacts.

SUMMARY

Radiographic film consists of an emulsion containing silver halide crystals coated on a polyester base. Exposure to x-rays and visible light produces changes in the silver halide crystals to form a latent image. The latent image is the distribution of exposed and unexposed silver halide crystals on the film. Developing the film changes the latent image into a permanent visible image. Film development converts exposed silver halide crystals to black metallic silver and removes the unexposed crystals. The transmission of light through a radiographic film is described by the film's optical density. Optical density is a measure of the degree of darkness of the film. A plot of the optical density versus log radiation exposure is known as the characteristic curve of a film. The characteristic curve shows the speed, contrast, and latitude of the film. Higher-speed films require less exposure to produce a given density. High-contrast films produce large density differences for small differences in exposure. Films with wide latitude produce acceptable image densities over a wide range of exposures. Orthochromatic film is sensitive to green light and requires a special deep red safelight filter. Radiographic film is sensitive to light, temperature, humidity, radiation, and pressure during storage and handling. Improper storage and handling can produce artifacts and fog that produce unwanted densities on the film.

QUESTIONS

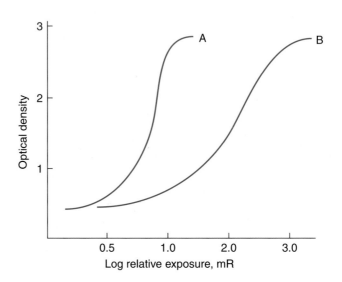

USE THE FIGURE ABOVE TO ANSWER QUESTIONS 1 TO 4.

1. _____ Which film is faster?
2. _____ Which film has the greater contrast?
3. _____ Which film is slower?
4. _____ Which film has the greater latitude?
5. A characteristic curve of a film relates
   a. optical density to the light transmitted through the film.
   b. subject contrast to tissue density.
   c. optical density to developer temperature.
   d. optical density to log relative exposure.
6. The straight-line portion of the characteristic curve is
   a. the usable optical density region.
   b. a measure of contrast.
   c. the usable exposure region.
   d. all of the above.
7. The film base
   a. provides support for the film emulsion.
   b. is clear so that the image can be seen on the view box.
   c. provides support during development.
   d. is/does all of the above.

8. The sensitivity speck is a sensitive region
   a. in the polyester film base.
   b. in the film cassette.
   c. on the silver halide crystal.
   d. in the developer solution.
9. The latent image is the distribution of
   a. exposed and unexposed crystals in the undeveloped film.
   b. blackened silver halide crystals after development.
   c. blackened silver halide crystals in the developer solution.
   d. blackened and unexposed silver halide crystals on the undeveloped x-ray film.
10. Optical density
    a. relates the transmitted light to the incident light.
    b. is the logarithm of the ratio of incident to transmitted light.
    c. measures the darkness of the film.
    d. is/does all of the above.
11. The useful range of optical densities is
    a. 0.2 to 3.0.
    b. 0.5 to 2.5.
    c. 1.0 to 3.0.
    d. 2.5 to 5.0.
12. The contrast of a film
    a. is the slope of the straight-line portion of the characteristic curve.
    b. relates the optical density and the radiation exposure.
    c. is measured by the gamma of the film.
    d. is/does all of the above.
13. A high-contrast film has a _____ latitude.
    a. wide
    b. narrow
14. The optical density of a film is measured with a
    a. sensitometer.
    b. densitometer.
    c. opticometer.
    d. optidensitometer.
15. Film with an optical density of 0.3 would appear
    a. very light.
    b. in the useful range.
    c. very dark.

In the characteristic curve shown below, identify the regions (use for Questions 16 to 19).

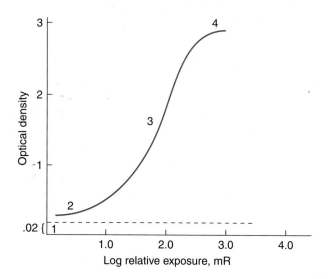

16. The shoulder region of the curve is
    a. 1.
    b. 2.
    c. 3.
    d. 4.
17. The toe region of the curve is
    a. 1.
    b. 2.
    c. 3.
    d. 4.
18. The base plus fog region of the curve is
    a. 1.
    b. 2.
    c. 3.
    d. 4.
19. The straight-line region of the curve is
    a. 1.
    b. 2.
    c. 3.
    d. 4.
20. A wide-latitude film provides a _____-contrast image.
    a. low
    b. high

21. Film with an optical density of 1.5 would appear
    a. very light.
    b. in the useful range.
    c. very dark.
22. Film with an optical density of 3.0 would appear
    a. very light.
    b. in the useful range.
    c. very dark.

For Questions 23 to 28, indicate whether the property is described by the characteristic curve. Answer a for true or b for false.

23. _____ Resolution
24. _____ Contrast
25. _____ Base plus fog level.
26. _____ Latitude
27. _____ Speed
28. _____ Focal spot size

ANSWERS TO CHAPTER 11 QUESTIONS

1.	a		15.	a
2.	a		16.	d
3.	b		17.	b
4.	b		18.	a
5.	d		19.	c
6.	d		20.	a
7.	d		21.	b
8.	c		22.	c
9.	a		23.	b
10.	d		24.	a
11.	b		25.	a
12.	d		26.	a
13.	b		27.	a
14.	b		28.	b

12

Film Processors

At the completion of this chapter, the student will be able to

1. Identify the stages in film processing.
2. Identify the components and describe the operation of automatic film processors.
3. Describe the effect of temperature and time on speed, contrast, latitude, and base plus fog.
4. Identify the requirements for a radiographic darkroom.

INTRODUCTION

After the invisible latent image is formed on the film, it is necessary to develop the film. This involves reducing the exposed silver halide crystals of the latent image to metallic silver and dissolving away the unexposed silver halide crystals. This development is a chemical process that is usually done in an automatic film processor. It is important for the student to recognize how changes in film processing can change the appearance of the final image.

AUTOMATIC FILM PROCESSING

Processing a film transforms the invisible latent image into a permanent visible image. The visible image is produced by reducing silver ions in the exposed crystals to black metallic silver. The metallic silver on the film appears black instead of the familiar shiny silver color because the silver crystals are so small

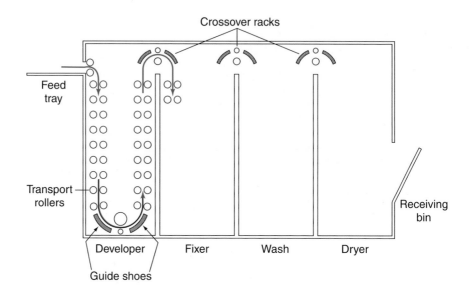

Figure 12.1 Schematic view of automatic processor stages.

that they scatter light instead of reflecting it. Film processing consists of four
stages: development, fixing, washing, and drying.

Automatic processors can transport a film through the four processing
stages in 90 seconds (s) or less. Figure 12.1 shows a schematic view of an automatic processor.

The transport system takes the film from the feed tray through a series of
rollers into the development tank, the fixer tank, the wash tank, and finally the
drying chamber. Each stage of processing is essential in the production of a diagnostic-quality radiograph.

> *The four stages of film processing are development, fixing, washing,*
> *and drying. These can be accomplished in an automatic film processor*
> *in 90 s or less.*

DEVELOPER

The **developer** is a water-based solution containing chemicals that will reduce
the exposed silver halide crystals to metallic silver without changing the unexposed silver halide crystals. The latent image is a distribution of exposed and
unexposed silver halide crystals in the emulsion. The surface charge on the exposed crystals is lower near the sensitivity speck. The surface charge on the
unexposed crystals is unchanged. The reducing agents in the developer are
electronegative and are repulsed by the negative charges around the unex-

posed silver halide crystals. The lower negative charge near the sensitivity speck of the exposed crystals permits the reducing agents to interact with these crystals and reduce them to black metallic silver. Figure 12.2 shows how the developer's reducing agent acts primarily on the exposed crystals.

As the film enters the developer tank, the warm, water-based developer solution soaks into the emulsion, softening it and causing it to swell. The developer consists of two reducing agents, **hydroquinone** and **phenidone.** These reducing chemicals add electrons to the silver ions, converting them to silver atoms. This reducing reaction releases bromine ions into the developer solution.

The developer solution is effective only in a basic, or alkaline, environment. The acidity of a solution is described by its pH. Basic solutions have pH values greater than 7; acidic solutions have pH values less than 7. The pH of the developer must be greater than 7. Sodium carbonate is added to the developer solution to maintain the proper pH.

All developer solutions are caustic and can cause chemical burns. If any developer solution is spilled or splashed on the skin, it should be immediately washed off. Eye protection must be worn whenever the developer solution is changed.

Development is a chemical reaction whose speed depends on time, temperature, and concentration. If the development time, the temperature, or the concentration is increased, more crystals will be reduced to black metallic silver. Potassium bromide is added to the developer as a restrainer to inhibit the action of the developer on the unexposed silver halide crystals. The restrainer is not completely effective, so as development proceeds, some unexposed crystals may be developed. The development of unexposed silver halide crystals is a major contributor to fog.

Oxygen from the air weakens the reducing action of the developer. **Sodium sulfite** is added to the developer solution to remove oxidizing agents and maintain the chemical activity of the developer. Developer supply tanks have lids to prevent oxidation by the air.

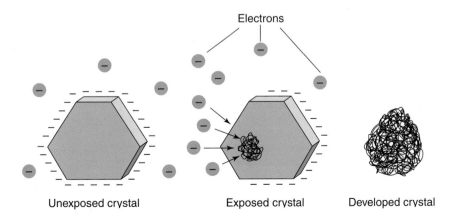

Figure 12.2 **Action of developer on silver halide crystals.**

Glutaraldehyde is added to the developer to control the amount of swelling of the emulsion. If the emulsion swells too much, it becomes soft and sticks to the processor rollers. Glutaraldehyde also hardens the emulsion during the drying process to improve the storage and handling characteristics of the processed film. If the glutaraldehyde concentration in the developer solution is depleted, wet and sticky films will result.

Development of the latent images changes the exposed silver halide crystals to metallic silver while leaving the unexposed crystals unchanged. The basic developer solution, which is caustic, contains two reducing agents, hydroquinone and phenidone. The speed of development depends on the concentration of the chemicals, the temperature of the developer solution, and the amount of time the film is left in the solution. Glutaraldehyde is added to the developer solution to prevent excessive swelling of the emulsion in the warm solution and to aid in hardening the emulsion during drying.

FIXER

The action of the developer must be stopped before the film can be exposed to light. This is done by the fixer. The **fixer** stops the reducing action of the developer and removes the unexposed silver halide crystals. The fixer solution is also called the hypo solution or clearing agent because it removes unexposed silver halide crystals from the emulsion. The clearing agent in the fixer solution is **ammonium thiosulfate.** The fixer solution also contains acetic acid, which gives the fixer its vinegarlike smell. The acid ensures that the fixer solution is acidic rather than basic, and thus stops the action of the developer. Sodium sulfite is added to the fixer solution to remove oxidizing agents and maintain the chemical activity of the fixer. Sodium sulfite is the only chemical used in both the developer and fixer solutions. The fixer solution also contains potassium alum to shrink and harden the emulsion after the unexposed crystals have been removed. After the film leaves the fixer solution, it is washed with water. Table 12.1 lists the chemicals contained in the developer and fixer solutions and their functions.

The acetic acid fixer solution stops development action, which can proceed only in a basic solution. The ammonium thiosulfate dissolves away the unexposed silver halide crystals. Sodium sulfite is added to both the developer and the fixer to counteract the effects of oxygen, which weakens both solutions.

Table 12.1

Chemicals Contained in the Developer and Fixer Solutions and Their Functions

Chemical	Function
Developer	
Hydroquinone	Reducing agent
Phenidone	Reducing agent
Sodium carbonate	Maintain proper pH
Sodium sulfite	Preservative
Potassium bromide	Restrainer
Glutaraldehyde	Hardener
Water	Solvent
Fixer	
Ammonium thiosulfate	Clearing agent
Acetic acid	Maintain proper pH
Potassium alum	Hardener
Sodium sulfite	Preservative
Water	Solvent

WASHING

Developer or fixer chemicals that are left in the emulsion will slowly be oxidized by the air and will turn the film brown. The washing stage removes all chemicals remaining in the emulsion. The incoming wash water is filtered before it enters the wash tank. The water is constantly circulated and drained to ensure that it is clean. Unremoved fixer can combine with metallic silver crystals to form silver sulfide or dichroitic stains. Incomplete removal of the fixer solution is known as hypo retention. Degradation of the image quality of stored films as a result of incomplete washing will appear only after several years.

DRYING

Most of the wash water is removed by the processor rollers as the film is transported into the drying chamber. The final drying of the film is done by currents of hot air. Drying removes the remnants of the water on the film. It also shrinks and hardens the emulsion and seals the supercoat to protect the film during handling and storage.

CONTAMINATION

Contamination of the basic developer by the acid fixer lowers the pH, reducing the effectiveness of the developer and producing lower-contrast, "washed-out" images. Contamination can occur when new chemicals are added or during the cleaning of film transport components. Drops of warm fixer can condense and contaminate the developer solution when the processor is turned off. For this reason, the lid of the processor should always be lifted and propped partially open when the processor is turned off. This will allow vapors to escape and reduce cross contamination and corrosion of processor parts.

Contamination of the fixer by the developer is not a problem. Some developer is inevitably carried along when the film is transferred into the fixer tank. The processor system is designed to compensate for this contamination.

RECIRCULATION AND REPLENISHMENT

The developer and fixer solutions must be constantly mixed to ensure that their chemical strength is uniform. Mixing also ensures that fresh chemicals come in contact with the emulsion. This mixing or agitation is produced by circulation pumps. A microswitch on the first set of transport rollers senses each film as it enters the processor and turns on the transport system and the pumps to replenish the developer and fixer solutions.

The processing of each film uses up small amounts of the developer and fixer chemicals. The replenishment system automatically maintains the correct chemical concentration. Each time a film is processed, the microswitch activates the replenishment pumps to add developer and fixer solutions. The replenishment solutions are contained in large replenishment tanks located near the processor.

Copy films are different from conventional film. Replenishment rates adjusted for conventional double-emulsion films will not maintain the proper chemical concentrations after a large number of copy films have been processed because copy film has only a single emulsion layer. This is especially important if the processor is also used to develop mammography films, which require critical control of processor chemistry.

Automatic processors have a standby switch that turns the transport roller drive motor off after a few minutes of inactivity. This motor must be restarted before another film can be processed.

The film must be washed after it leaves the fixer solution because residual fixer can lead to fading of the image over a period of years. The processor rollers remove most of the wash water, but the remainder is removed by currents of warm, dry air. The processing of each film weakens the chemical strength of the developer and fixer, so replenishment pumps add developer and fixer chemicals to maintain proper concentrations. Contamination of the developer solution by the fixer should be avoided by taking care during the addition of chemicals and during cleaning of the film transport system and by opening the processor lid at the end of the day when the processor is turned off.

FILM TRANSPORT SYSTEM

The film transport system carries the film through the developer, fixer, and wash tanks and through the dryer chamber. The feed tray at the entrance to the automatic processor guides the film into the processor. Rollers 1 inch (in.)

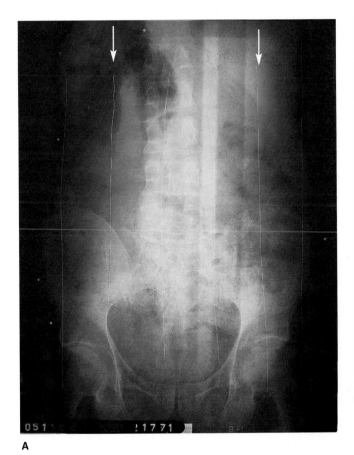

A

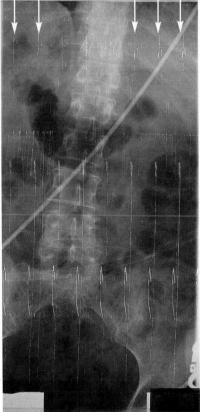

B

Figure 12.3 **Guide-shoe artifact.**

in diameter grip the film and move it through the developer, fixer, wash, and dryer stages. The rollers for the various stages are connected by gears in a vertical rack assembly. The rack can be removed for cleaning. The speed of film transport through the processor is controlled by the motor driving the rollers through a series of gears. In some processors, the transport speed can be changed from normal (90 s) processing to either rapid (45 s) or extended [3 minutes (min)] processing. At the bottom of each vertical rack there is a turnaround assembly containing **guide shoes** that hold the film against the bottom roller while the film reverses direction. The guide shoes have ribs to reduce friction and keep the film in alignment. Guide-shoe misalignment can remove some of the soft emulsion, causing processor artifacts, which appear as white scratch lines in the directions of film travel. Figure 12.3A and B show artifacts produced by misaligned guide shoes.

At the top of each tank, the film is carried across to the next tank by **crossover racks.** The crossover racks also contain rollers and guide shoes. The rollers squeeze out the chemicals in the emulsion prior to the film entering the next tank. After washing, the film passes through the dryer and is deposited in the output bin. Figure 12.4 shows an expanded view of the transport system guide shoes and crossover rack. The transport system drive motor and gears are usually set for 90-s processing. The film transport rollers, crossover racks, and guide shoes must be periodically cleaned to maintain good-quality images.

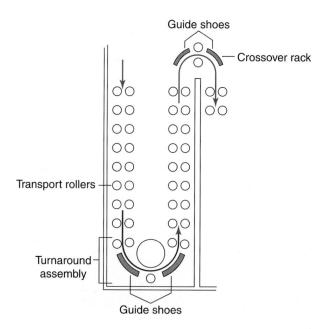

Figure 12.4 Film transport system.

EFFECT OF CONCENTRATION, TIME, AND TEMPERATURE

Any change in developer concentration, developing time, or developing temperature will change the speed, contrast, and base fog of the image. An increase in time, temperature, or concentration will increase the film speed and base fog. An increase in the time, temperature, or concentration will also increase the contrast of the film.

The speed of the transport motor controls the amount of time the film is immersed in the developer, fixer, and wash tanks. Time and temperature are inversely proportional; as one is increased, the other must be decreased to maintain the same optical density for the same exposure.

A **thermostat** controls heating elements to maintain the developer and fixer at the proper temperature. The thermostat is set to maintain the developer temperature in the range between 92 and 95°F. Developer temperatures below this range result in slower chemical reactions and an underdeveloped film with decreased density and low contrast. Temperatures above this range result in rapid chemical reactions, overdeveloped film, increased image density, and a high-contrast, narrow-latitude image.

RAPID PROCESSING

By increasing the temperature and chemical concentrations, the total processing time can be reduced to 45 s. The sensitometric characteristics of rapid processing films are designed to be identical to conventional 90-s processed film.

EXTENDED PROCESSING

Extended processing is used in mammography to increase the film contrast and speed and reduce the patient dose. Standard chemicals and temperatures are used, but the processing time is extended to 3 min by slowing the film transport speed.

PROCESSOR QUALITY ASSURANCE

Processing is the last in a long series of careful steps designed to produce a diagnostic-quality image. Any error in processing will prevent the production of high-quality radiographs. Processor cleanliness, temperature, and chemical effectiveness must be maintained within strict limits. The rollers and gears must be periodically inspected for wear and replaced before their degradation affects image quality.

Processor quality assurance is covered more completely in Chap. 20.

Extended processing increases film contrast and speed by slowing the film transport system to increase the time the film is immersed in the developing solution. Increasing the temperature and chemical concentration allows rapid processing of images. The processor operation should be monitored daily, and the processor should be cleaned periodically.

THE DARKROOM

The darkroom is an essential part of a radiology department. The darkroom entrance should be designed so that entry does not inadvertently expose films. Lightproof mazes, rotating doors, interlocks, and double entry doors are used to eliminate the possibility of exposure of undeveloped film to light. The darkroom temperature and humidity must be controlled to avoid artifacts.

DARKROOM SAFELIGHTS

An exposed film is much more sensitive than an unexposed film because some silver halide crystals may have been partially exposed. Darkrooms do not have to be totally dark, but the light level must be very low. **Safelights** provide low-level illumination without exposing the film. A safelight contains a low-wattage light bulb with a special filter to maintain low light intensity. An amber filter is used with blue-sensitive film. The **GBX filter** produces a deep red light. Red light from the GBX filter has low energy and is safe for green-sensitive orthochromatic films.

A test can be performed to determine the amount of safelight fogging. Half of a uniformly exposed but undeveloped film is covered with a piece of cardboard, and the film is left on the darkroom table under the safelight for 2 min. The film is then developed in the usual way. After processing, the difference in optical density between the covered and uncovered side should be less than 0.05 optical density. Figure 12.5 shows a darkroom safelight test.

Figure 12.5 **Test for darkroom safelight fog.**

SILVER RECOVERY

The final processed film contains only about half the silver contained in the original emulsion. Silver is classified as a toxic heavy metal by the Environmental Protection Agency. Environmental laws restrict the amount of silver discharged in waste liquid to less than 5 parts per million. Therefore, the silver must be removed from the fixer solution before that solution is discarded as waste. The most common method of silver removal is the electrolytic recovery system. This system is attached to the drain or waste line of the fixer tank; the used fixer solution circulates through the recovery system, where an electric current removes the silver ions from the fixer solution and converts them into metallic silver. The recovered silver can be sold to commercial companies.

DAYLIGHT PROCESSING SYSTEMS

With daylight processing systems, a darkroom is not required in order to load and unload the film cassettes. All film handling is done automatically inside the daylight processor. An exposed cassette is placed in the entrance slot, and the cassette is drawn into the daylight processor and opened. The film is removed from the cassette and started through the processing cycle. The cassette is then reloaded with an unexposed film, which is stored in a bulk magazine inside the daylight processor, and returned ready for another exposure. The daylight processor has a storage magazine for each size film used by the department. The development, fixing, washing, and drying cycles are the same as in a conventional automatic processor. Figure 12.6 shows a daylight process-

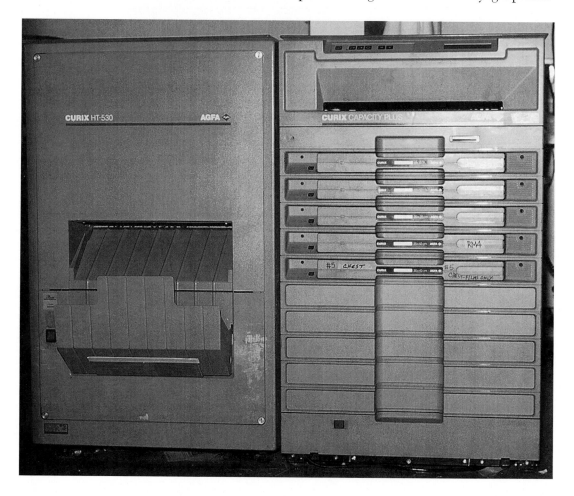

Figure 12.6 Daylight processing system.

ing system. Of course, a darkroom is still needed to load the daylight processor magazines.

DRY PROCESSING FILM

Dry processing film is used to permanently record digital images from computed tomography, magnetic resonance imaging, ultrasound, and digital radiographic systems. The digital image data are transferred onto a special film, which is then processed using heat to fix the image on the film.

The safelights in the darkroom must be checked at least annually and whenever a bulb is changed to ensure that the safelight does not cause fogging of the film. Special GBX filters on the safelight are needed for orthochromatic film. Unexposed silver is dissolved away during the developing process. It can be recovered from the fixer solution and recycled. Daylight processors permit the development of exposed film without the need to open the exposed cassette in a darkroom. Dry film systems do not require developing solutions; instead, they use heat to fix the image on the film.

SUMMARY

Film processing consists of developing, fixing, washing, and drying. Film processing converts the latent image in the emulsion into a permanent visible image by reducing the exposed silver halide grains to black metallic silver. Chemical agents in the basic developer solution include two reducing agents, hydroquinone and phenidone. The fixer is an acidic solution that stops the developer action. It contains ammonium thiosulfate, which dissolves away the unexposed silver halide crystals. Changing the developer chemical concentrations, the time, or the temperature will change the speed, contrast, and base fog of the final image. Film must be processed in the dark, either in a darkroom or in a daylight film processor. The darkroom safelight and filter must match the characteristics of the film used. The processing chemicals are classified as hazardous materials and must be disposed of in an approved manner. Daylight processors permit the development of exposed film without the need to open the exposed cassette in a darkroom. Dry film systems do not require developing solutions; instead, they use heat to fix the image on the film.

QUESTIONS

1. The developer solution
   a. softens the emulsion.
   b. reduces the exposed silver halide crystals to black metallic silver.
   c. is basic.
   d. is/does all of the above.
2. The fixer solution
   a. stops the action of the developer.
   b. hardens the emulsion.
   c. dissolves the unexposed silver halide crystals.
   d. is/does all of the above.
3. The developer solution
   a. is acidic.
   b. is basic.
   c. is neutral.
4. The order of the film processing stages is
   1. Fixing
   2. Drying
   3. Developing
   4. Washing
   a. 1, 2, 3, 4.
   b. 3, 4, 1, 2.
   c. 3, 1, 4, 2.
   d. 3, 4, 1, 4, 2.
5. The fixer solution
   a. is acidic.
   b. is basic.
   c. is neutral.
6. Contamination of the _____ solution by the _____ solution will result in lower-contrast, "washed-out" radiographs.
   a. fixer; developer
   b. developer; fixer
   c. developer; wash
   d. wash; fixer
7. Increasing the development time or the developer concentration or temperature will _____ the speed of the film.
   a. increase
   b. decrease
   c. not change
8. Increasing the development time or the developer concentration or temperature will _____ the contrast of the film.
   a. increase
   b. decrease
   c. not change

9. Increasing the development time or the developer temperature or concentration will _____ the base fog of the film.
   a. increase
   b. decrease
   c. not change
10. Increasing the developer concentration or temperature will _____ the latitude of the film.
    a. increase
    b. decrease
    c. not change
11. Increasing the developer concentration will _____ the spatial resolution of the film.
    a. increase
    b. decrease
    c. not change

For Questions 12 to 15, will decreasing the temperature, time, or concentration of the developer have the given effect? Answer a for true or b for false.

12. _____ Decrease the film contrast
13. _____ Increase the film speed
14. _____ Decrease the film latitude
15. _____ Increase the base plus fog
16. The purpose of the guide shoes in an automatic processor is to
    a. draw the film into the processor.
    b. maintain the film alignment during transport of the film into the next tank.
    c. press the developer out of the emulsion.
    d. agitate the chemicals.
17. The purpose of the guide shoes in an automatic processor is to
    a. draw the film into the processor.
    b. agitate the chemicals.
    c. transport the film into the next tank.
    d. press the chemicals out of the emulsion.
18 Silver recovery systems remove silver from used
    a. developer solution.
    b. fixer solution.
    c. wash water.
    d. film.
19. Replenishment systems in automatic processors replenish
    a. unexposed film emulsion.
    b. developer and fixer solutions.
    c. used wash water.
    d. drying racks.

20. Which of the following chemicals is used to remove the unexposed silver from the film?
    a. Sodium sulfite
    b. Glutaraldehyde
    c. Ammonium thiosulfate
    d. Acetic acid

21. Replenishment of the chemicals in the processor is done automatically
    a. when the film enters the dryer.
    b. when the film enters the processor.
    c. after the 3:00 P.M. shift change.
    d. when the film enters the fixer.

22. The replenishment system is controlled by a
    a. crossover rack.
    b. timer.
    c. drive motor.
    d. microswitch.

23. If the development time is increased, the temperature of the developer should be _____ to keep the optical density the same for the same exposure.
    a. increased
    b. decreased
    c. unchanged

24. The undeveloped silver crystals are removed from the film emulsion during the _____ stage of processing.
    a. developing
    b. fixing
    c. washing
    d. drying

25. Film development is achieved
    a. by an oxidizing agent in an acid solution.
    b. by an oxidizing agent in a basic solution.
    c. by a reducing agent in an acid solution.
    d. by a reducing agent in a basic solution.

26. Replenishment rates are based on the
    a. speed of the transport roller motor.
    b. size of the processor tanks.
    c. amount and size of the films processed.
    d. frequency of processor maintenance.

27. The principal purpose of the circulation pumps is to
    a. agitate the film.
    b. agitate the chemical solutions.
    c. replenish the chemicals.
    d. change the solution temperature.

28. Which of the following is a reducing agent?
    a. Glutaraldehyde
    b. Hydroquinone
    c. Acetic acid
    d. Alum
29. The purpose of the rollers in an automatic processor is to
    a. maintain film alignment.
    b. agitate the chemicals.
    c. start replinishment pumps.
    d. press the chemicals out of the emulsion.

ANSWERS TO CHAPTER 12 QUESTIONS

1.	d	16.	b
2.	d	17.	c
3.	b	18.	b
4.	c	19.	b
5.	a	20.	c
6.	b	21.	b
7.	a	22.	d
8.	a	23.	b
9.	a	24.	b
10.	b	25.	d
11.	c	26.	c
12.	a	27.	b
13.	b	28.	b
14.	a	29.	d
15.	b		

13

Intensifying Screens

OBJECTIVES

At the completion of this chapter, the student will be able to:

1. Describe the purpose and construction of intensifying screens.
2. Describe the characteristics of rare earth screens.
3. Identify the factors that affect screen speed and spatial resolution.

INTRODUCTION

X-rays that are able to penetrate through a thick patient will easily pass through a film emulsion only a fraction of a millimeter thick. This means that there are not many interactions in the film. To increase the number of x-rays absorbed and reduce the patient dose, intensifying screens convert x-rays into light, which then exposes the film emulsion. This chapter covers the construction and characteristics of intensifying screens.

INTENSIFYING SCREENS

The purpose of an **intensifying screen** is to increase the efficiency of x-ray absorption and decrease the dose to the patient. An intensifying screen converts a single x-ray into thousands of lower-energy light photons, which expose

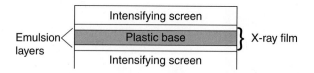

Figure 13.1 **Intensifying screens are located on either side of the film.**

the film. Most x-rays that are able to pass through a 30-centimeter (cm)-thick patient have no trouble passing through a film emulsion that is less than 1 millimeter (mm) thick. Only about 1 percent of the film's optical density is produced by x-rays; the other 99 percent results from intensifying screen light. This light is produced when an x-ray interacts with the phosphor crystals in the screen. Today essentially all radiographic images are formed using intensifying screens. The x-ray film is held in a lightproof cassette between two intensifying screens. Figure 13.1 shows a typical cassette with the film located between its intensifying screens.

The conversion of x-ray energy into light energy reduces the amount of radiation required to produce an acceptable image. Figure 13.2 illustrates the steps involved in converting a single x-ray into many visible light photons.

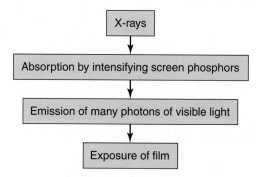

Figure 13.2 **Steps in the intensifying-screen process of converting a few x-rays into many photons of visible light.**

INTENSIFYING SCREEN CONSTRUCTION

An intensifying screen consists of a plastic base supporting a reflective layer, a phosphor layer, and a protective layer. Figure 13.3 illustrates the construction of a typical intensifying screen.

Screen Base

A 1-mm-thick plastic screen base provides support for the other components of the screen. It is flexible but, unlike the film base, is not transparent.

Reflective Layer

The screen phosphor crystals emit light in all directions. Less than half the light produced by the screen phosphor crystals is directed toward the film. The reflective layer redirects the light from the phosphor toward the film. Figure 13.4 shows how the reflective layer redirects screen light toward the film.

The Phosphor Layer

The **phosphor** layer is made up of crystals embedded in a clear plastic support medium. The phosphor crystals convert x-rays into visible light by means

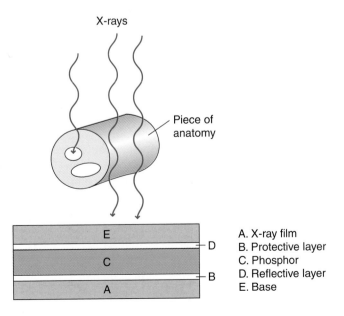

Figure 13.3 Intensifying screen construction.

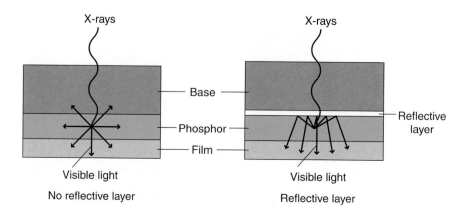

Figure 13.4 The reflective layer on the screen base redirects light from the phosphors back onto the film.

of two mechanisms, **fluorescence** and **phosphorescence.** Fluorescence is the production of light during the stimulation of the phosphor by the x-rays; phosphorescence is the continuation of light emission after the stimulation ceases. Most of the light output from intensifying screens is due to fluorescence.

The material, size, and distribution of the phosphor crystals and the thickness of the phosphor layer determine the speed and resolution of the intensifying screen. There is a trade-off between speed, patient dose, and resolution. Thicker screens have higher speed and require a lower patient dose but have poorer spatial resolution. Different film/screen combinations are chosen for different clinical applications.

Phosphor Materials

Intensifying screens are made of higher atomic number (higher Z) phosphors to increase x-ray interaction. About 5000 light photons are produced by each x-ray absorbed by a phosphor crystal. The number of light photons produced by one x-ray is described by the **conversion efficiency.** This is a measure of the screens' efficiency in converting x-ray energy into light energy.

The intensifying screens developed by Thomas Edison in the early 1900s used calcium tungstate ($CaWO_4$) crystals as the phosphor. Calcium tungstate crystals give off blue light and are 3 to 5 percent efficient in converting x-ray energy into light. They were in common use until the mid 1970s, when rare earth screens were introduced. **Rare earth screens** use elements from the rare earth section (Z = 57 to 70) of the periodic table. Rare earth elements used in intensifying screens include gadolinium, lanthanum, and yttrium. They are 15 to 20 percent efficient in converting x-ray energy into light because their K absorption edges are closer to the average energy of diagnostic x-ray beams.

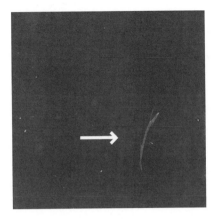

Figure 13.5 White-line artifact caused by a scratch on the intensifying screen.

Protective Layer

The protective layer is a thin plastic layer about 0.01 mm thick that protects the phosphor layer from abrasion when the film is inserted into and removed from the cassette. The protective layer cannot withstand scratches from fingernails, rings, or hard objects. Scratches that remove the protective layer also remove the phosphor, layer producing white, negative-density artifacts. Figure 13.5 illustrates an artifact produced by a scratch on the intensifying screen.

The intensifying screen converts a few highly penetrating x-rays into many visible light photons to increase the efficiency of the detection process. Phosphor materials are coated on a reflective layer supported by a flexible plastic base.

SPECTRAL MATCHING

Spectral matching refers to matching the wavelength or color of the light from the screen to the film sensitivity. Figure 13.6 compares the light output from calcium tungstate and rare earth screens.

Different screen phosphors emit light of different colors or wavelengths. The response of the film must be matched to the light wavelength of the intensifying screen. There are two classes of intensifying screens, those that emit blue light and those that emit green light. Calcium tungstate $(CaWO_4)$ and

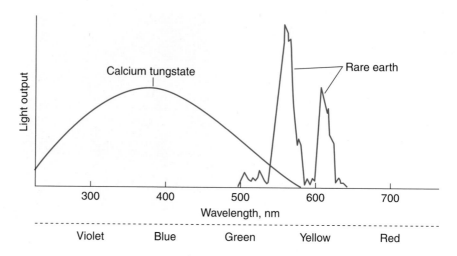

Figure 13.6 **Light output from calcium tungstate and typical rare-earth screen materials.**

some rare earth materials emit blue light. Other rare earth materials emit green light. There are two general groups of film, whose sensitivities are designed to match the light from the different types of intensifying screens. Blue-sensitive, or **panchromatic,** film is used with calcium tungstate and other blue-light-emitting screens. Green-sensitive, or **orthochromatic,** film is used with green-emitting rare earth intensifying screens. A mismatch between intensifying screen and film results in reduced efficiency and increased patient dose. Table 13.1 presents representative screen materials, their K-absorption-edge energy, and the color of light emitted. Recall that the average x-ray energy is about one-third the applied kVp.

Table 13.1
Screen Materials and Their Characteristics

Phosphor Material	K-edge Energy	Emitted Light Color
Calcium tungstate	70	Blue
Gadolinium	50	Green
Lanthanum	39	Blue
Yttrium	17	Blue

SCREEN SPEED

Screen speed is a term used to describe how much light is obtained from a given x-ray exposure. Standard speed is set at 100. Film/screen systems range in speed from 50 to 1000.

There are three types of screens: detail, medium-speed, and high-speed. **Detail** screens are used for higher-resolution imaging, such as extremity examinations. **Medium-speed screens,** formally called par-speed screens, are used for routine imaging. **High-speed screens** are used for examinations that require short exposure times. Table 13.2 gives the speed ranges associated with each of these screen types. The mAs must be changed to compensate for a change in screen speed. The amount of change is given by the ratio of the screen speeds.

Changing from a high-speed to a detail screen requires an increase in mAs to maintain the same optical density. As an example, if a 400-speed screen is replaced by a 50-speed screen, if the original mAs was 5 mAs with the 400-speed screen, what is the new mAs for the 50-speed screen?

$$mAs_2 = mAs_1 \times (\text{old screen speed/new screen speed})$$
$$mAs_2 = mAs_1 \times (400/50)$$
$$mAs_2 = mAs_1 \times 8$$
$$mAs_2 = 5 \times 8$$
$$mAs_2 = 40 \text{ mAs}$$

The mAs_2 is the new mAs, and the mAs_1 is the old or original mAs used.

The automatic exposure circuit (AEC) must be calibrated for a particular film/screen combination. Using a cassette with a screen speed other than that for which the AEC is set will produce an image with improper density. For example, if a detail screen is used with an AEC set for medium-speed screens, the image will appear too light because the detail screen speed would require a higher exposure than produced by the AEC.

Thicker screens have more phosphor crystals available for interaction with the x-rays and are faster because they absorb more x-rays. Fewer x-rays are

Table 13.2

Screen Types and Speeds

Screen Type	Speed
Detail	50
Medium-speed	100
High-speed	400–1000

needed to produce the same optical density when faster screens are used, resulting in lower patient dose.

> *High-speed screens require less exposure to produce the same optical density. The size, shape, and type of the phosphor material determine the efficiency of the conversion of x-rays to light. Rare earth materials are more efficient, but some give off light with a different wavelength (color). The response of the film must be matched to the light emitted by the screens. Faster screens reduce the dose to the patient. Screen speed ranges from 50 to 1000.*

ABSORPTION AS A FUNCTION OF X-RAY ENERGY

Photoelectric absorption in the screen depends on the x-ray energy and the K-shell binding energy of the phosphor material. The K-shell absorption energy refers to x-ray energy just high enough to remove a K-shell electron from its orbit. Figure 13.7 shows the absorption of x-rays for calcium tungstate and for typical rare earth materials plotted as a function of x-ray energy.

The sharp rise in x-ray absorption occurs at the K-edge binding energy. X-rays with energies above the K-shell binding energy have enough energy to interact with and remove a K-shell electron. X-rays with energies below the K-shell binding energy can remove only L-, M-, or N-shell electrons. If the x-ray energy is above the K-edge energy, absorption is much higher. Rare earth phosphor materials are chosen because their K-edge energies occur in the diagnostic energy range. Today rare earth screens are used extensively in diagnostic radiology.

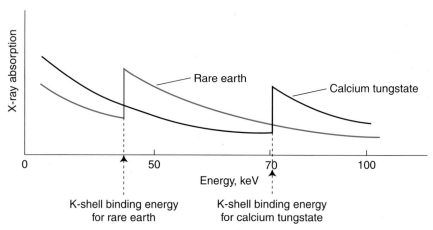

Figure 13.7 **Absorption of x-rays by calcium tungstate and typical rare-earth screen materials.**

RADIOGRAPHIC NOISE OR QUANTUM MOTTLE

Radiographic noise or **quantum mottle** is a random speckled appearance of an image. It is similar to the "salt and pepper" or "snow" seen with poor TV reception. It is caused by the statistical fluctuations in x-ray interactions. Radiographic noise or quantum mottle depends on the number of x-rays interacting with the phosphor crystals in the screen. Images produced with a smaller number of x-rays have higher quantum mottle or radiographic noise. It is especially noticeable when the number of x-rays forming the image is too low. Technical factors that influence the amount of quantum mottle include mAs, kVp, and screen speed. Screens with greater conversion efficiency convert more x-rays into light, so they require fewer x-rays and produce images with more noise. Faster screens have more quantum mottle because they require fewer x-rays to produce the same optical density. High-speed screens used with high-kVp, low-mAs techniques result in images with increased quantum mottle.

Intensifying screen phosphors are highly absorbing for x-rays with energies just above their K-shell binding energy. This sharp rise in absorption is called K-edge absorption. High-speed screens reduce the dose to the patient but increase quantum mottle by reducing the number of x-rays reaching the detector.

INTENSIFICATION FACTOR

The efficiency of the screen is described by the **intensification factor.** The intensification factor is the ratio of the mAs values required to produce the same optical density without and with the screen. Typical intensification factors range from 25 to several hundred. High-speed screens have higher intensification factors than slower-speed screens.

SPATIAL RESOLUTION

Spatial resolution is the minimum separation between two objects at which they can be recognized as two separate objects. Spatial resolution is measured using a line pair test pattern and has units of line pairs per millimeter (lp/mm). Spatial resolution depends on the thickness of the screen and the phosphor size. Thicker screens have poorer spatial resolution because the light spreads sideways and blurs out the edges of an image. Figure 13.8 illustrates why thicker screens have poorer spatial resolution. Thicker high-speed screens have poorer spatial resolution than thinner slower-speed screens.

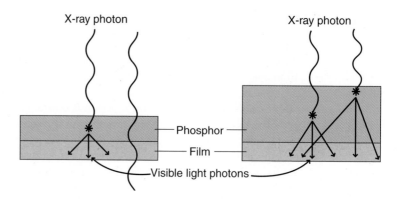

Figure 13.8 **Thicker intensifying screens are faster because they have more interactions, but they have poorer spatial resolution because the light spreads out further before it reaches the film.**

FILM/SCREEN CASSETTES

Diagnostic films are held inside of **film cassettes.** A cassette has a pair of intensifying screens glued to the interior front and back. The purpose of the cassette is to provide a lightproof holder for the film. Proper film/screen contact is necessary to achieve good image detail. The front side of the screen is constructed of low atomic number material to reduce attenuation of the x-rays entering the cassette. The cassette also contains a thin layer on the back to attenuate exit radiation. For this reason, the tube side is always indicated on the cassette. Film cassettes come in a variety of sizes. Standard sizes are given in Table 13.3.

A cassette opens like a book, and the film fits into the recessed half of the cassette. It is important to use the correct film size. There is an area of the cassette used for image identification that has no intensifying screen. This identification area has a sliding cover that is opened when the cassette is placed in the ID camera. Patient information is recorded on the film in this area.

Table 13.3
Standard Cassette Sizes

Size in Centimeters	Size in Inches
18 × 24	8 × 10
24 × 30	10 × 12
28 × 35	11 × 14
35 × 43	14 × 17

A

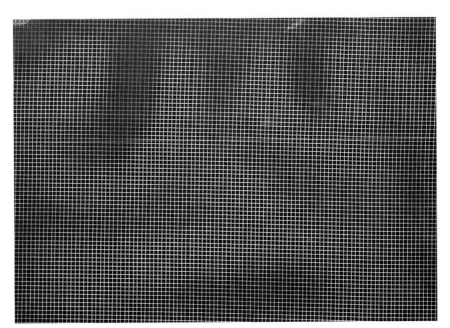

B

Figure 13.9 Examples of good *(A)* and poor *(B)* film/screen contact.

FILM/SCREEN CONTACT

Poor film/screen contact destroys detail and spatial resolution because the light from the screen diffuses before it reaches the film. Many cassettes have a slight curve on the door side of the cassette so that pressure is applied when the cassette is closed. This extra pressure ensures good film/screen contact. Film/screen contact can be evaluated using the wire mesh test. A screenlike wire mesh embedded in plastic is placed over the film cassette to be tested. After exposure, the film is developed. Any areas of poor film/screen contact appear as blurred or unsharp areas on the image. Figure 13.9 shows an image of a wire mesh test pattern showing good (Fig. 13.9A) and poor (Fig. 13.9B) film/screen contact.

CASSETTE CARE

Every screen cassette has an identification number. This number appears on every exposed film and can be used to trace artifacts to a particular cassette. For example, a series of fogged films caused by a light leak due to a dropped cassette, or a white area on the film caused by removal of the intensifying phosphor by a scratch on the screen, can be readily traced to the damaged cassette. Screens should be cleaned regularly and whenever artifacts appear on the images. Dirt on the screens will result in white or negative density spots on the image. Areas of darker density are called positive densities.

The intensification factor is the ratio of the mAs value required to produce the same optical density without the screen to the mAs with the screen. Cassettes must be handled carefully to avoid damaging them. Scratches on the intensifying screens can remove the phosphor coating, leading to negative density artifacts. Film/screen contact is tested with a wire mesh and must be adequate to prevent loss of spatial resolution.

SUMMARY

Intensifying screens convert x-ray energy into light energy. Modern intensifying screens utilize rare earth phosphors whose K absorption edges are matched to diagnostic x-ray energies. These phosphors emit green or blue light, which is matched to the spectral sensitivity of the film. There are three classes of screen speeds: high-speed, medium-speed, and detail. High-speed screens require fewer x-rays, resulting in lower patient doses, but have more quantum noise. Detail screens produce superior spatial resolution but require increased patient doses. Cassettes, which provide a light-tight container for the film, must be cleaned and checked regularly for good film/screen contact.

QUESTIONS

1. Spectral matching of film and screen refers to matching of the
   a. film crystal size to the phosphor crystal size.
   b. emulsion thickness to the phosphor thickness.
   c. color of the cassette to the film sensitivity.
   d. film sensitivity to the color of the light emitted by the phosphor.
2. When a medium-speed screen system is substituted for a detail screen,
   a. the patient dose is reduced.
   b. spatial resolution is improved.
   c. quantum mottle will be decreased.
   d. patient motion artifacts will generally increase.
3. In order to increase the spatial resolution of a film/screen system, the most important factor would be to
   a. change to a faster film.
   b. change to a faster-speed screen.
   c. change to a slower-speed screen.
   d. change to extended processing.
4. Changing from a 200-speed screen to a 50-speed detail screen requires a(n) _____ in mAs.
   a. increase by a factor of 2
   b. increase by a factor of 4
   c. decrease by a factor of 2
   d. decrease by a factor of 4
5. Which of the following film/screen combinations would require the highest mAs?
   a. Detail
   b. Medium-speed
   c. High-speed
6. Film/screen contact is evaluated by a
   a. line pair test.
   b. densitometer.
   c. wire mesh test.
   d. sensitometer.
7. Scratches on the screen will appear as _____ artifacts.
   a. negative
   b. positive

8. Which of the following are rare earth phosphor materials?
   1. Calcium tungstate
   2. Gadolinium
   3. Lanthanum
   4. Yttrium
   a. 1, 2, and 3
   b. 2, 3, and 4
   c. 1, 3, and 4
   d. 1, 2, 3, and 4

9. Which of the following is *not* related to the construction of an intensifying screen?
   a. Plastic base
   b. Phosphor layer
   c. Emulsion layer
   d. Reflective layer

10. Which type of film should be used with green-emitting rare earth screens?
    a. Panchromatic
    b. Orthochromatic
    c. Duplicating
    d. 105-mm spot

11. When changing from a detail screen to a high-speed screen, the mAs should be
    a. increased.
    b. decreased.
    c. not changed.
    d. none of the above.

12. Which screen type will result in the poorest spatial resolution?
    a. Detail
    b. Medium-speed
    c. High-speed

13. Quantum mottle depends on the
    a. K-shell absorption.
    b. intensification factor.
    c. film/screen contact.
    d. number of x-rays interacting in the phosphor.

14. Radiographic noise or quantum mottle can be reduced by using
    a. high kVp and a small focal spot.
    b. low kVp and high mAs.
    c. high kVp and low mAs.
    d. low mAs and a large focal spot.

15. Using detail screens with the AEC calibrated for medium-speed screens will result in _____ density.
    a. increased
    b. decreased
    c. unchanged

ANSWERS TO CHAPTER 13 QUESTIONS

1. d
2. a
3. c
4. b
5. a
6. c
7. a
8. b

9. c
10. b
11. b
12. c
13. d
14. b
15. b

14

Grids and Scatter Reduction

OBJECTIVES

At the completion of this chapter, the student will be able to

1. Describe the effect of scatter on radiographic contrast.
2. Identify the factors that affect the amount of scatter.
3. Identify methods of scatter reduction.
4. Describe the construction of an antiscatter grid.

INTRODUCTION

Most of the x-rays entering a patient undergo scattering before they exit the patient. Only those x-rays that do not have an interaction in the patient are useful in forming the diagnostic image. Scattered x-rays, or scatter, contain no useful information. Removing the scattered x-rays from the beam before they reach the image receptor greatly improves image contrast. Grids are the most widely used antiscatter devices in radiology. They eliminate scatter by removing x-rays that do not come directly from the focal spot.

EXIT RADIATION

Exit radiation is the combination of transmitted and scattered radiation that passes through the patient. Transmitted radiation undergoes no interac-

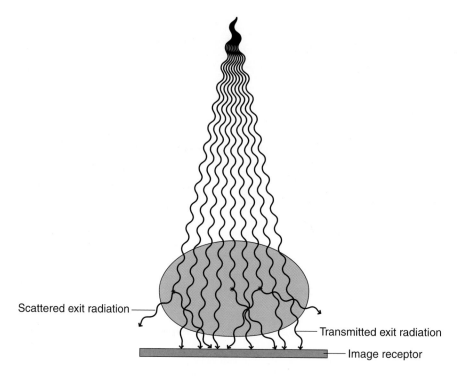

Scattered exit radiation

Transmitted exit radiation

Image receptor

Figure 14.1 **Transmitted and scattered exit radiation leaving a patient.**

tion in the patient. It passes through the patient with no change in direction or loss of energy. Scattered radiation has undergone at least one Compton scattering interaction. Scattered radiation changes direction and loses energy before leaving the patient. Scattered radiation has lower energy and is emitted from the patient in all directions. Scattered radiation is the source of exposure to personnel in the room during fluoroscopy and portable examinations. Figure 14.1 illustrates how exit radiation is made up of transmitted and scattered radiation.

EFFECT OF SCATTER ON CONTRAST

Scattered radiation reduces radiographic contrast by adding a general background density over the entire image. Scattered radiation provides no diagnostic information. The presence of scatter lowers image contrast and makes objects more difficult to see in the radiographic image.

FACTORS THAT AFFECT THE AMOUNT OF SCATTER

Scatter depends on patient or part thickness, x-ray energy, and field size. It does not depend on SID or focal spot size. The technologist can change the x-ray energy by changing the kVp and the field size by adjusting the collimator to reduce scatter. Careful selection of the field size and kVp can significantly reduce the amount of scatter and improve image quality.

Patient Thickness

An increase in tissue thickness increases the amount of scatter because there are more atoms available for interactions in the thicker tissue. The greater number of interactions produces more scatter. With some examinations, it is possible to reduce the part thickness, which reduces the amount of scatter. In mammography, for example, compression reduces tissue thickness and scatter. Figure 14.2 illustrates the increase in scatter as the patient thickness increases.

X-ray Beam Energy

The kVp is the factor that controls x-ray energy or the penetrability of the beam. Increasing the kVp results in more forward scatter exiting the patient and striking the image receptor. Decreasing the kVp decreases the x-ray beam energy and the amount of scatter. However, lower-energy x-rays have decreased penetration and result in higher patient doses because more x-rays are absorbed in the patient. The kVp selected must be tailored to the body part under examination.

Field Size

Larger field sizes produce more scatter because the larger area results in more tissue's being radiated. Decreasing the field size decreases the area of tissue available for x-ray interactions. Smaller field sizes result in less scattered radiation and higher image contrast.

COLLIMATION

The purpose of collimation is to define the size and shape of the primary x-ray beam that strikes the patient and to provide a visible light field in the same location as the x-ray field. Figure 14.3 shows a schematic view of a light-localizing collimator.

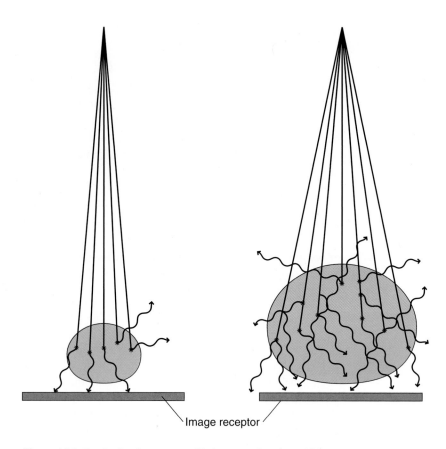

Image receptor

Figure 14.2 **Scattering increases with increased patient thickness.**

A light-localizing collimator consists of two pairs of lead shutters that are adjusted to intercept x-rays outside the desired x-ray field. Some collimators have an iris-like shutter that can approximate a circular field. A light source is located off the x-ray beam axis, and a mirror directs the light through the shutters. The x-ray beam passes through the mirror with very little attenuation. The distance from the mirror to the light source is equal to the distance from the mirror to the tube focal spot, so the light and radiation fields are the same distance from the patient surface. The collimator adjustment controls have indicators to show the field size in centimeters or inches at different source to image receptor distances (SIDs).

Positive beam limitation (**PBL**) collimators automatically adjust the x-ray beam to the size of the image receptor. Sensors in the cassette holder (sometimes called the Bucky tray) detect the size of the image receptor and adjust the collimator shutters to match the cassette size. A PBL collimator

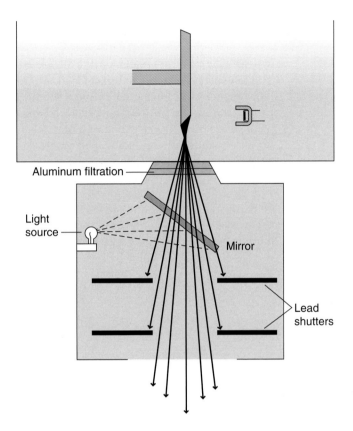

Figure 14.3 **Schematic view of a light-localizing collimator.**

prevents the selection of a field larger than the image receptor, but the field size can be reduced to limit the field to the area of interest and decrease scatter.

Exit radiation is the combination of transmitted and scattered radiation leaving the patient. Scatter reduces image contrast. It increases with increased patient thickness, beam energy, and field size.

SCATTER REDUCTION TECHNIQUES

The two most important methods of reducing scatter are beam collimation and grids. Reducing scatter radiation improves radiographic contrast. Reducing the field size reduces the amount of scatter.

GRIDS

A **grid** consists of alternating strips of radiopaque and radiolucent materials. The radiopaque material is usually lead. A grid removes scatter from the exit radiation before it reaches the image receptor. The grid is located between the patient and the image receptor. Scattered x-rays are preferentially attenuated by the lead strips, because they are not parallel to the grid interspaces. The interspaces, which are the radiolucent spaces between the lead strips, are made of plastic or aluminum. The radiolucent materials allow transmitted x-rays to reach the image receptor while the lead strips intercept the scatter. Figure 14.4 illustrates the construction of a typical grid and the absorption of scatter. Only x-rays that are almost parallel with the interspaces pass through the grid. When to use a grid is a matter of professional judgment. Grids are usually employed when the body part is greater than 10 centimeters (cm) thick.

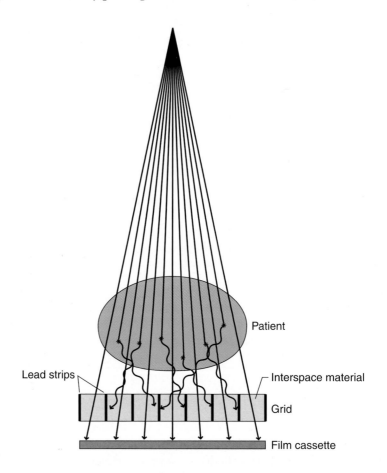

Figure 14.4 Scatter absorption with a typical grid.

Grid Ratio

The amount of scattered radiation removed by the grid depends on the height of and the distance between the lead strips. The amount of scatter eliminated, often called the scatter cleanup, depends on the grid ratio. The **grid ratio** is the ratio of the height of the lead strips to the distance between the lead strips or the thickness of the interspace:

$$GR = h/D$$

Figure 14.5 illustrates the grid ratios of two different grids.

EXAMPLE 1:

What is the grid ratio of a grid that has lead strips 4 millimeters (mm) in height and 0.5 mm apart?

ANSWER:

$$GR = h/D$$
$$GR = 4/0.5$$
$$GR = 8$$

The grid ratio is 8:1.

Grid ratios typically range from 5:1, pronounced "five to one," to 16:1. Grids with higher grid ratios remove more scattered radiation but are much more difficult to align properly. For this reason, portable examinations are usually taken using grid ratios of less than 12:1.

Grid Frequency

The grid frequency is the number of lead strips per centimeter or per inch. Grids with thinner strips have higher grid frequencies and are less visible on the radiographic image. Typical grid frequencies range from 24 to 80 lines per centimeter (60–200 lines per inch).

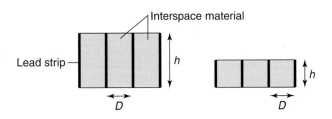

Figure 14.5 Grid ratio *h/D* for two grids.

Bucky Factor

The **Bucky factor** measures how much scatter is removed by the grid and how the technical factors must be adjusted to produce the same optical density. Scattered radiation accounts for a significant portion of the density of the final radiograph. If a grid removes some scatter, the exposure factors must be increased to compensate for the decrease in x-rays reaching the image receptor. The Bucky factor is the ratio of the mAs required with the grid to the mAs required without the grid to produce the same optical density. It is always greater than 1. The Bucky factor depends on the grid ratio and the grid frequency but is usually in the range of 3 to 5. This means that adding a grid requires an increase in mAs by a factor of 3 to 5 to obtain the same optical density as with a nongrid technique. The use of a grid increases the patient dose by the Bucky factor. The Bucky factor is used to calculate the necessary change in mAs when a grid is added or when changing to a grid with a different grid ratio. Table 14.1 gives the Bucky factors for different grid ratios. A non-grid technique has a Bucky factor of 1.

EXAMPLE 2:

What change in mAs must be made to change from a nongrid technique to one using an 12:1 grid?

$$mAs_2 = mAs_1 \times (\text{new Bucky factor/old Bucky factor})$$

ANSWER:

The required increase in mAs is given by the Bucky factor. From Table 14.1, the Bucky factor for a 12:1 grid is 5. The mAs must be increased by a factor of 5.

$$mAs_2 = mAs_1 \times 5$$

Table 14.1

Grid Ratios and Associated Bucky Factors

Grid Ratio	Bucky Factor
None	1
5:1	2
6:1	3
8:1	4
12:1	5
16:1	6

EXAMPLE 3:

A portable examination taken at 75 kVp and 6 mAs without a grid gives an acceptable optical density but very little contrast as a result of scatter. What mAs should be used if a 8:1 grid is added before the repeat exposure?

ANSWER:

$$mAs_2 = mAs_1 \times (\text{new Bucky factor/old Bucky factor})$$

From Table 14.1, the Bucky factor of an 8:1 grid is 4.

$$mAs_2 = 6 \times 4/1$$
$$mAs_2 = 24 \text{ mAs}$$

Required Change in mAs Following a Change of Grids

If a grid with a different grid ratio is used in a follow-up examination, the change in mAs is given by the ratio of the Bucky factors.

EXAMPLE 4:

An examination taken in the department used 30 mAs with a 12:1 grid. What mAs should be used for a follow-up portable examination taken with an 8:1 grid?

$$mAs_2 = mAs_1 \times (\text{new Bucky factor/old Bucky factor})$$
$$mAs_2 = 30 \times (4/5)$$
$$mAs_2 = 30 \times 0.8$$
$$mAs_2 = 24 \text{ mAs}$$

Grids remove scatter by intercepting scattered x-rays that deviate from the straight path through the patient. The grid ratio is the ratio of the height of the lead strips to the distance between the lead strips. Grids with higher grid ratios remove more scatter but are more difficult to align. The Bucky factor relates the mAs with and without the grid. It is the amount of mAs increase required to compensate for the introduction of the grid and maintain the same optical density.

TYPES OF GRIDS

There are two types of grids, parallel and focused. **Parallel grids** have parallel lead strips. **Focused grids** have the lead strips angled toward a fixed distance from the front surface of the grid. This distance is known as the focal distance of the grid. The divergent rays transmitted from the x-ray source pass through the focused grid interspaces, while the scattered x-rays are intercepted.

PARALLEL GRID CUTOFF

Parallel grid cutoff arises because parallel grids are constructed with the lead strips parallel to the central axis of the x-ray beam, but x-rays diverge from the focal spot. **Grid cutoff** is the interception of transmitted x-rays by the radiopaque strips of a grid. It occurs because x-rays near the edge of the field are not parallel to the lead strips and so are attenuated. To reduce grid cutoff, smaller field sizes and larger SIDs should be used with parallel grids. Parallel grid cutoff produces a film that has the correct optical density in the center but is lighter at both edges. Figure 14.6 illustrates parallel grid cutoff.

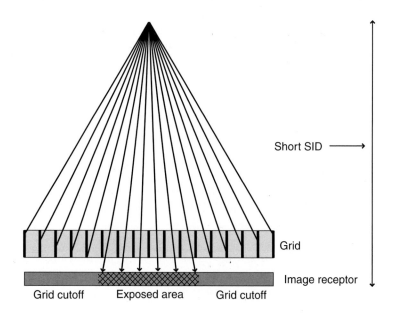

Figure 14.6 **A parallel grid cutoff due to short SID and large field size.**

FOCUSED GRIDS

Focused grids eliminate grid cutoff at the edges of the field because the lead strips are angled toward the center and converge at the focal distance. When the x-ray source is in line with the center of the grid and located at the grid focal distance, there is no grid cutoff because the transmitted radiation passes through the radiolucent interspaces. Focused grids are recommended for examinations that must use large fields or short SIDs. Typical focused grid distances are 100 and 180 cm. Focused grids can be used at distances within about ±5 cm of the focal distance with no noticeable grid cutoff. Figure 14.7 illustrates the construction of a focused grid.

Focused Grid Cutoff

Focused grids that are used at other than the proper SIDs will show grid cutoff. Focused grids that are used outside the focal range or upside down show a correct density in the central portion of the image, but decreased density toward both edges. Focused grids that are located off center or not perpendicular to the central ray show reduced density on only one side of the image.

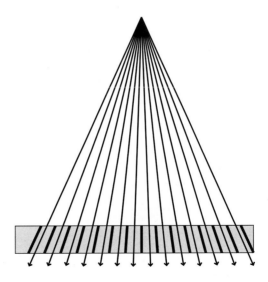

Figure 14.7 **The construction of a focused grid.**

GRID ALIGNMENT

Improper positioning of the grid will always produce grid cutoff. The grid must be placed perpendicular to the central ray to eliminate grid cutoff. The central ray can be angled to the grid provided that it is angled along the long axis of the grid strips, but not across or perpendicular to the strips. Figure 14.8 shows how an improperly positioned grid produces grid cutoff.

Grid cutoff rarely occurs in the radiology department, where fixed cassette holders or Bucky trays are routinely used. Grid alignment is more critical with high grid ratios and can be a serious problem with portable radiographs. Careful positioning of grids during portable examinations is especially important because even slight misalignments will produce noticeable grid cutoff. Grid cutoff during portable examinations is a major cause of retakes.

Table 14.2 gives the appearance of different forms of grid cutoff and the possible causes.

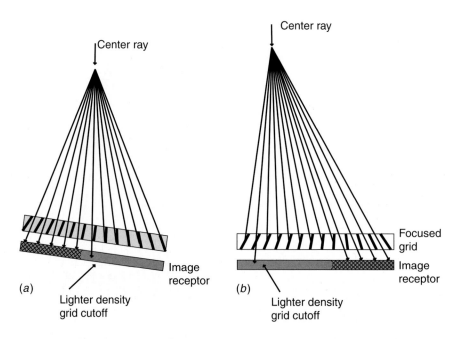

Figure 14.8 Two conditions that produce grid cutoff and lighter densities on one side of the image: (a), a misaligned (nonperpendicular) focused grid; (b), an off-center focused grid.

Table 14.2
Grid Artifact Appearances and Their Possible Causes

Optical Density	Possible Causes
Correct density in the center, lower density on both sides of image	Parallel grid at too short SID Upside-down focused grid Focused grid outside focal distance range
Correct density in the center and on one side, low density on one side	Grid center not aligned with central axis Grid not perpendicular to central axis

MOVING OR BUCKY GRIDS

Stationary grids with low grid frequencies produce noticeable grid lines on the final image. One way to eliminate these grid lines is to move the grid during the exposure. This motion of the grid blurs out the grid lines so that they are not noticeable. Moving grids are called **Bucky grids,** named after one of the inventors, Gustaf Bucky. Bucky grids are located under the table above the image receptor. Bucky grids are also called reciprocating grids because they move back and forth in front of the film cassette. A selector at the control panel activates the grid motor. If the motor is not activated, the grid will be stationary during exposure and grid lines will be apparent on the image.

AIR GAP TECHNIQUE

The **air gap technique** is an alternative method of scatter reduction that can be used instead of a grid. This technique uses an increased object to image distance (OID) to reduce the scatter reaching the image receptor. It is used in lateral cervical spine radiographs. The increased OID causes much of the scattered radiation to miss the image receptor. The air does *not* filter out the scattered x-rays. This eliminates the need to use a grid to reduce scatter. Figure 14.9 illustrates how the air gap technique reduces scatter. An OID of at least 6 inches (in.) is required for effective scatter reduction with the air gap technique. When the OID is increased, there is an increase in magnification and a reduction in detail. To compensate for this, a longer SID is utilized with a small focal spot size. Because of the larger SID, the mAs must be increased, but the patient dose does not increase because the inverse square decrease of the x-ray intensity offsets the increased mAs.

Parallel grid cutoff arises when the field size is so large that the direct beam can no longer pass through the parallel grid openings. Grid cutoff appears as a lighter density near the edges of the image. Focused

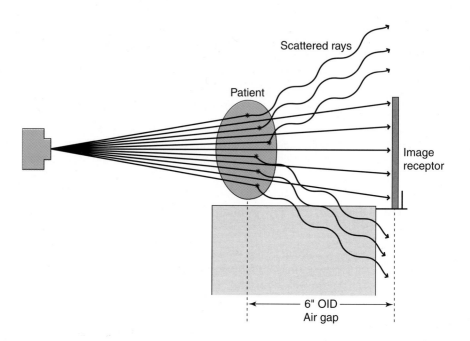

Figure 14.9 **Air-gap scatter-reduction technique.**

grids, which are designed to reduce grid cutoff, must be used at a specific distance. Bucky grids move the grid during the exposure to remove the appearance of grid lines on the image. An air gap can also reduce the scatter reaching the image receptor.

SUMMARY

Radiation leaving the patient is a combination of transmitted and scattered radiation. Scatter decreases contrast and depends on field size, patient thickness, and beam energy or kVp. The primary methods of scatter reduction are a reduction in field size and the use of a grid. In special applications such as cervical spine imaging, an air gap can be used to reduce scatter. Grids are constructed of alternating strips of a radiopaque material such as lead and a radiolucent material such as aluminum or plastic.

Using a grid with a higher grid ratio increases the patient dose, increases the Bucky factor, increases the film contrast, and requires an increase in mAs. The Bucky factor is the ratio of mAs with the grid to mAs without the grid. High grid ratios are not used in portable imaging because the alignment is very critical.

QUESTIONS

1. Exit radiation consists of
   a. transmitted radiation.
   b. scattered radiation.
   c. transmitted plus scattered radiation.
   d. transmitted minus scattered radiation.
2. Increasing the field size will _____ the amount of scatter.
   a. increase
   b. decrease
   c. not change
3. Increasing the x-ray beam energy will _____ the amount of scatter.
   a. increase
   b. decrease
   c. not change
4. A decrease in patient thickness will _____ the amount of scatter.
   a. increase
   b. decrease
   c. not change
5. Changing from a large to a small focal spot will _____ the amount of scatter.
   a. increase
   b. decrease
   c. not change
6. A grid is made of
   a. alternating strips of muscle and fat.
   b. alternating strips of lead and plastic.
   c. alternating strips of gelatin and emulsion.
   d. alternating strips of paper and plastic.
7. The grid ratio is the ratio of the
   a. height of the lead strips to the distance between the lead strips.
   b. height of the lead strips to the width of the lead strips.
   c. height of the plastic strips to the width of the plastic strips.
   d. thickness of the grid to the width of the film cassette.
8. Grid cutoff can result from
   a. a focused grid used at the wrong SID.
   b. using small SIDs with a parallel grid.
   c. an upside-down focused grid.
   d. all of the above.
9. When a grid with a higher grid ratio is used, the radiation dose to the patient will _____ and the radiographic contrast will _____.
   a. increase; decrease
   b. increase; increase
   c. decrease; increase
   d. decrease; decrease

10. When a grid with a lower grid ratio is substituted for one with a higher grid ratio,
    1. the mAs must be increased.
    2. the mAs must be decreased.
    3. the radiographic contrast will increase.
    4. the radiographic contrast will decrease.
    a. 1
    b. 2
    c. 2 and 3
    d. 2 and 4
11. The number of lead strips per centimeter is called the
    a. Bucky factor.
    b. grid ratio.
    c. grid frequency.
    d. grid focal factor.

A radiographic examination using a focused grid produces images with densities that are lighter toward both edges. In Questions 12 to 16, is the factor a possible cause of the problem? Answer a for true or b for false.

12. _____ Patient motion
13. _____ Incorrect SID
14. _____ Poor film/screen contact
15. _____ SID in focusing range
16. _____ Grid placed upside down
17. Which of the following are used to improve contrast and reduce scatter?
    a. Collimation and filtration
    b. Grids and collimation
    c. Filtration and grids
    d. High kVp and long SID
18. An increase in patient thickness will increase the amount of scatter.
    a. True
    b. False
19. An exposure of 70 kVp, 10 mAs without a grid produces an acceptable density with too much scatter. A second exposure using a 12:1 grid is to be made. What should the new mAs be?
    a. 2 mAs
    b. 25 mAs
    c. 50 mAs
    d. 100 mAs
20. Increasing the grid frequency will make the grid lines on the final radiographic image.
    a. more visible.
    b. less visible.
    c. have the same visibility.

21. A focused grid
    a. is always used with thin body parts.
    b. must be used at the correct SID.
    c. requires a decrease in mAs compared to the no-grid mAs.
    d. has a Bucky factor of zero.
22. The Bucky factor
    a. indicates how much the mAs must be decreased from that used with nongrid techniques.
    b. indicates how fast the grid is moving.
    c. indicates how much the mAs must be increased over that used with nongrid techniques.
    d. indicates how much scattered radiation is present.
23. The grid is located
    a. between the patient and the image receptor.
    b. between the tube and the patient.
    c. behind the image receptor.
    d. between the patient and the transformer.
24. The air gap technique is utilized to reduce scatter
    a. with the use of a grid.
    b. without the use of a grid.
    c. with a short OID.
    d. with air filtering out the scatter.

ANSWERS TO CHAPTER 14 QUESTIONS

1.	c	13.	a
2.	a	14.	b
3.	a	15.	b
4.	b	16.	a
5.	c	17.	b
6.	b	18.	a
7.	a	19.	c
8.	d	20.	b
9.	b	21.	b
10.	d	22.	c
11.	c	23.	a
12.	b	24.	b

Unit IV

Special Imaging Techniques

15

Fluoroscopy

OBJECTIVES

At the completion of this chapter, the student will be able to

1. Identify the components of a fluoroscopic system.
2. Identify the components of an image intensifier.
3. Describe the purpose of an automatic brightness control circuit.
4. Identify the factors that influence patient dose during fluoroscopy.

INTRODUCTION

Fluoroscopy is a dynamic x-ray technique used to image moving structures and to localize potential abnormalities without recording the images on film. It gives a real-time or dynamic image as the x-rays pass through the patient. An **image intensifier** converts x-ray energy into visible light energy. The image intensifier is used during fluoroscopy for increased sensitivity and brightness; this reduces the patient dose. Inside the image intensifier, the pattern of x-rays is converted into an electron pattern, and the electrons are accelerated onto an output phosphor and converted into a brighter visible light image. In this chapter we cover the construction and application of an image intensifier and the automatic brightness circuit of a fluoroscopic system.

FLUOROSCOPY

Fluoroscopy is a dynamic imaging modality designed to observe moving structures in the body, in contrast to conventional radiography, which produces

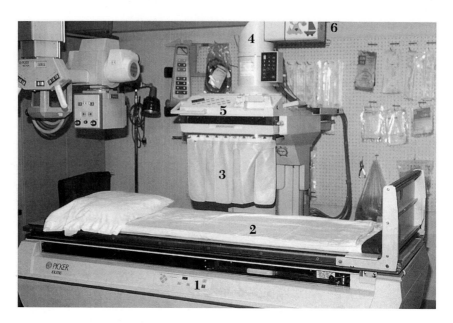

Figure 15.1 **A fluoroscopic imaging system. 1, Undertable tube; 2, tabletop; 3, lead drape; 4, image-intensifier tower; 5, spot film cassette slot; 6, TV camera.**

static images of body structures. During fluoroscopy, a radiologist views the fluoroscopic image and obtains a diagnosis. Spot films of the fluoroscopic image can be obtained whenever a permanent record is needed. Figure 15.1 shows a typical fluoroscopic room. Most fluoroscopic rooms also have an overhead tube for conventional radiography and are called "R and F" rooms.

X-RAY TUBE

Fluoroscopic x-ray tubes have the same design and construction as conventional x-ray tubes, but they are operated for many minutes at much lower milliampere (mA) values. Typical fluoroscopic tube currents are 1 to 5 mA, whereas radiographic tube currents are 50 to 500 mA. The fluoroscopic tube is usually located beneath the patient support table. Tube shielding and beam-limiting collimators are also located in the tube housing beneath the table. The collimators adjust the size of the x-ray beam and restrict x-rays to the image receptor, which is the image intensifier. The source to skin distance (**SSD**) of a fixed fluoroscopic tube must be at least 38 centimeters (cm) [15 inches (in)], and portable C-arm fluoroscopic units must have an SSD of at least 30 cm (12 in). This is to limit the radiation dose to the skin during fluoroscopic procedures.

TABLE

The table that supports the patient can be rotated into a vertical position for upright examinations. Some tables are constructed of carbon fiber material to reduce attenuation of the x-ray beam by the tabletop, thus reducing patient exposure.

IMAGE INTENSIFIER TOWER

The image intensifier tower contains the image intensifier and a group of controls that allow the operator to adjust the field size, move the x-ray tube and table, and make spot film exposures. A lead drape hangs from the image intensifier tower to attenuate radiation scattered from the patient. The spot film camera and TV camera are mounted at the top of the image intensifier tower. The tower is connected to the x-ray tube mount, so that both move together as a unit. The x-ray beam is always directed at the image intensifier.

EYE PHYSIOLOGY

The first fluoroscope was invented by Thomas Edison. Early fluoroscopic systems employed a phosphor coating on a lead glass plate. The image brightness of these systems was so low that they could be viewed only with a dark-adapted eye. The retina of the human eye has two types of light receptors, rods and cones. Cone vision requires bright light; rod vision is used in dim light. Cone vision has excellent spatial resolution with high visual acuity because the cones are concentrated near the center of the retina. Rod vision has poor spatial resolution and is color blind. The image intensifier was developed to increase the brightness of the image so that the image could be viewed with cone vision. Figure 15.2 shows a cross-sectional view of a typical image intensifier tube.

Image intensification increases the brightness of the fluoroscopic image so that cone vision can be used to view the image. The image intensifier is usually mounted in a tower above the patient support table. The x-ray tube is mounted beneath the table with a minimum SSD of 38 cm for fixed units. Typical filament currents in the continuously operating x-ray tube in the fluoroscopic mode are 1 to 5 mA, as compared to typical tube currents in the radiographic mode, which are 50 to 500 mA.

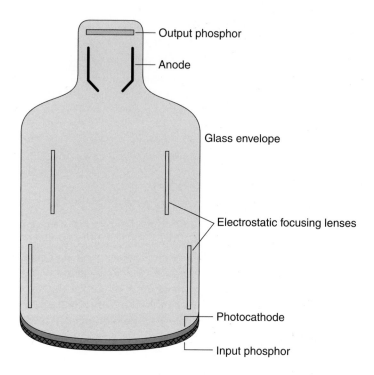

Figure 15.2 **Cross-section of an image-intensifier tube and its components.**

IMAGE INTENSIFIER COMPONENTS

Input Phosphor

The input phosphor of the image intensifier tube is made of cesium iodide (CsI) crystals because CsI has high x-ray absorption and light emission characteristics. The interactions in the input phosphor are similar to the interactions in an intensifying screen. The input phosphor absorbs about 60 percent of the exit radiation leaving the patient. Each x-ray produces between 1000 and 5000 light photons.

Photocathode

The **photocathode** is located just behind the input phosphor. The photocathode is made of a special material that emits electrons when it is struck by light. Light from the input phosphor ejects electrons from the photocathode. The number of electrons is proportional to the amount of light striking the photocathode. Bright regions of the phosphor cause the photocathode to emit many electrons. Dark regions of the phosphor result in the emission of few electrons. The pattern of x-rays at the input phosphor is converted into a similar pattern of electrons leaving the photocathode.

Focusing Electrodes

Electrodes inside the image intensifier focus the negative electrons from the photocathode onto the output phosphor. Electrostatic lenses can change the magnification of the image by changing the focal point of the electrons.

Anode and Output Phosphor

Electrons from the photocathode are accelerated toward the anode by high voltage. The electrons pass through the anode and strike the output phosphor. The output phosphor is made of zinc cadmium sulfide (ZnCdS), which efficiently converts electron energy into visible light. The light intensity from the output phosphor is much greater than that from the input phosphor.

BRIGHTNESS GAIN

The total gain in brightness comes from a combination of acceleration of the electrons, called flux gain, and compression of the image size, called minification gain.

Flux gain is produced by the conversion of the electron energy into light energy. Typical flux gains are 50 to 100. The electron energy comes from the accelerating voltage between the photocathode and the anode.

Minification gain is produced by concentrating the light from the larger input phosphor onto the smaller output phosphor. Minification gains vary from 40 to 90. Changing the collection area of the input phosphor changes the minification gain.

Brightness gain is obtained by multiplying flux gain by minification gain. Typical image intensifiers have brightness gains of 5000 to 30,000.

EXAMPLE 1:

What is the total brightness gain if the flux gain is 70 and the minification gain is 81?

ANSWER:

Brightness gain = flux gain × minification gain
Brightness gain = 70 × 81
Brightness gain = 5670

The output image at the output phosphor is over 5000 times brighter than the image at the input phosphor.

The input phosphor converts the incident x-rays into light. The photocathode converts the light into electrons, which are focused and accelerated toward the anode. The electrons striking the output phosphor produce the final bright image. The total brightness gain is made up of the flux gain, produced by the acceleration of the electrons, and the minification gain, produced by the reduction of image size.

AUTOMATIC BRIGHTNESS CONTROL

The **automatic brightness control (ABC)** circuit maintains the fluoroscopic image at a constant brightness by regulating the radiation output of the x-ray tube. This circuit is also known as the automatic brightness stabilizer (ABS). A detector monitors the brightness level of the image intensifier output phosphor. The ABC adjusts the fluoroscopic mA to maintain a constant output brightness regardless of the thickness or density of the body part being examined.

MAGNIFICATION

Dual- or multiple-mode image intensifiers provide different magnifications for different applications. **Magnification,** an increase in the image size of an object, allows for better visualization of small structures. The operator can change the magnification through the controls on the image intensifier tower. Selection of a smaller portion of the input phosphor produces a magnified image but results in a higher patient dose because there is less minification gain in the magnification mode. The ABC circuit increases the fluoroscopic mA to compensate for the reduced minification gain. Figure 15.3 illustrates the image intensifier focusing for a normal and a magnified image.

LAST IMAGE HOLD

Some fluoroscopic units can display the last image when x-ray production is stopped. This is also known as "freeze frame" capability. The output image is digitized and continuously displayed on the output monitor. Most portable

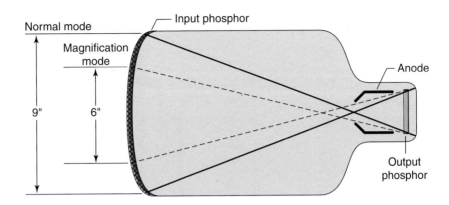

Figure 15.3 Image-intensifier magnification mode and normal mode focusing.

C-arm fluoroscopic units have this capability. It allows the operator to study the image without continuously exposing the patient and staff to additional radiation.

> *The automatic brightness control maintains a constant output brightness regardless of the thickness or density of the portion of the patient's anatomy being viewed. The ABC circuit monitors the brightness of the image intensifier and changes the mA as required to maintain constant brightness. Dual-mode image intensifiers can provide different levels of magnification through the selection of only a portion of the input phosphor for display on the output phosphor. In the magnification mode, the ABC increases the mA to compensate for the lower minification gain. Freeze frame or last image hold fluoroscopic systems continuously display the last image without the necessity for continuing to irradiate the patient.*

FLUOROSCOPIC DISPLAYS

The image at the output phosphor of the image intensifier can be coupled to a TV camera for TV monitor viewing or to a spot film camera or cine camera. A closed-circuit TV system is used for dynamic imaging; cine and spot film images provide permanent records of the examination. Figure 15.4 illustrates how the output phosphor of the image intensifier can be viewed or recorded in different ways. A beam-splitting mirror sends the output phosphor image to both the spot film camera and the TV system.

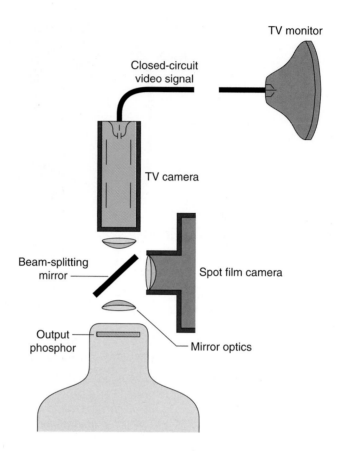

Figure 15.4 Viewing and recording images from the image intensifier.

Television

The image intensifier output phosphor is viewed with a TV camera and displayed on a TV monitor. A TV camera is mounted on the image intensifier tower to view the image intensifier output phosphor. The TV camera is similar to a home video camera. The TV camera converts the light image from the output phosphor into electrical signals, which are displayed on a standard TV monitor.

Standard TV screens in the United States have 525 lines in a horizontal direction. This limits the resolution to about 2 line pairs per millimeter (lp/mm). The resolution of the image intensifier output phosphor is about 5 lp/mm, so the TV display is the weak link in the imaging chain. Some fluoroscopic systems are equipped with 1000-line display monitors to match the display to the resolution of the output phosphor.

Recording the Fluoroscopic Image

Fluoroscopic images can be recorded using a conventional spot film camera, a cine camera, a standard videocassette recorder (**VCR**), or a digital image recorder. VCRs and cine cameras record dynamic images. VCR images are analog images recorded on magnetic tape. Cine cameras record the images on 35-mm movie film. Spot films provide a permanent static record of findings viewed during fluoroscopy. Fluoroscopic images can also be digitized and stored as digital data.

Spot Films

Spot images can be recorded on conventional radiographic film or 105-mm roll film. When a conventional film is desired, the cassette is moved in front of the image intensifier, an exposure is made, and the cassette is moved out of the way. The x-ray tube must be switched from fluoroscopic mA (low) to radiographic mA (high) before the exposure can be made. A second method of providing a permanent record of the fluoroscopic image is with a spot film camera that uses 105-mm roll film. The spot film camera is mounted near the output phosphor of the image intensifier and records from one to several frames per second. The radiation dose to the patient is less with 105-mm spot film images than with conventional cassette images because the image is taken from the output phosphor rather than with an intensifying screen.

Conventional Film Cassettes

The image intensifying tower has a slot that accepts a film cassette. It is located between the image intensifier and the patient and has a grid in place between the patient and the cassette. The image format can be selected so that there can be multiple exposures or images on one film—for example, one on one, two on one, or four on one. The images are obtained using the automatic exposure control (AEC) and conventional radiographic mA. When an image is obtained using a film-loaded cassette, the x-ray tube is switched from a low fluoroscopic mA to a higher radiographic mA, such as 200 or 300 mA. This results in an increased patient dose compared to spot films obtained with a camera from the image intensifier image. The image intensifier should be positioned close to the patient to reduce patient exposure and decrease magnification.

Videocassette Recording

Videocassette recording makes a permanent record of the dynamic fluoroscopic images on magnetic tape. These images are the same as those displayed on the TV monitor and can be played back on a VCR unit similar to a home VCR player.

Cine Recording

Fluoroscopic images can also be recorded on 35-mm movie film. Such recording is referred to as cinefluorography, or simply **cine.** The output phosphor image is directed to the cine camera by a beam-splitting mirror. Cine image recording uses 35-mm film at 30 or 60 frames per second. Special x-ray tubes and generators that pulse the x-rays so that the x-ray beam is on only when the cine film is in position and the camera shutter is open are required. Cine imaging is common in angiography and cardiac catheterization. The principal advantage of cine recording is the improved spatial resolution; however, radiation exposure rates are about ten times greater than in conventional fluoroscopy.

Digital Recording

A majority of the new fluoroscopic units have digital recording capabilities. The fluoroscopic images are obtained in the conventional manner and then processed and stored as digital data in a manner similar to that used in computed tomography (CT) and magnetic resonance imaging (MRI). The digital images can be enhanced by changing the contrast or density prior to printing a hard copy. Analog images from the TV camera are converted to digital images and entered into computer files for later viewing. Digital imaging is discussed further in Chap. 17.

> *Fluoroscopic images are usually displayed on a TV monitor. Individual images can be recorded on 105-mm spot film, a conventional film cassette, a VCR tape, or as digital data.*

MOBILE C-ARM FLUOROSCOPY

Mobile C-arm units are portable fluoroscopy systems that are used in the operating room, the emergency room, and many other areas when it is not possible to bring the patient to the radiology department. Figure 15.5 shows a typical C-arm unit. The name comes from the physical connection between the x-ray tube and the image intensifier, which looks like a "C." The tube and image intensifier can be moved to provide anteroposterior, posteroanterior, or lateral fluoroscopic examinations as needed. C-arm fluoroscopes are equipped with last image hold and digital recording capabilities.

PATIENT DOSE

The patient dose during fluoroscopy depends on the patient thickness, the exposure rate, and the duration of exposure. Higher exposure rates, thicker patients, and longer fluoroscopic examinations produce higher patient doses.

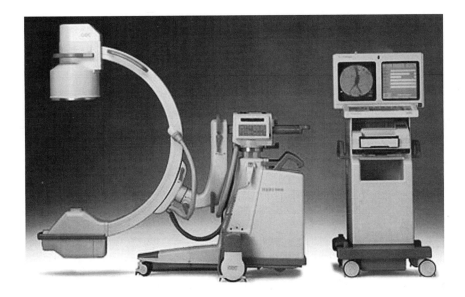

Figure 15.5 **Typical C-arm unit. (*Courtesy of GE Medical Systems. With permision.*)**

The exposure of the patient depends on the thickness and density of the body part being examined, the distance from the image intensifier to the patient, and the image intensifier magnification. A change in any of these factors changes the exposure rate because the ABC circuit adjusts the mA to maintain a constant output brightness. This mA adjustment changes the patient dose. Thicker, dense body parts are more difficult to penetrate and require higher exposure rates, resulting in higher patient doses.

The x-ray intensity at the image intensifier depends on the source to image receptor distance (SID). Moving the image intensifier closer to the patient decreases the SID and increases the beam intensity at the surface of the input phosphor. This results in the ABC's decreasing the mA and producing a lower patient dose.

Mobile C-arm fluoroscopic units make it possible to take the fluoroscope to the patient rather than bringing the patient to the fluoroscopic unit. The patient dose during fluoroscopy varies with patient size, magnification, and length of examination. The image intensifier should be located as close as possible to the patient, as this results in a decreased patient dose and improved image quality.

FLUOROSCOPIC TIMER

All fluoroscopic systems are equipped with a 5-minute (min) timer as required by law. The timer must audibly indicate when 5 min of fluoroscopy has elapsed. There is no limit to the number of times the timer may be reset. Some departments record the total fluoroscopy time in the patient's record so that the dose due to fluoroscopy can be calculated if necessary.

SUMMARY

Fluoroscopy is a method of viewing dynamic moving structures. A fluoroscopic system contains an x-ray tube, a patient support table, and an image intensifier. The image intensifier produces a brighter image by converting x-rays into visible light at the input phosphor, converting visible light into electrons at the photocathode, accelerating and focusing the electrons onto the output phosphor, and finally converting the electrons into visible light at the output phosphor. An automatic brightness control circuit maintains the brightness of the output phosphor at a constant level by adjusting the fluoroscopic mA. Brightness gain is a combination of flux gain and minification gain. The output phosphor is brighter than the input phosphor because of brightness gain. Flux gain is produced by the acceleration of electrons in the image intensifier tube. Minification gain is produced because the output phosphor is smaller than the input phosphor. A TV camera views the output phosphor image and displays the image on a standard TV monitor. Fluoroscopic images can be recorded on spot films, videotape, or cine film. Patient dose is affected by patient size, the amount of magnification, and the distance between the patient and the image intensifier input surface. All fluoroscopic systems must have a timer to audibly indicate when 5 min of fluoroscopy have elapsed.

QUESTIONS

For Questions 1 to 4, when a fluoroscope is switched from the standard to the magnification mode the _____ factor increases. Answer a for true or b for false.

1. _____ Minification gain
2. _____ Patient dose
3. _____ Small structure visualization
4. _____ mA

5. The input phosphor of an image intensifier is made of _____, and the output phosphor is made of _____.
   a. zinc cadmium sulfide (ZnCdS); cesium iodide (CsI)
   b. calcium tungstate ($CaWO_4$); zinc cadmium sulfide (ZnCdS)
   c. cesium iodide (CsI); zinc cadmium sulfide (ZnCdS)
   d. cesium iodide (CsI); calcium tungstate ($CaWO_4$)
6. The input phosphor of an image intensifier
   a. converts electron energy into light photons.
   b. converts x-ray energy into light photons.
   c. converts light photons into electrons.
   d. forces electrons to converge on the input phosphor.
7. The output phosphor of an image intensifier
   a. converts electron energy into light photons.
   b. converts x-ray energy into light photons.
   c. converts light photons into electrons.
   d. forces electrons to converge on the input phosphor.
8. The focusing electrodes of an image intensifier
   a. convert electron energy into light photons.
   b. convert x-ray energy into light photons.
   c. convert light photons into electrons.
   d. force electrons to converge on the input phosphor.
9. The photocathode of an image intensifier
   a. converts electron energy into light photons.
   b. converts x-ray energy into light photons.
   c. converts light photons into electrons.
   d. forces electrons to converge on the input phosphor.
10. Changing from standard to magnification mode on an image intensifier
    1. increases the patient dose.
    2. decreases the patient dose.
    3. produces a magnified image.
    4. decreases the minification gain.
    5. increases the flux gain.
    a. 2, 3, and 4
    b. 1 and 3
    c. 1, 3, and 4
    d. 2 and 4
11. In an image intensifier tube, the _____ gain arises because the input diameter is larger than the output diameter.
    a. minification
    b. confiscation
    c. flux
    d. radiation

12. _____ gain is due to the acceleration of electrons with the focusing voltage.
    a. Magnification
    b. Confiscation
    c. Flux
    d. Radiation
13. Brightness gain is the product of the _____ gains.
    a. magnification and minification
    b. minification and flux
    c. flux and magnification
    d. confiscation and flux
14. The ABC detector is located
    a. behind the film cassette.
    b. at the input to the image intensifier tube.
    c. at the output of the image intensifier tube.
    d. behind the x-ray tube.
15. The purpose of the ABC is to maintain a constant
    a. brightness at the output phosphor.
    b. brightness at the input phosphor.
    c. mA regardless of patient thickness.
    d. patient thickness.
16. The ABC circuit adjusts _____ to maintain _____.
    a. constant brightness; constant mA
    b. mA; constant brightness
    c. mA; constant patient thickness
    d. patient thickness; constant brightness.
17. The area of the eye in which nerves detect an image is known as the
    a. lens.
    b. cornea.
    c. retina.
    d. iris.
18. The _____ are very sensitive and are used for viewing in dim light.
    a. rods
    b. cones
19. The _____ have good spatial resolution and are used for viewing in bright light.
    a. rods
    b. cones
20. Cinefluorography is used primarily for
    a. gastrointestinal studies.
    b. urinary studies.
    c. cardiac studies.
    d. orthopedic studies.

21. The film most commonly used in spot film imaging is
    a. 16-mm.
    b. 35-mm.
    c. 70-mm.
    d. 105-mm.
22. Fluoroscopic mA currents are in the range from
    a. 1 to 5 mA.
    b. 50 to 100 mA.
    c. 100 to 200 mA.
    d. 300 to 400 mA.
23. The minimum distance between the source and the patient skin surface for a fixed fluoroscopic unit is _____ cm.
    a. 15
    b. 30
    c. 38
    d. 42
24. An image intensifier increases
    a. motion.
    b. electricity.
    c. brightness.
    d. voltage.
25. The fluoroscopic timer indicates when _____ min of fluoroscopy time have elapsed.
    a. 2
    b. 5
    c. 10
    d. 15

ANSWERS TO CHAPTER 15 QUESTIONS

1.	b	17.	c
2.	a	18.	a
3.	a	19.	b
4.	a	20.	c
5.	c	21.	d
6.	b	22.	a
7.	a	23.	c
8.	d	24.	c
9.	c	25.	b
10.	c		
11.	a		
12.	c		
13.	b		
14.	c		
15.	a		
16.	b		

16

Mammography

OBJECTIVES

At the completion of this chapter, the student will be able to

1. Describe the purpose of mammography.
2. Describe the x-ray spectra used in mammography.
3. Describe the film/screen systems used in mammography.
4. State the reason for compression in mammography.

INTRODUCTION

Mammography is the radiographic examination of the breast and is utilized for the early detection of cancer. It is one of the most challenging radiographic examinations because it requires imaging of both small, high-contrast calcifications and large, low-contrast masses. For this reason, special x-ray tubes and films are used.

The differential absorption of fat, glandular tissue, fibrous tissue, and cancerous tissue is very similar. Small microcalcifications are often associated with cancer. All these tissues must be clearly imaged on a single film. The technical factors of the examination must be tightly controlled to produce diagnostic-quality mammograms. The federal Mammographic Quality Standards Act **(MQSA)** sets out strict guidelines to ensure high-quality mammographic examinations. Only specially trained technologists are permitted to perform mammographic examinations. Mammography uses low-kVp values, in the range from 20 to 35 kVp. This voltage is lower than that for conventional radiography to increase differential absorption and improve subject contrast. The poor penetration of the low-energy x-rays is not a disadvantage because most breasts are less than 10 centimeters (cm) thick. Figure 16.1 shows a schematic illustration of a typical mammographic unit.

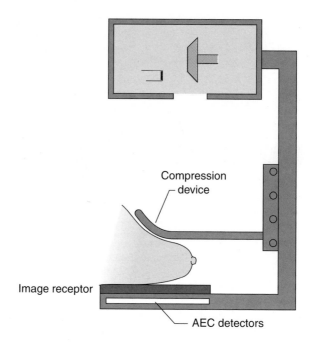

Figure 16.1 **Schematic of a typical mammographic unit.**

X-RAY TUBE

Special mammographic x-ray units have molybdenum anodes to produce low-energy x-ray beams that are optimized for breast imaging. The **molybdenum** anode produces K characteristic x-rays with energies of 17.4 and 19.9 kiloelectron volts (keV). Changing the applied kVp does not change the energy of the K characteristic x-rays.

Some mammographic units have provision to select a **rhodium** anode and/or a rhodium filter. The binding energies of the K and L shells in rhodium are slightly higher than those of molybdenum. Rhodium produces K characteristic x-rays with energies of 20 and 22 keV. The beam from a tube with a rhodium filter and a molybdenum anode has slightly higher penetration than a beam from a molybdenum anode with a molybdenum filter. Rhodium filters and anodes are used for patients with extremely dense or thick breasts. The patient dose and image contrast are decreased with the use of rhodium filters or anodes. Tungsten anode tubes with aluminum filters are not used in mammography.

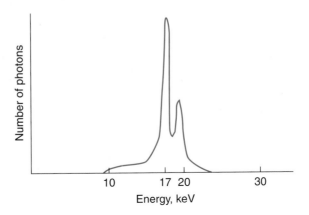

Figure 16.2 **X-ray spectrum from a tube with a molybdenum anode and a 0.03-mm molybdenum filter.**

FILTRATION

The purpose of mammographic filters is to remove low- and high-energy x-rays. Lower-energy x-rays do not penetrate through the breast but increase the patient dose. Higher-energy x-rays decrease image contrast. A 0.03-millimeter (mm) molybdenum filter allows the molybdenum characteristic x-rays to pass through while filtering out both higher- and lower-energy x-rays. Some tubes with molybdenum anodes can be switched from molybdenum to rhodium filters when imaging thick or dense breasts. The half-value layer (HVL) of mammographic x-ray units is typically 0.3 to 0.4 mm aluminum (Al) equivalent. Note that the HVL is expressed in millimeters of aluminum, even though the filter itself is made of molybdenum. Figure 16.2 illustrates the spectrum from a molybdenum anode tube with a 0.03-mm molybdenum filter.

HEEL EFFECT

Mammographic x-ray tubes are oriented with the cathode-anode axis perpendicular to the chest wall, with the cathode at the chest wall side. This orientation produces an image with a more uniform density because the heel effect produces greater intensity at the thicker chest wall and less intensity toward the nipple. Figure 16.3 shows the orientation of the cathode-anode axis in relation to the chest wall.

Special mammographic tubes have molybdenum or rhodium anodes, which provide higher-intensity low-energy x-rays from their K

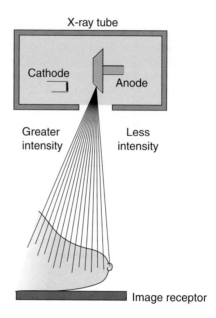

X-ray tube

Cathode

Anode

Greater
intensity

Less
intensity

Image receptor

Figure 16.3 Orientation of the cathode-anode axis along the breast uses the heel effect to produce a more uniform film density.

characteristic x-rays. Most mammographic tubes have 0.03-mm-thick molybdenum filters. The tubes are aligned with the tube axis perpendicular to the chest wall, with the cathode at the chest wall and the anode at the nipple to take advantage of the heel effect.

FOCAL SPOT SIZES

Mammographic tubes have two focal spot sizes, a large (0.3-mm) focal spot for routine mammography and a small (0.1-mm) focal spot for magnification mammography. MQSA requirements state that a mammographic system must be able to image at least 13 line pairs per millimeter (lp/mm) in the direction parallel to the cathode-anode axis and 11 lp/mm in the direction perpendicular to the cathode-anode axis. The effective focal spot is smaller than the actual focal spot because of the line focus principle. The effective focal spot is smaller toward the anode, or nipple, side because the anode is tilted.

GRIDS

The purpose of grids is to remove scatter and improve image contrast. Moving grids are used for routine mammographic examinations. Grid ratios of about 4:1 and grid frequencies of 10 lines per centimeter are routinely employed in screening mammography. Using a grid in mammography both improves contrast and increases the patient dose by about a factor of 2.

COMPRESSION

Compression of the breast with a radiolucent compression device improves image quality by reducing patient motion and providing more uniform tissue thickness. The decreased breast thickness reduces scatter and patient dose. Compression of the breast by 1 cm reduces the dose by a factor of 2 because the HVL in tissue is about 1 cm for mammographic energies.

Mammographic tubes are equipped with two focal spot sizes, usually a 0.3-mm large focal spot and a 0.1-mm small focal spot. Because the breast is not as thick as many other body parts, a grid with a lower grid ratio can be used. Typical mammographic grids have 4:1 grid ratios. Compression makes the breast thickness more uniform, reduces motion artifacts, and reduces the radiation dose to the patient.

FILM/SCREEN COMBINATIONS

In mammography, single-emulsion film with a single-screen cassette is generally used to maintain high detail imaging. A high-speed rare earth screen is used to reduce exposure time, patient motion, and radiation dose. The film is positioned in front of the screen so that the exit radiation from the breast strikes the film before reaching the intensifying screen. If the film/screen order were reversed, the interactions in the screen would be further from the film, and light diffusion through the greater distance would degrade image resolution because the spreading of light blurs edges.

Special double-emulsion mammographic films have been developed to further reduce exposure time and patient dose. These films are used with half-thickness front screens and full-thickness back screens. Double-emulsion films have almost twice the speed of a single-emulsion film with nearly the same detail resolution.

FILM PROCESSING

Mammographic film can be developed using conventional or extended automatic processing. Extended processing uses the same chemicals and temperatures as regular processing, but the film processing time is increased. Total processing time is increased from 90 seconds (s) to 3 minutes (min) by increasing the film transport time. Extended processing increases film speed and contrast and allows for a decrease in patient dose. However, extended processing results in reduced film latitude, requiring careful selection of exposure factors to eliminate retakes.

Single-emulsion film is used in mammography because it has superior spatial resolution compared with conventional double-emulsion film. It can be developed using conventional or extended processing in an automatic film processor. Extended processing increases the processing time from 90 s to 3 min and increases the contrast and speed of the film but decreases film latitude.

MAGNIFICATION MAMMOGRAPHY

Magnification images are used to examine suspicious areas of the breast. The source to image receptor distance (SID) is fixed in mammographic units, so magnified images are obtained by decreasing the source to object distance (SOD) while increasing the object to image distance (OID). A 0.1-mm focal spot is used to achieve good detail resolution. Magnification factors of 1.5 to 2 are obtained using the 0.1-mm focal spot. The air gap between the breast and the film cassette reduces scatter and eliminates the need for a grid. Magnification mammography has a limited field of view and is not able to image the entire breast.

AUTOMATIC EXPOSURE CONTROL

The correct selection of mAs exposure factors is critical in producing a high-quality mammographic image. The automatic exposure control (**AEC**) circuit achieves proper image density by measuring the amount of exit radiation and terminating the exposure at the proper time. The AEC detector is placed behind the film cassette to prevent imaging of the detector. Mammographic units have provisions for changing the position of the AEC detector along the chest wall–nipple axis. The AEC detector should be positioned under the portion of the breast with the greatest density, to avoid underexposed regions. Figure 16.4 illustrates the possible positions of the AEC detector cells.

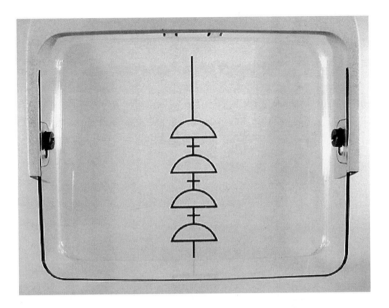

Figure 16.4 **Possible positions of the AEC detector cells.**

RADIATION DOSE

The radiation dose to the breast is reported as an average glandular dose. Glandular breast tissue is the tissue at risk for radiation-induced breast cancer. MQSA regulations require that the average dose to the breast be less than 3 milligray (mGy) [300 millirad (mrad)] per view. The average glandular dose for each view imaged using a grid is usually about 1.4 mGy (140 mrad). Typical screening examinations consist of a craniocaudad and a mediolateral view, resulting in a dose to each breast of 2.8 mGy (280 mrad) per examination.

Magnification images are used to examine small suspicious areas of the breast. A 0.1-mm focal spot is used to obtain good detail resolution. The AEC detector is located behind the film cassette holder to avoid imaging of the detector. It should be placed beneath the average thickness of the breast to obtain a proper-density exposure. The radiation dose to the breast is limited to less than 3 mGy per view.

SUMMARY

Mammography forms images of breast tissues with low differential absorption and small microcalcifications using a low-kVp technique. Mammographic tubes have special molybdenum anodes with 0.3- and 0.1-mm focal spots. The K characteristic x-rays of molybdenum have energies of 17.4 and 19.9 keV. The 0.03-mm molybdenum filter passes the molybdenum K characteristic x-rays and removes both higher- and lower-energy x-rays. Single-screen cassettes are used with single-emulsion films to obtain high-detail images. Moving grids with 4:1 ratios remove scatter and improve image contrast. The AEC circuit, whose detectors are placed behind the film cassette, terminates the exposure to produce the correct image density. Compression of the breast during mammography improves image quality by decreasing scatter and reducing patient motion. Magnification mammography is used to study suspicious breast regions. Extended processing increases image contrast and speed while reducing film latitude and patient dose. The typical glandular dose is about 2.8 mGy for a typical two-view examination.

QUESTIONS

1. Mammographic tubes have _____ anodes and _____ filters.
   a. tungsten; molybdenum
   b. molybdenum; molybdenum
   c. molybdenum; aluminum
   d. aluminum; molybdenum
2. Typical mammographic tube filtration placed in the beam is
   a. 0.03 mm molybdenum.
   b. 0.3 mm aluminum.
   c. 0.3 mm molybdenum.
   d. 0.3 mm aluminum.
3. Mammographic units must have HVLs greater than
   a. 0.03 mm molybdenum.
   b. 0.03 mm aluminum.
   c. 0.3 mm molybdenum.
   d. 0.3 mm aluminum.
4. The _____ of a mammographic x-ray tube is placed toward the chest wall to take advantage of the heel effect.
   a. cathode
   b. anode
5. Typical focal spot sizes for mammographic tubes are
   a. 0.01 and 0.03 mm.
   b. 0.1 and 0.3 mm.
   c. 1 and 3 mm.
   d. 10 and 30 mm.

6. The K characteristic x-rays from a molybdenum anode tube have energies of _____ and _____ keV.
   a. 15.4; 17.9
   b. 17.4; 19.9
   c. 19.4; 21.9
   d. none of the above

7. The kVp range used for mammography is
   a. 20 to 25 kVp.
   b. 20 to 35 kVp.
   c. 35 to 40 kVp.
   d. 60 to 90 kVp.

8. Increasing the kVp in a mammographic unit will _____ the energy of the characteristic x-rays.
   a. decrease
   b. increase
   c. not change

9. Increasing the kVp in a mammographic unit will _____ the contrast of the image.
   a. decrease
   b. increase
   c. not change

10. Compression of the breast during mammography
    a. reduces patient motion.
    b. reduces scatter.
    c. reduces patient dose.
    d. does all of the above.

11. Extended processing of mammographic films
    a. decreases contrast.
    b. decreases latitude.
    c. increases patient dose.
    d. decreases speed.

12. Exit radiation passes through the _____ first after exiting the breast.
    a. intensifying screen
    b. film
    c. AEC
    d. cathode

13. A screening mammography examination uses the _____ views.
    1. craniocaudad
    2. mediolateral
    3. lateromedial
    4. anteroposterior
    a. 1 and 2
    b. 1 and 3
    c. 1 and 4
    d. 2 and 4

14. Magnification mammography
    a. uses a 0.3-mm focal spot.
    b. is used for screening.
    c. is used to examine suspicious areas.
    d. is/does all of the above.
15. The AEC detector is located
    a. in front of the cassette.
    b. behind the cassette.
    c. above the patient's breast.
16. The radiation dose from a typical screening examination is _____ mrad per breast.
    a. 140
    b. 280
    c. 450
    d. 600

ANSWERS TO CHAPTER 16 QUESTIONS

1.	b	9.	a
2.	a	10.	d
3.	d	11.	b
4.	a	12.	b
5.	b	13.	a
6.	b	14.	c
7.	b	15.	b
8.	c	16.	b

17

Digital Imaging

OBJECTIVES

Upon completion of this chapter, the student will be able to

1. Describe how a matrix of pixels is used to form a digital image.
2. Identify the relation between matrix size, pixel size, and field of view.
3. Identify the components of a digital imaging system.
4. Describe the operation of a computed radiography system.

INTRODUCTION

Digital images are used throughout radiology. They appear as computed tomographic (**CT**), magnetic resonance (**MR**) ultrasound (**US**), mammography, computed radiography (**CR**), direct radiography (**DR**), fluoroscopy, nuclear medicine (**NM**), and diagnostic images. Unlike film images, whose contrast, speed, and latitude are fixed during manufacturing, the appearance of digital images can be altered after they have been recorded and stored. Changes in the processing and display of the digital data can enhance information and suppress noise in the final image. An understanding of digital imaging systems will aid in producing diagnostic-quality digital images. The advantages of digital imaging include the ability to adjust the contrast after the image has been recorded, to process the image to emphasize important features, and to transfer the images to a remote site.

PICTURE ELEMENTS OR PIXELS

A digital image is a **matrix** of picture elements or **pixels.** A matrix is a group of numbers arranged in rows and columns. Digital images typically have between 25,000 and 1 million pixels. There are three numbers associated with each pixel, two to define its location and the third to represent the intensity of the image at that location. An image is formed by a matrix of pixels. The size of the matrix is described by the number of pixels in the rows and columns. A small matrix has a small number of pixels, and a large matrix has a larger number of pixels. For example, a matrix with 256 pixels in each row and column is called a 256 by 256 matrix (written 256×256); one with 512 pixels in each row is called a 512 by 512 matrix. Figure 17.1 shows how a matrix of numbers can be used to form a digital image.

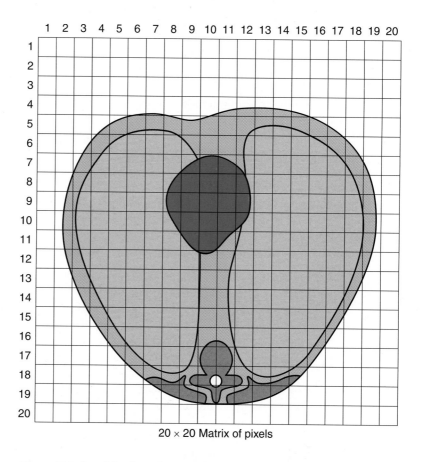

20 × 20 Matrix of pixels

Figure 17.1 **A matrix of numbers used to form a digital image.**

FIELD OF VIEW

The field of view (**FOV**) describes how much of the patient is imaged in the matrix. A 200-mm field of view means that a 200-mm-diameter portion of the patient is imaged. The matrix size and the field of view are independent. The matrix size can be changed without affecting the field of view, and the field of view can be changed without changing the matrix size. Changes in either the field of view or the matrix size will change the pixel size.

RELATION BETWEEN FIELD OF VIEW, MATRIX SIZE, AND PIXEL SIZE

EXAMPLE 1:

Original Image Size: What is the pixel size in millimeters (mm) of a 256×256 matrix for an image with a 20-centimeter (cm) field of view?

ANSWER:

$$20 \text{ cm} = 200 \text{ mm}$$
$$200 \text{ mm}/256 \text{ pixels} = 0.8 \text{ mm/pixel}$$

If the field of view is changed and the matrix size stays the same, the pixel size changes.

If the field of view increases and the matrix size remains the same, the pixel size increases. If the field of view decreases and the matrix size remains the same, the pixel size decreases.

If the field of view remains the same and the matrix size changes, the pixel size changes. An increase in the matrix size results in a decreased pixel size.

EXAMPLE 2:

Change of Field of View from 20 to 30 cm: What is the pixel size in millimeters of a 256×256 matrix for an image with a field of view of 30 cm?

ANSWER:

$$30 \text{ cm} = 300 \text{ mm}$$
$$300 \text{ mm}/256 \text{ pixels} = 1.2 \text{ mm/pixel}$$

EXAMPLE 3:

Change of Matrix Size from 256×256 to 512×512: What is the pixel size in millimeters of a 512×512 matrix for an image with a field of view of 20 cm?

ANSWER:

$$20 \text{ cm} = 200 \text{ mm}$$
$$200 \text{ mm}/512 \text{ pixels} = 0.4 \text{ mm/pixel}$$

Digital images are made up of many pixels arranged in rows and columns in a matrix. Each pixel contains location and intensity information.

SPATIAL RESOLUTION AND PIXEL SIZE

Spatial resolution describes the minimum separation between two objects at which they can be distinguished as two separate objects in the image. Digital images with smaller pixel sizes have better spatial resolution. Spatial resolution is measured in line pairs per millimeter (lp/mm). Two pixels are required in order to image one line pair because a line pair consists of one bright and one dark line. Increasing the matrix size decreases the pixel size and improves spatial resolution, because there are more, but smaller, pixels in the matrix. Figure 17.2 shows how the spatial resolution and appearance of a digital image change as the matrix size and pixel size change. Typical matrix sizes in diagnostic radiology are 256, 512, and 1024, with some matrices as small as 64×64 or as large as 2048×2048.

The relationship between field of view, matrix size, pixel size, and spatial resolution is given in Table 17.1.

Table 17.1

Relationship between Field of View, Matrix Size, Pixel Size, and Spatial Resolution

Field of View	Matrix Size	Pixel Size	Spatial Resolution
Increases	Remains constant	Remains constant	Decreases
Decreases	Remains constant	Remains constant	Increases
Remains constant	Increases	Decreases	Increases
Remains constant	Decreases	Increases	Decreases

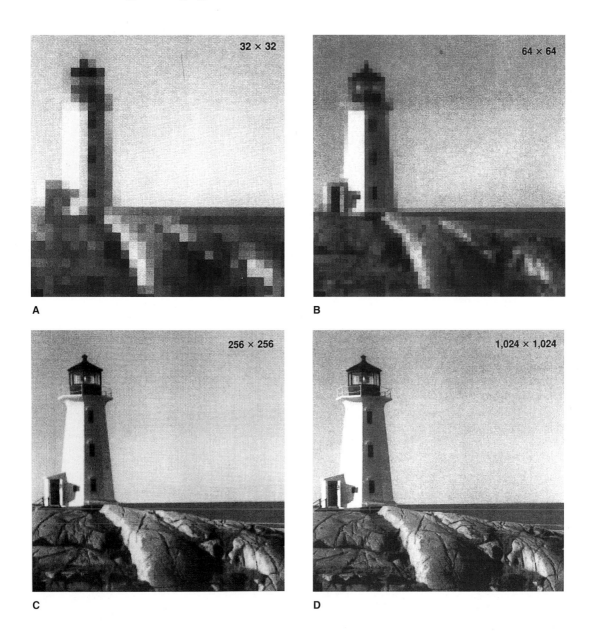

Figure 17.2 The spatial resolution and appearance of a digital image change as the matrix size and pixel size change. A, 32 X 32. B, 64 X 64. C, 256 X 256. D, 1024 X 1024. *(Balter, S: Fundamental properties of digital images.* Radiographics, *1993. With permission.)*

CONTRAST RESOLUTION

Contrast resolution describes the minimum density difference between two tissues that can be detected in an image as different densities. Contrast resolution depends on the size of the pixels. Images with larger pixels have better contrast resolution because the pixels cover a large area and have more information. The contrast of an image is described by the number of densities between black and white. A high-contrast image has few densities between black and white; a low-contrast image has many densities between black and white. An image with only two densities, black and white, has the highest contrast; pixels in the image are either black or white. An image with four densities has pixels in the image that are black, dark gray, light gray, and white. High-contrast images are short-scale contrast images. They have superior contrast resolution because it's easy to discriminate between different densities. However, the image is useful only over a limited range of densities. Figure 17.3 shows four images with different numbers of densities. Figure 17.3*A* is a high-contrast image with only two densities; Fig. 17.3*B* is an image with four densities; Fig. 17.3*C* has 16 densities; Fig. 17.3*D* is a low-contrast image with 256 densities.

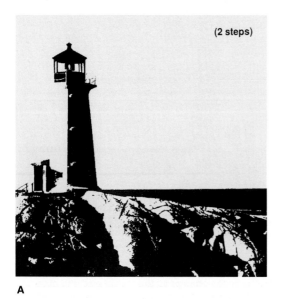
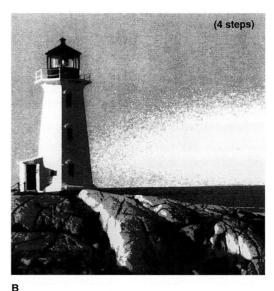

A

B

Figure 17.3 **Four images having different numbers of contrast densities.** *(Balter, S: Fundamental properties of digital images. Radiographies, 1993. With permission.)*

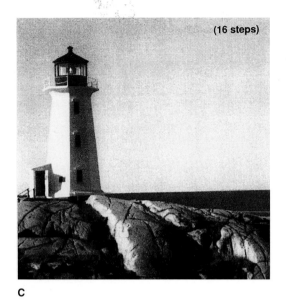

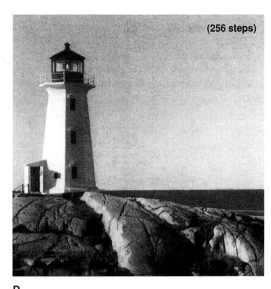

C

D

Figure 17.3 *(continued)*

LEVEL AND WINDOW CONTROLS

Figure 17.4*A* shows an abdominal image with high contrast (*A*) and low contrast (*B*). Figure 17.4*C* and *D* shows a high-contrast (*D*) and a low-contrast image (*C*) of the thorax. The contrast scale of a digital image can be electronically altered by changing the level and window controls. The **level control** sets the density value displayed as the center of the window or density range. The **window control** sets the number of density differences between black and white that are displayed. Narrow window settings produce short-scale contrast, high-contrast images because there are few density differences between black and white. Figure 17.4 shows the effect on image appearance of changing the window and level controls.

Larger matrices have smaller pixels and superior spatial resolution. The level control sets the density value that is displayed as the central density; the window control sets the number of densities between black and white. Narrow windows produce short-scale contrast images with high contrast and few densities between black and white.

Figure 17.4
How changing
the window and
the level control
affect image
appearance.
A. High-contrast
abdominal image.
B. Low-contrast
abdominal image.
C. Low-contrast
thorax.
D. High-contrast
thorax.

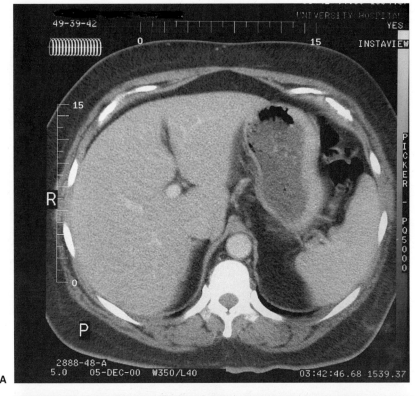

A

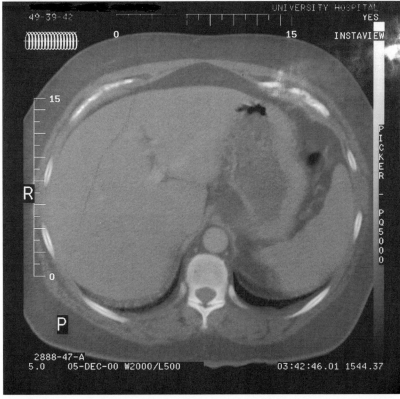

B

Figure 17.4
(continued)

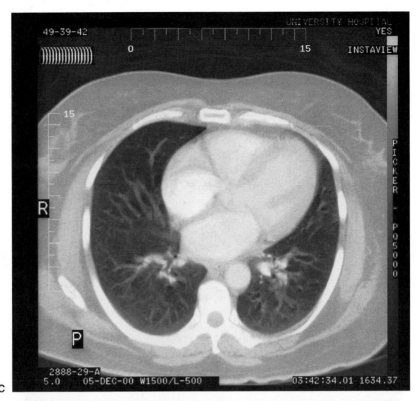

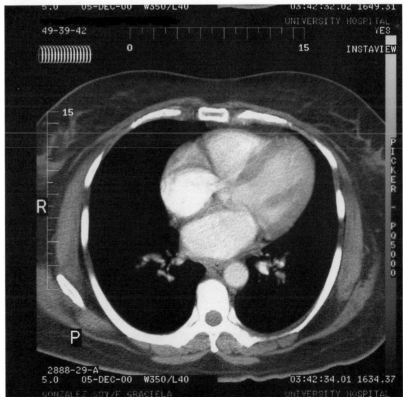

Table 17.2
Sources of Digital Images

1	Directly from MR, CT, or NM
2	Digitized fluoroscopic images
3	Computed radiographic plates
4	Direct radiography
5	Digitized conventional film images

DIGITAL IMAGING SYSTEMS

After the primary x-ray beam passes through the patient, the exit radiation is detected, and the signal data are processed, displayed, and stored. Figure 17.5 shows the basic components of a digital imaging system.

The five major sources of digital images are shown in Table 7.2.

Systems such as computed radiography, magnetic resonance, and computed tomography collect image data directly as digital data. These are known as direct digital systems. If the imaging system does not provide digital data di-

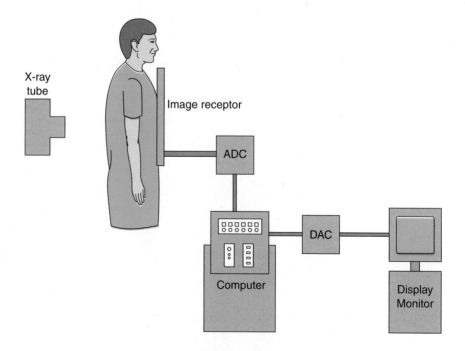

Figure 17.5 **Basic components of a digital imaging system.**

rectly, it is necessary to convert the analog data to digital data. One of the earliest detectors for digital systems, and one that is still widely used, is an image intensifier tube connected to a fluoroscopic imaging system. Most portable C-arm fluoroscopes and modern fixed fluoroscopic units convert image intensifier images into digital data. It is also possible to convert a conventional film/screen image into a digital image using a film digitizer.

ANALOG-TO-DIGITAL SYSTEMS

All direct digital systems initially convert the analog signal from the detector to a digital signal using an analog-to-digital converter (**ADC**). The digital data are then available for processing, display, and storage.

Imaging detectors produce continuously varying signals called analog signals. Digital systems represent the signal by a series of discrete values. A digital signal can have either one value or the next value, but no value in between. Analog-to-digital converters convert analog signals to digital signals. Digital-to-analog converters (**DACs**) convert digital signals to analog signals. Figure 17.6 shows an analog signal and the corresponding digital signal. Digital signals

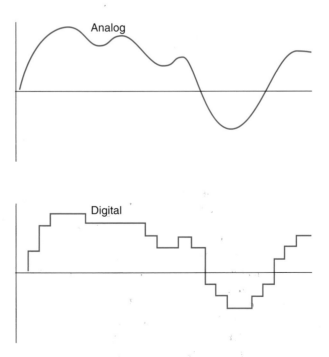

Figure 17.6 An analog signal and the corresponding digital signal.

with finer digitization (more discrete values) will more closely represent the analog signal. Conventional cable TV is an analog signal because the voltage signal is continuously changing. Digital satellite TV is sent from the satellite to the home as a digital signal and then converted into an analog signal at the input to the home TV set.

COMPUTED RADIOGRAPHY

Computed radiography (**CR**) uses a special solid-state detector plate instead of a film inside a cassette. The exterior dimensions and appearance of the CR cassette are the same as those of a conventional film cassette. The CR cassette is placed in the Bucky tray and exposed in the same manner as a conventional film cassette. Most CR systems are set up to have the same response as a 200-speed film/screen system, although this can be changed. The resolution of CR systems depends on the pixel size but is not as good as that of conventional film/screen systems. The contrast resolution of CR is superior to that of conventional film/screen systems.

The CR cassette contains a solid-state plate that responds to radiation by trapping energy in the locations where the x-rays strike. More x-rays in a location result in more energy being trapped at that location. This distribution of trapped energy forms the latent image.

Figure 17.7 diagrams the steps in forming and developing a CR image. After the exposure, the CR cassette is placed in the processing module to produce a visible image. A laser scans the detector plate, releasing the trapped energy to form the pixel data. These pixels are displayed as the visible image.

The processing module opens the CR cassette and scans the detector plate with a low-intensity laser. This prescan is used to determine the exposure level and to set the processing parameters. After the prescan is completed, a high-intensity laser beam scans back and forth across the detector plate while the plate is moved under the laser. The laser beam converts the trapped energy to visible light, which is detected by a photomultiplier tube. The light intensity and the position of the laser beam are stored as digital data for each pixel.

After the entire plate has been scanned, a high-intensity light source releases any remaining trapped energy to prepare the plate for reuse. The cassette is then closed and returned to the ready bin for reuse. The entire processing cycle requires about 60 seconds (s). It is never necessary to open the CR cassette or to handle the detector plate.

The CR detector plate is made of a thin, glasslike material and is extremely fragile. CR plates and cassettes can be reused many thousands of times, but will break if dropped. The radiation dose from a CR exposure is usually set to correspond to a comparable film/screen exposure.

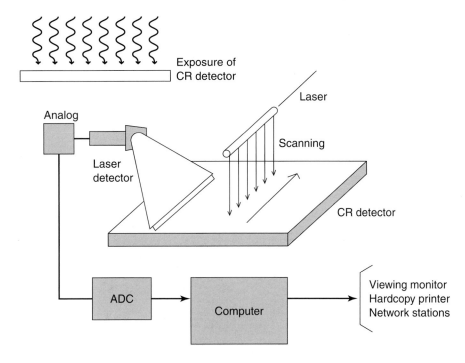

Figure 17.7 The steps in forming a computed radiographic image (CR).

DIRECT RADIOGRAPHY

Direct radiography (**DR**) uses an array of small solid state detectors to provide data directly to form the digital image. The major advantage of the direct radiography system is that no handling of a cassette is required. The image data is transferred directly to the computer for processing. There are two forms of direct radiography systems: one uses a linear array of detectors, which sweeps across the area to be imaged; the other has an array of detectors formed into a matrix. The linear array records the position of the array and the signal from each detector to form the image. In the matrix system, each detector provides data for one pixel. The linear array requires fewer detectors but a longer time to form each image. This increases the tube heat load and the possibility of patient motion artifacts. A matrix array system requires many more detectors than a linear array system to achieve the same spatial resolution. For example, to image a 5×5-m field with a 5-lp/mm resolution requires 250,000 detectors, whereas a linear array requires only 500 detectors for the same resolution. Film screen systems typically have resolutions of 8-lp/mm.

FILM DIGITIZATION

Any image recorded using a conventional film/screen cassette can be converted into a digital image by a film digitizer. A film digitizer measures the light transmitted at each location on the film, converts the light intensity to a digital value, and records the location and intensity values as an image pixel. The film is introduced into the feed tray and transported through the digitizer while the image is scanned for digitization. After digitization, the image can be processed, displayed, or transmitted just any other digital image. Figure 17.8 shows a film digitizer.

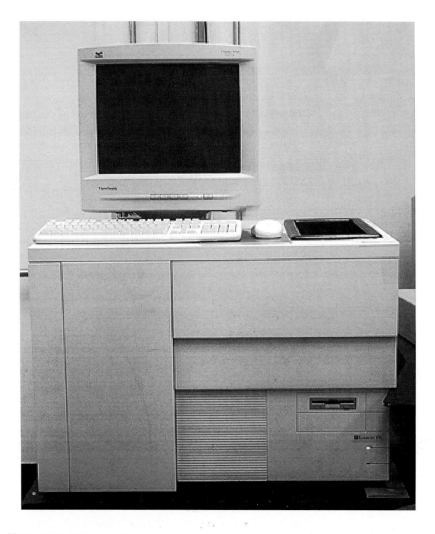

Figure 17.8 **A film digitizer.**

PICTURE ARCHIVING AND COMMUNICATIONS SYSTEM AND TELERADIOLOGY

No matter how the digital image is obtained, it can be sent over either a dedicated line or conventional telephone lines to other display sites in the hospital or elsewhere. There is no limit to the number of monitor stations that can display the same image simultaneously. Images of a trauma victim can be sent to the radiology, emergency, and surgery departments at the same time. Such distribution of images within a hospital is part of a **picture archiving and communications system (PACS).** It is also possible to send images across the street, state, or country. Once the image has been digitized there is no limit to the distance it can be sent. Sending images to remote sites is called **teleradiology.**

HARD COPY PRODUCTION

Diagnostic interpretation can be made from the display monitor, called a soft copy display, or the image can be printed on film, called a hard copy. Hard copies are produced on multiformat cameras or laser printers.

A multiformat camera takes a picture of the display screen. It is called a multiformat camera because multiple images can be produced on a single sheet of film. A laser printer scans a laser beam across a sheet of film to expose the image. The intensity of the laser beam, and hence the density of the image, is controlled by the digital data. The laser printer can also produce multiple images on the same film. Both the laser printer and the multiformat camera are connected to an automatic film processor, so their images are ready for immediate interpretation after the film is developed. The digital image data are stored in a computer and can be retrieved whenever required to produce additional hard copies or replace lost films.

DRY FILM PROCESSORS

Images from digital data can be formed using dry film processors that process and print the image in a single step. Dry film processors require no chemical solutions to produce a ready-to-interpret image on film. The special dry film can be loaded into the holding magazine with the room lights on, because it is processed by a thermal printer head. When a hard copy of the digital data is formed in the dry processor, a sheet of the special film is removed from the holding magazine and transported past the thermal head, which blackens the film. Pixel locations with higher-intensities are displayed as darker areas on the film. The special thermal film cannot be processed in a conventional automatic processor and can be used only with digital data. Because the special dry film is activated by heat and is insensitive to room lights, no darkroom is needed with a dry film processor.

DATA COMPRESSION

Data compression reduces the number of pixels that are stored or processed in an image. Compression algorithms can reduce the size of the data in an image matrix by a factor of 30 or more, while maintaining the diagnostic content of the image. Compressed images require less storage space and can be transmitted more rapidly. This means that an original image requiring 30 minutes (min) to transmit can be sent in 1 min in a compressed form.

SUMMARY

A digital image is formed by a matrix of numbers called pixels. Each pixel specifies a unique location and contains information about the image intensity at that location. The field of view describes how much of the patient is imaged. The spatial resolution of the digital image is limited by the pixel size. Smaller pixels provide better spatial resolution. The contrast resolution of a digital image is established by the number of discrete values stored in the pixels. The window control determines the number of density differences between black and white in the display. The level control sets the center density value in the display. A small number of densities produces a high-contrast image. Digital imaging systems include CR, DR, MR, CT, NM, and fluoroscopic units. Detectors used in digital imaging include fluoroscopic image intensifiers, gas-filled ionization chambers, and scintillation crystals. Images on film can be digitized and then processed and transmitted in PACS or teleradiology systems. An analog-to-digital converter changes analog signals into digital signals. Computed radiography employs a thin solid-state detector plate inside a special CR cassette that is the same size and shape as a conventional film/screen cassette and can be used in the same Bucky holders. Data compression reduces the size of the image matrix and reduces the time required to transmit, process, and retrieve the images and the memory space required to store the images. Digital data can be displayed for interpretation on display monitors, called soft displays, or printed on film, called hard copies. Hard copies of digital data can be produced by multiformat cameras, laser printers, or dry film processors.

QUESTIONS

1. A digital image is made up of
   a. a pixel of matrices.
   b. a matrix of pixels.
   c. a vortex of pixels.
   d. a matrix of vortices.
2. Which matrix size has the smallest pixels?
   a. 128×128
   b. 256×256
   c. 512×512
   d. 1024×1024
3. What is the pixel size in millimeters of a 256 matrix with a 25-cm field of view?
   a. 0.1
   b. 1.0
   c. 10
   d. 100
4. What is the pixel size in millimeters of a 512 matrix with a 30-cm field of view?
   a. 0.06
   b. 0.6
   c. 6.0
   d. 60
5. What is the pixel size in millimeters of a 256 matrix with a 15-cm field of view?
   a. 0.06
   b. 0.6
   c. 6.0
   d. 60
6. If the field of view increases and the matrix size remains unchanged, the contrast resolution will be
   a. improved.
   b. degraded.
7. If the field of view remains unchanged and the matrix size increases, the spatial resolution will be
   a. improved.
   b. degraded.
8. How many pixels are required to image one line pair?
   a. 1
   b. 2
   c. 3
   d. 4

9. Spatial resolution describes
   a. the maximum separation of two objects that can be distinguished as separate objects on the image.
   b. the minimum density difference between two tissues that can be distinguished as separate tissues.
   c. the maximum density difference between two tissues that can be distinguished as separate tissues.
   d. the minimum separation of two objects that can be distinguished as separate objects on the image.
10. Contrast resolution describes
    a. the maximum separation of two objects that can be distinguished as separate objects on the image.
    b. the minimum density difference between two tissues that can distinguished as separate tissues.
    c. the maximum density difference between two tissues that can be distinguished as separate tissues.
    d. the minimum separation of two objects that can be distinguished as separate objects on the image.
11. The window control sets the
    a. number of density differences in the display.
    b. number of pixels in the matrix.
    c. number of matrices in the pixel.
    d. density value in the middle of the display.
12. PACS stands for
    a. primary access of compressed studies.
    b. picture archiving and computer system.
    c. picture archiving and communications system.
    d. picture access to communications system.
13. Dry film processors
    a. use dry chemicals to produce the image.
    b. use holding magazines that must be loaded in a darkroom.
    c. use heat to produce the image.
    d. use fragile detector plates.
14. Computed radiographic systems use
    a. detector plates that are read by a scanning laser beam.
    b. detector plates of dry chemicals.
    c. detector plates that are read by a thermal head.
    d. conventional screen cassettes.
15. Data compression
    a. results in faster processing.
    b. produces faster transmission times.
    c. requires less storage space.
    d. does all of the above.

ANSWERS TO CHAPTER 17 QUESTIONS

1.	b	9.	d
2.	d	10.	b
3.	b	11.	a
4.	b	12.	c
5.	b	13.	c
6.	a	14.	a
7.	a	15.	d
8.	b		

18

Computed Tomography

OBJECTIVES

At the completion of this chapter, the student will be able to

1. Describe the operation of a computed tomography (CT) scanner.
2. Identify the components of a CT scanner.
3. Define CT numbers.
4. Identify the factors that influence spatial and contrast resolution.

INTRODUCTION

The invention of the CT scanner revolutionized radiographic examinations because of the difference in appearance and sensitivity of CT scans. CT scanners produce cross-sectional images of the body with the tissues and organs displayed separately, instead of superimposed as in a conventional radiograph. CT scans are much more sensitive to small differences in tissue composition than are conventional radiographs. Conventional radiographs are plain shadowgrams with the images of all the tissues and organs superimposed. CT views are perpendicular to the body axis and are called transaxial images. The term *CAT scan* comes from the words *computed axial tomographic scan.*

CT scanners measure the transmission of the x-ray beam through the body. Figure 18.1 shows a schematic view of a CT scanner. The x-ray tube rotates in a circle around the patient, and a thin x-ray beam slices through the body to produce the image data. The support table and patient advance and the tube again rotates around the patient to generate data for the next image. Typical axil CT examinations consist of 10 or more slices and require only several minutes to complete. Spiral CT examinations can be completed in less than one minute.

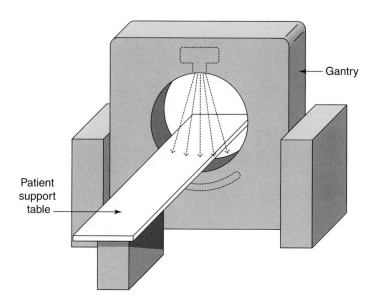

Figure 18.1 Schematic of a CT scanner.

The exit radiation is detected and converted into a digital signal. Data from many different entrance angles are processed in a computer to determine the transmission and attenuation characteristics of the tissues in the slice under examination. The data are stored in a matrix of pixels. The digital pixel data are processed in a digital-to-analog converter (DAC) before being displayed. The DAC converts the digital data into an analog signal for display.

COMPONENTS OF A CT SCANNER

A CT scanner consists of a doughnut-shaped gantry, a patient support table, a computer system, and an operator's console with display. Figure 18.2 shows the gantry and patient support table of a modern CT scanner.

THE GANTRY

The gantry is a doughnut-shaped structure containing the x-ray circuit, the x-ray tube, and the radiation detectors. Inside the gantry cover is a large ring that holds the detectors and the track for the x-ray tube while it rotates around the patient.

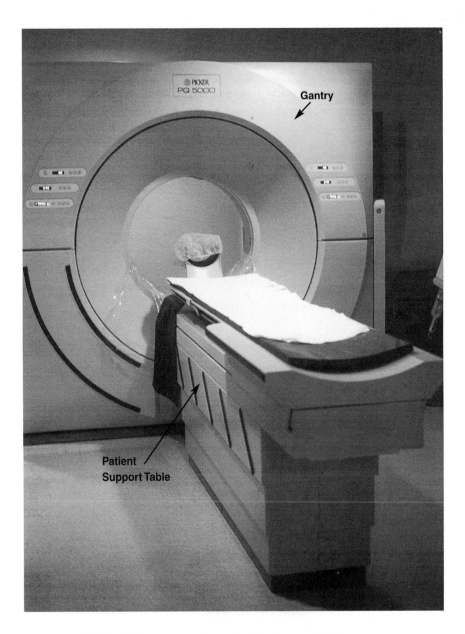

Figure 18.2 **Modern CT scanner gantry and patient support table.**

X-ray Circuit

There are two kinds of x-ray circuits: one operates at low frequency [60 hertz (Hz)] and is about the size of a large office desk, and the other is a high-frequency circuit (3000 Hz) about the size of a suitcase. The 60-Hz circuit, because of its size, must be located outside the gantry in the CT room and is connected to the rotating x-ray tube by flexible high-voltage cables. The cables prevent the tube from rotating more than 360° without rewinding so axial CT examination collect data one slice at a time.

The high frequency circuit is small enough to be mounted with the x-ray tube on the rotating frame inside the gantry. Both the tube and the circuit rotate together around the patient. The input voltage is connected to the circuit through slip rings that allow the circuit and the x-ray tube to continuously rotate. Continuous rotation is necessary for spiral CT scanning.

X-ray Tube

The x-ray tube is a high-heat-capacity tube that is capable of operating at more than 400 milliamperes (mA) and 150 kilovolts peak (kVp) for several seconds. Many CT tubes are designed with heat capacities greater than 1 million heat units. The x-ray beam is collimated into a fan-shaped beam. The thickness of the beam is set by adjustable collimators located at the exit of the x-ray tube housing. The thickness of the beam determines the amount of tissue irradiated and the volume of each pixel element. The volume element is called a **voxel.** The collimator and detector geometry prevents most scattered x-rays from reaching the detectors. Figure 18.3 shows a fan-shaped beam from a CT scanner and the relationship between an individual pixel and voxel.

Radiation Detectors

The radiation detectors in the gantry can be mounted either in a stationary ring around the gantry or on a support frame that rotates in a circle around the patient opposite the x-ray tube. In either system, the detectors measure the exit radiation transmitted through the patient at different angles around the patient. Systems with stationary detectors utilize more than 4000 detectors. Rotating detector systems use enough detectors to intercept the entire fan beam. The image quality, resolution, and efficiency of the stationary and rotating detector systems are effectively the same.

Figure 18.4 shows the detector arrangements for stationary and rotating detector systems.

CT scanners employ scintillation crystals, gas-filled ionization chambers, or solid-state detectors as radiation detectors. The image quality and detection efficiency of the different types of detectors are approximately the same.

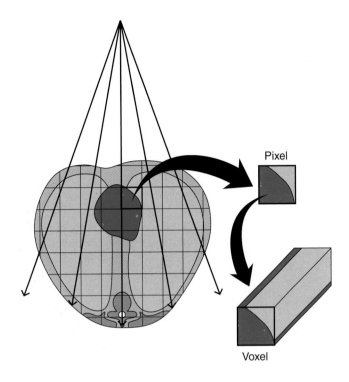

Figure 18.3 **A fan beam from a CT scanner and the relationship between a pixel and a voxel.**

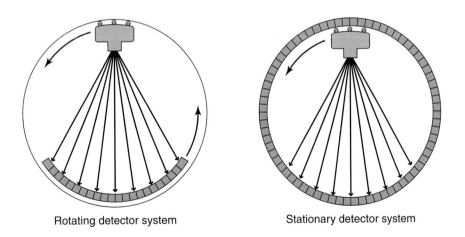

Figure 18.4 **Arrangement of rotating and stationary detector systems.**

Scintillation Detectors

Scintillation detectors are special crystals that give off a flash of light when an x-ray interacts with the crystal. More radiation produces more light. The light from the scintillation crystal is detected by a **photomultiplier** tube, which converts light into an amplified electrical signal.

Gas-Filled Ionization Detectors

Gas-filled ionization chambers produce an electrical signal when x-rays pass through the chamber. Electrodes in the ionization chamber produce an electric field across the gas-filled chamber. X-rays produce ionization in the gas. The electric field pulls the negative ions to the positive electrode and the positive ions to the negative electrode. This flow of electrons is an electric current. The current produced is proportional to the ionization in the chamber and the radiation passing through the chamber.

Solid-State Detectors

A **solid-state detector** functions in the same way as a gas-filled ionization detector, except that the electric field and ionization are produced in a solid. The ionizations occur in the solid rather than in a gas.

The arrangement and type of detectors used in a particular CT scanner are selected by the manufacturer for commercial reasons. The processing of the signal from any type of detector is essentially the same in all CT scanners. The image quality of all modern CT scanners is effectively the same.

PATIENT SUPPORT TABLE

The patient support table is constructed of low atomic number materials to reduce attenuation of the x-ray beam. It is constructed to support patients weighing as much as 450 pounds. The positioning of the table is called **indexing.** Table indexing must be accurate and reproducible within 1 millimeter (mm). In conventional axial CT scanning, the tube rotates around the patient to collect data for one slice, the table indexes into the gantry at a preset distance, and the tube rotates again to collect data for the next slice. The x-ray beam is on only during tube rotation. In a typical axial CT examination involves collecting data from 10 or more slices and requires several minutes to complete. In spiral scanning, the support table moves steadily through the gantry while the tube continuously rotates around the table and patient the entire spiral CT examination can be completed in less than one minute.

A CT scanner consists of a circular gantry containing the x-ray tube and radiation detectors, a high-voltage x-ray circuit, and a patient support table. The x-ray tube has collimators to set the size of the x-ray beam and a high-heat-capacity rotating anode. Scintillators or gas or solid-state detectors intercept the radiation passing through the patient. The high-voltage circuit is connected to the tube through thick cables if it operates at 60 Hz, or is mounted on the rotating ring with the tube if it is a high-frequency circuit. The support table moves the patient through the gantry continuously or at specified increments to produce separate scans.

SPATIAL RESOLUTION

Spatial resolution is defined as the minimum separation of two objects that can be distinguished in the image as two separate objects. Digital images with smaller pixel sizes have better spatial resolution. Spatial resolution is measured in line pairs per millimeter (lp/mm). Typical CT resolution depends on the design of the unit but is generally between 0.6 and 1.0 lp/mm. Two pixels are required to image one line pair. Increasing the matrix size decreases the pixel size and improves spatial resolution but increases the time required for processing and storing the images. Spatial resolution in CT scanning depends on a combination of factors, including focal spot size, beam collimation, detector size, matrix size, and pixel size. Larger matrices with smaller pixels have better spatial resolution. Utilizing small focal spots and narrow collimation provides better spatial resolution.

COMPUTER SYSTEM

The computer system calculates the attenuation of the individual voxels using the x-ray exit radiation data collected at many different tube positions around the patient. These transmission data are converted into attenuation data for each voxel. The computer programs used to perform these calculations are called algorithms. The calculations of the CT numbers must be very fast to produce images for immediate viewing. The digital data are stored for later recall.

OPERATOR'S CONSOLE

The operator's console contains the controls that turn the CT scanner on and off and controls to select the indexing of the table motion and scan thickness, the scan time, and the level and width of the displayed image. The focal spot size usually cannot be selected from the operator's console. It is preprogrammed with the kVp and mA values for individual anatomic sites. Patient information, all scan parameters, and the image data are stored in a data file. Hard copy images are printed on film using a multiformat camera or laser printer. These images are reviewed for diagnostic interpretation by the radiologist.

CT NUMBERS

The CT number of each voxel is calculated from the transmission data collected as the beam passes through the patient at many different angles. The relative attenuation characteristics of a voxel are reported as a CT number, sometimes referred to as Hounsfield units. Changing the size of either the pixel or the voxel may change the CT number because different tissues may be included in the voxel. The CT number of a tissue is always calculated relative to the attenuation of water. The CT number of a tissue is given by

$$\text{CT number of tissue} = [(\mu_{\text{tissue}} - \mu_{\text{H}_2\text{O}})/\mu_{\text{H}_2\text{O}}] \times 1000$$

where μ_{tissue} is the linear attenuation coefficient of the tissue and $\mu_{\text{H}_2\text{O}}$ is the linear attenuation coefficient of water. Because the CT number is based on the difference between the tissue attenuation coefficient and the attenuation coefficient of water, the CT number of water is always equal to zero. Tissues with densities greater than that of water have positive CT numbers; tissues with densities less than that of water have negative CT numbers. If a tissue floats in water, it has a negative CT number. Usually tissues with negative CT numbers are displayed as darker objects. Tissues with positive CT numbers appear as lighter densities. Table 18.1 shows the CT numbers of some common tissues.

Table 18.1
CT Numbers of Various Tissues

Tissue	CT number or Hounsfield Number
Air	−1000
Lung	−300
Fat	−50
Water	0
White matter	+30
Gray matter	+35
Blood	+40
Muscle	+50
Liver	+60
Dense bone	+1000

CONTRAST RESOLUTION

One of the major advantages of CT scanning is its ability to image tissues with similar attenuation characteristics. Contrast resolution is the ability to distinguish two objects with similar attenuation values. For example, blood and liver are very close in attenuation characteristics but have different appearances on a CT scan of the abdomen. Figure 18.5 demonstrates the difference in appearance between blood in the aorta and liver tissue in a CT examination of the abdomen.

Contrast resolution is determined by the number of density differences stored in each pixel. A low-contrast image has many density differences. A high-contrast image has few density differences.

CT examinations using iodinated contrast media are performed to image both arterial and venous phases of the circulatory system. Iodinated contrast

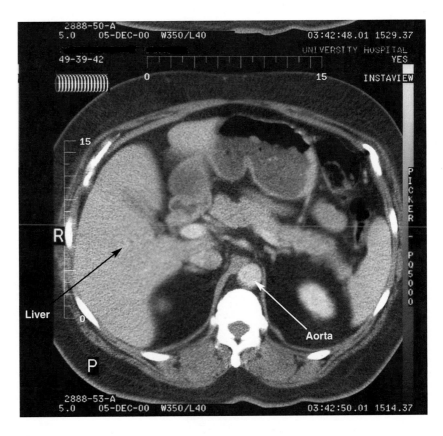

Figure 18.5 A CT scan of the abdomen can distinguish between blood and liver tissues.

media are injected either by hand or by a power injector. Power injectors, or automatic injectors, permit more accurate timing of contrast delivery. Power injectors are also used in cardiology and angiography to inject a known amount of contrast at a fixed rate. Typical CT contrast examinations are performed first without contrast, then scanned again after contrast injection. This permits observation of the structures under examination.

SPIRAL CT SCANNING

In spiral CT scanning, sometimes called helical scanning, the patient support table moves through the gantry continuously while the tube rotates around the patient. The attenuation data are collected continuously during the entire scan. Spiral scanning differs from conventional CT scanning in that the support table is not stopped at the center of each slice location while the data are collected. Figure 18.6 illustrates how the x-ray tube of a spiral CT scanner rotates around the patient while the patient support table moves through the CT scan plane. The acquisition time is the time required to collect the CT data. The acquisition time for conventional axial CT scans is typically several seconds per slice. The acquisition time for spiral scans is about 30 s. The examination time is the total time required to collect CT data. For spiral scanning, the acquisition time and the examination time are the same. For conventional axial CT scanning, the ex-

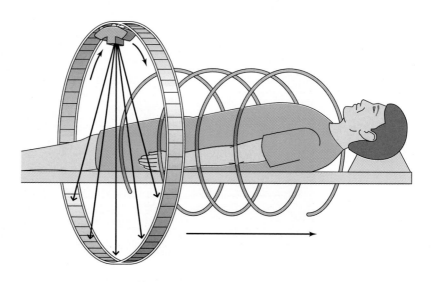

Figure 18.6 **Operation of a spiral CT scanner.**

amination time includes the time for both data acquisition and table indexing to the next slice position. A conventional axil CT examination requires several minutes to complete, which is much longer than a spiral CT examination.

Special algorithms are used to calculate the individual pixel values and form the spiral CT images. Factors that influence the image in spiral CT scanning are the rate of table advance and the section thickness. The ratio of these factors is known as the pitch. The pitch is the rate of table advance per revolution divided by the section thickness. The tube typically rotates at one revolution per second. The section thickness can be set at values between 1 and 10 mm. For example, if the section thickness is 5 mm and the table moves at 5 mm/s (5 mm/revolution), the pitch is 1. If the table moves at a rate of 10 mm/s with a section thickness of 5 mm, the pitch is 2. The extent of a spiral scan is the distance from the top to the bottom of the scan. A scan with a pitch of 2 has an extent twice as great as a scan with a pitch of 1. Typical spiral scans have a pitch between 1 and 2.

CT FLUOROSCOPY

Spiral CT allows the continuous imaging of a section of the body, or real time CT fluoroscopy. CT fluoroscopy is used for lesion drainage and biopsies. The tube continuously rotates around the patient and the physician can control the position of the support table to move anatomy in or out of the field. Entrance exposure rates are 2-3 times higher than conventional fluoroscopy.

RADIATION DOSE FROM CT SCANNING

The radiation dose per slice is about 15 milligray (mGy) [1500 millirads (mrad)]. This is delivered to a point in the patient. The contribution due to scatter from adjacent slices in a multislice examination doubles this dose. The dose to a point in the middle of a 10-slice examination is about 30 mGy (3000 mrad). The dose from conventional and spiral CT scans is approximately the same.

The spatial resolution of CT scans depends on the focal spot size, pixel size, and matrix size. Smaller pixel sizes give better spatial resolution. The CT number of a tissue describes the difference in density between the tissue and water. The CT number of water is always 0. The CT numbers of fat and lung are less than 0; those of muscle and bone are greater than 0. In most CT displays, air is dark and bone is white. Contrast resolution describes how close in density two tissues can be and still be recognized as separate tissues. High mA CT scans with large pixels have superior contrast resolution because they have more x-ray counts in each pixel. In spiral CT scanning, the tube and detectors rotate continuously while the support table and patient are moved into the gantry. Spiral CT scans produce a complete examination in a shorter time because the tube rotates continuously around the patient instead of starting and stopping for each slice. Typical radiation doses for a CT scan are from 30 to 50 mGy (3000 to 5000 mrad) per examination.

SUMMARY

CT scanners provide cross-sectional images, also called transaxial images, of the body by measuring the x-ray transmission through the body. The x-ray tube is mounted on a circular frame inside the gantry together with the radiation detectors. Scintillators, gas-filled chambers, or solid-state detectors are used as radiation detectors in CT scanners. The detectors are mounted either on a stationary ring or on a support frame that rotates opposite the x-ray tube. A thin x-ray beam is transmitted through the patient and detected by the radiation detectors. The patient support table moves the patient through the gantry at preset increments, in conventional CT scanning, or continuously, in spiral CT scanning. Computer algorithms convert the transmission data from the detectors into CT numbers. These CT numbers describe the attenuation characteristics of the tissues within the transaxial slices. CT numbers range from 1000 for air to +1000 for compact bone, with water always set at 0. The major advantage of CT scanning is its high-contrast resolution. Contrast resolution is the ability to distinguish tissues with small differences in attenuation characteristics. CT fluoroscopy is the continuous imaging at a section of the body.

QUESTIONS

1. CT scanning provides a(n) _____ view of the body.
   a. axial
   b. linear
   c. longitudinal
   d. transaxial
2. The gantry of a spiral CT scanner contains
   a. the tube.
   b. the detectors.
   c. high-voltage circuit.
   d. all of the above.

3. An x-ray tube in a CT scanner has
   a. two cathodes.
   b. a high heat capacity.
   c. a high-frequency anode.
   d. a stationary anode.
4. The x-ray beam in a CT scanner is shaped into a _____ beam.
   a. pencil
   b. circular
   c. fan
   d. hypocyclodial
5. The thickness of a CT slice is controlled by the
   a. target angle.
   b. filament size.
   c. patient thickness.
   d. adjustable collimators.
6. A voxel is
   a. a picture element.
   b. a volume element.
   c. a data storage element.
   d. the volume control element.
7. Detectors used in CT scanners are
   a. solid-state.
   b. gas-filled.
   c. scintillation.
   d. all of the above.
8. The detector that gives off a flash of light when irradiated is
   a. solid-state.
   b. gas-filled.
   c. a scintillation.
   d. all of the above.
9. The detector that employs a photomultiplier tube in the detection circuit is
   a. solid-state.
   b. gas-filled.
   c. scintillation.
   d. all of the above.
10. The patient support table
    a. is made of low-attenuation material.
    b. moves the patient through the x-ray beam.
    c. indexing must be accurate within 1 mm.
    d. is/does all of the above.

11. Spatial resolution describes the _____ of two objects that can be distinguished as separate objects.
    a. maximum separation
    b. minimum separation
    c. maximum size
12. Contrast resolution describes the ability to distinguish the _____ of two objects.
    a. separation
    b. attenuation difference
    c. motion
    d. size
13. Indexing refers to the
    a. amount of table movement.
    b. tube rotation speed.
    c. rotations per centimeter of patient motion.
    d. changes in high voltage.
14. In spiral CT scanning, pitch is the ratio of
    a. the rotation speed to the patient motion per revolution.
    b. the amount of table advance per revolution to the section thickness.
    c. the section thickness to the revolutions per second.
    d. the section thickness to the revolutions per patient motion.
15. Computer programs that calculate the CT numbers are called
    a. Pym programs.
    b. soft contrast diagrams.
    c. hard-wired.
    d. algorithms.
16. The CT number of water is
    a. −1000.
    b. −50.
    c. 0.
    d. 1000.
17. The CT number of fat is
    a. −1000.
    b. −50.
    c. 0.
    d. 1000.
18. The CT number of bone is
    a. −1000.
    b. −50.
    c. 0.
    d. 1000.

19. Fat has _____ CT number than (as) water.
    a. a greater
    b. a smaller
    c. the same
20. In _____ CT scanning, the table moves continuously through the gantry.
    a. conventional
    b. spiral
21. In _____ CT scanning, the table is indexed into the gantry at preset distances.
    a. conventional
    b. spiral
22. The major advantage of CT scanning is its
    a. high count rate.
    b. small pixel sizes.
    c. accurate indexing of table motion.
    d. high contrast resolution.

ANSWERS TO CHAPTER 18 QUESTIONS

1.	d	12.	b
2.	d	13.	a
3.	b	14.	b
4.	c	15.	d
5.	d	16.	c
6.	b	17.	b
7.	d	18.	d
8.	c	19.	b
9.	c	20.	b
10.	d	21.	a
11.	b	22.	d

19

Magnetic Resonance Imaging

OBJECTIVES

At the completion of this chapter, the student will be able to

1. State the physical process involved in magnetic resonance imaging.
2. Identify the components and describe the operation of a magnetic resonance unit.
3. Identify the difference between T1 and T2 relaxation times.
4. Describe some safety hazards present near a magnetic resonance unit.

INTRODUCTION

The human body is more than 85 percent water, which consists of two hydrogen atoms and one oxygen atom (H_2O). Magnetic resonance imaging (**MRI**) uses radio frequency signals from hydrogen protons in the body to form images of body structures. It does not use x-rays or any other form of ionizing radiation. The magnetic resonance (**MR**) magnet provides a magnetic field to align the protons. This magnetic field is called the external or main magnetic field to distinguish it from the local magnetic fields in the immediate vicinity of the individual protons. The main magnetic field is given the symbol B_0. The protons in body tissues are aligned in the magnetic field and then moved out of alignment by radio frequency (**RF**) pulses. The frequency of the RF pulses is selected to resonate with the protons in the body. Only protons with the correct resonant frequency are moved out of alignment with the external magnetic field. As the out of alignment protons move back into alignment, they produce an RF signal, which is used to construct the MR image.

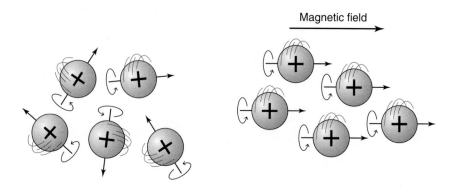

Figure 19.1 **Protons align themselves in a magnetic field. The protons used in MR imaging are hydrogen nuclei in the human body.**

MR PROTON ALIGNMENT

Hydrogen is the most abundant element in the body. Hydrogen nuclei, or protons, are constantly spinning. This spinning causes the protons to act like tiny magnets. In a magnetic field, the protons line up in the direction of the magnetic field, similar to the way a compass lines up in the earth's magnetic field. All the protons pointing in the direction of the magnetic field act together to produce a net magnetization, as if they were combined into one larger magnet. When a patient's body is placed in a magnetic field, the hydrogen protons line up in the direction of that magnetic field. The protons are not all perfectly aligned along the external magnetic field—some point in other directions—but there are more aligned with the magnetic field direction than in any other direction. Figure 19.1 shows how the protons line up in a magnetic field.

> *Hydrogen is the most abundant element in the human body. Hydrogen protons align with the magnetic field when the human body is placed in an MR magnet.*

RESONANCE

Resonance is the absorption or emission of energy only at certain specific frequencies. Radio and TV circuits are built to have selectable resonance frequencies. These circuits respond to a signal only at the selected resonance frequency and amplify only that signal. Resonance is used in TV sets to distinguish between, for example, signals from channel 4 and channel 5 because channel 4 and channel 5 have different frequencies.

Table 19.1

Larmor Frequency as a Function of Magnetic Field Strength

Magnetic Field Strength (T)	Larmor Frequency
0.5	21.1
1.0	42.3
1.5	63.4
2.0	84.6

The hydrogen protons in the body also have a resonance frequency called the **Larmor frequency.** The Larmor frequency depends on the magnetic field strength. Protons in stronger magnetic fields have higher resonance frequencies. Magnetic field strengths are measured in gauss (G) or tesla (T). The Larmor frequency of hydrogen is 42.3 megahertz per tesla (MHz/T). This means that a proton in a magnetic field with a strength of 1 T will have a resonant frequency of 42.3 MHz. Table 19.1 gives the Larmor frequency for hydrogen protons in different magnetic field strengths.

A hydrogen proton in a 1-T field will strongly absorb energy from only 42.3-MHz RF pulses. An **RF pulse** is a short burst of RF energy at a specific frequency. RF pulses at the Larmor frequency will rotate the protons out of alignment with the external magnetic field. When the protons move back into alignment with the external magnetic field, they give off RF signals, which are used to form MR images. Figure 19.2 shows how an external RF pulse (called the excitation pulse) can rotate the protons out of alignment with the external magnetic field.

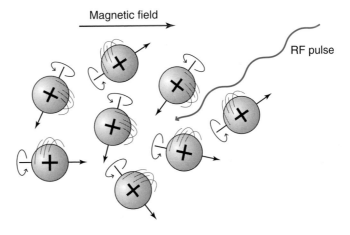

Figure 19.2 An external RF pulse can rotate protons out of alignment with magnetic field.

Hydrogen protons have a resonance frequency called the Larmor frequency. Hydrogen protons excited at the resonance frequency will absorb energy and rotate out of alignment with the external magnetic field. If the RF excitation pulse is not matched to the Larmor resonance frequency, the protons will not absorb energy and will remain aligned with the external magnetic field, and so will produce no signal.

PRECESSION

The hydrogen protons realign themselves into the direction of the external magnetic field by rotating around the magnetic field direction. This rotation, or **precession,** back into alignment with the magnetic field is similar to the spinning action of a child's top or gyroscope. The precession of the spinning top is around the direction of gravity; the precession of the protons is around the direction of the magnetic field. When these protons precess back into alignment with the external field, they give off RF energy at their Larmor frequency. This RF energy given off as the protons precess back into alignment makes up the signal used to form the magnetic resonance image. Figure 19.3 shows how protons precess back into alignment with the external magnetic field.

An RF pulse is used to rotate the protons out of alignment with the magnetic field. As the protons precess back into alignment, they give off RF energy at their Larmor frequencies. This RF energy given off as the protons precess back into alignment makes up the signal used to form the magnetic resonance image.

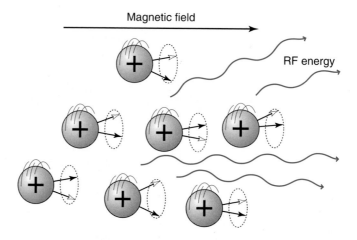

Figure 19.3 Protons precessing in a magnetic field.

Table 19.2

T1 and T2 Values for Various Organs at 1 T Magnetic Field Strength

Organ	T1 (ms)	T2 (ms)
Fat	220	90
Liver	440	50
Spleen	460	80
Muscle	600	40
White matter	700	90
Gray matter	820	100
Cerebrospinal fluid	2000	300
Blood	800	180
Water	2500	2500

T1 AND T2 RELAXATION TIMES

The time it takes for a proton to precess back into alignment with the external magnetic field is called the **T1 relaxation time.** Differences in T1 relaxation times depend on binding of the protons in different tissues. Protons in different types of tissues have different relaxation times because their elasticity and chemical bonds are different. These differences in T1 relaxation times are used to form T1-weighted MR images.

Protons in a magnetic field also have a second relaxation time, called T2. The **T2 relaxation time** depends on interactions between the protons in a small volume of tissue. When an RF excitation pulse rotates the protons out of alignment, all the protons start to precess back into alignment at the Larmor frequency. When the protons begin precessing, they all point in the same direction at the same time. They are said to be in phase. Because the local magnetic fields near the different protons are not exactly the same, some protons precess faster and some slower than the average. Because of these small differences in the local magnetic fields, the protons gradually lose phase and no longer point in the same direction at the same time. The T2 relaxation time of a tissue is the time it takes for the protons to lose their phase. The T2 relaxation time of a tissue is always shorter than its T1 relaxation time. Table 19.2 shows T1 and T2 for various tissues in a field strength of 1 T.

MR CONTRAST

MR images can be modified to emphasize either T1 or T2 by adjusting the RF excitation pulse. These modifications result in either T1- or T2-weighted im-

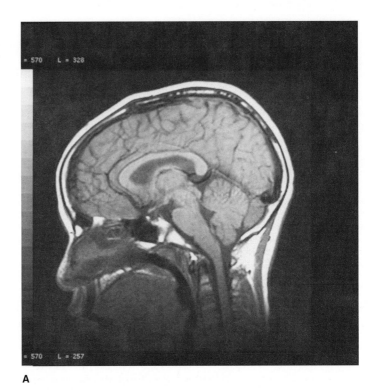

A

Figure 19.4 **A. TI-weighted image of the brain.**

ages. The same anatomy can have different appearances with T1- and T2-weighted images. The decision to obtain a T1- or T2-weighted image is based upon the structures to be imaged. Figure 19.4 shows the different appearances of T1- and T2-weighted images of the brain.

Soft tissue contrast with MRI is superior to that with computed tomography (CT) because of the T1 and T2 differences shown in Table 19.2. Intravenous MR contrast agents such as gadolinium DTPA are used to improve MR image contrast because they have T1 and T2 values that are very different from those of tissue.

Table 19.3 gives the appearance of some body tissues in T1- and T2-weighted images.

All tissues have two relaxation times, T1 and T2, and these are used to distinguish different tissues in the MR images. T1- and T2-weighted images of the same tissues often have different appearances. The selection of a T1- or T2-weighted image depends on the structures to be imaged.

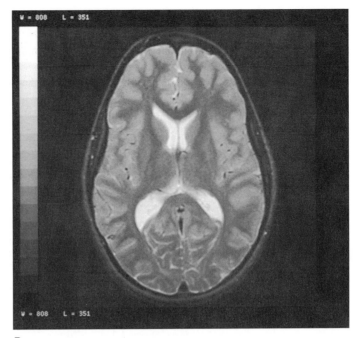

B

Figure 19.4 **B. T2-weighted image of the brain.**

MR EQUIPMENT

An MR imaging system consists of a magnet coil surrounding an opening called the **bore,** shim coils, gradient coils, surface coils, a patient support table, a computer, and a display system. The **main magnet coil** produces the external magnetic field used to align the hydrogen protons in the body. The main magnetic field is represented by B_0. **Shim coils** are used to improve the uniformity of the magnetic field near the edges of the bore. The patient is

Table 19.3

The Appearance of Some Body Tissues in T1- and T2-Weighted MR Images

Body Tissue	Appearance in T1-Weighted Image	Appearance in T2-Weighted Image
White matter	Bright	Dark
Gray matter	Dark	Bright
Spinal fluid	Dark	Bright
Hematoma	Bright	Dark

placed within the bore of the magnet during the scan. The table supports the patient within the magnetic field during the MR scan. The **gradient coils** are used to select the imaging plane. **Surface coils** detect the weak RF signals from the protons precessing back into alignment. The computer sets the times for the RF signals and processes the precession RF signal data to form the MR images. The display system allows viewing of the digital images on a TV monitor or recording them as hard copies.

MR Magnets

The two types of magnets used in MR units are superconducting magnets and permanent magnets. The strength of a magnetic field is measured in tesla or gauss. One tesla is equal to 10,000 gauss. The earth's magnetic field is about 0.5 G (5×10^{-5} T). A refrigerator magnet has a field strength of about 100 G. The external magnetic field used to align the protons can be produced by either a permanent magnet or a superconducting magnet. The external magnetic field must be uniform to ±50 microtesla (μT) so that a proton in a particular tissue has the same Larmor resonance frequency no matter where in the body it is located.

The magnetic field extending outside the bore is called the **fringe field.** The magnetic field that would extend out from the sides of the magnet is reduced almost to zero by special shielding coils.

Permanent Magnets

Permanent magnets are made of a ferromagnetic metal alloy that produces fields with strengths from 0.25 to 0.5 T. They require no current-carrying coils, need little maintenance, and have a large bore. This is an advantage in scanning large patients or individuals who have claustrophobia because most superconducting MR units have a 60-centimeter (cm) diameter bore and looks like a long tube. Permanent magnet MR units produce smaller RF signals, which may result in longer scan times. They are often installed in private clinics because they are less expensive to install and operate than superconducting MRI units.

Superconducting Magnets

Superconducting magnets employ coils made of a superconducting material to produce the magnetic field. The superconducting coils surround the bore of the magnet. Typical superconducting bore diameters are 50 to 60cm. The bore diameter limits the size of patients who can be scanned in a superconducting magnet. The superconducting coils operate in the same way as a conventional electromagnet to generate the magnetic field. Current flowing in the superconducting coils produces the magnetic field. The difference from conventional electromagnets is that superconducting coils allow the current to flow without any resistance at temperatures below 250°C (23 K). **Liquid helium** is employed to maintain this low temperature. The liquid helium is contained in a vacuum vessel called a **Dewar,** which surrounds the coils. The Dewar acts as a giant insulated Thermos bottle. Once the current is flowing in the superconducting coils, no additional electric power is needed to maintain the current

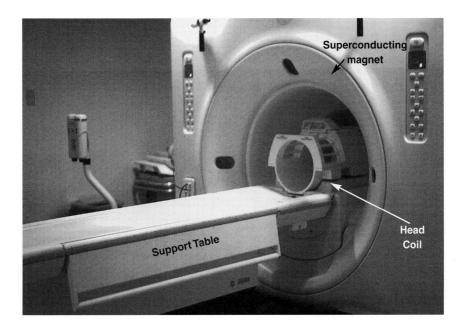

Figure 19.5 **A superconducting MR unit with a head coil on the support table. (Courtesy of GE Medical Systems. With permission)**

flow because the coils have zero resistance. The magnetic field of a superconducting unit is never turned off. Superconducting magnets produce magnetic fields from 1 to 1.5 T. Figure 19.5 shows a superconducting MRI unit with a surface coil designed for MR scans of the head on the support table.

> *MRI units employ either a permanent or a superconducting magnet to produce the external magnetic field. Superconducting magnets produce a constant magnetic field generated by superconducting coils. The superconducting coils, which have zero electrical resistance, are surrounded by liquid helium in a Dewar to maintain them at a temperature of 23 K.*

Shim Coils

Superconducting magnets employ shim coils to improve the uniformity of the external magnetic field and improve the quality of the MR images. The shim coils are mounted around the bore. Current in the shim coils improves the uniformity of the external magnetic field within the bore to ±50μT.

Gradient Coils

Gradient coils produce slight differences in the field strength at different locations in the patient. These slight differences in the field produce different Larmor frequencies at different locations in the body. By selecting the proper gradient field, a specific slice location and orientation can be chosen. Only the protons at the selected location are rotated out of alignment and contribute to the MR signal. Each image slice requires a separate gradient setting. During an MRI scan, the current through the gradient coils is automatically changed to collect data from the individual slices. The electronic indexing of the slice locations means that the patient is not moved during the scan.

Both permanent and superconducting MR units employ gradient coils to allow the operator to select the type and locations of imaging planes. Coronal, sagittal, transverse, or oblique sections can be selected. Pulsing of the gradient coils during image acquisition produces the familiar knocking or rapping noise heard during MR scanning.

Figure 19.6 shows the location of the gradient coils in a typical MR unit.

Surface Coils

Both permanent and superconducting MR units use surface coils to send the RF excitation pulses into the patient and to detect the RF signal from the pre-

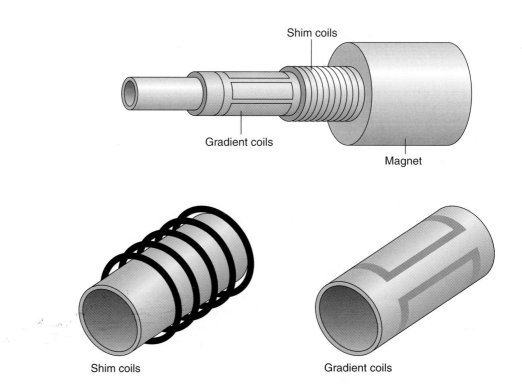

Figure 19.6 Schematic of gradient coil locations.

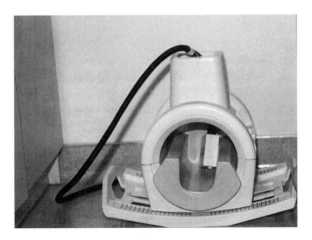

Figure 19.7 **Extremity surface coil.**

cessing protons. Surface coils are so named because they are placed on the surface of the patient. Surface coils are also called signal coils because they send and detect the signal. Surface coils are designed for imaging specific regions of the body. Figure 19.7 shows an extremity surface coil.

> *Shim coils improve the uniformity of the magnetic field. Gradient coils are used to select the different imaging planes. Surface coils are used to transmit the excitation pulse and collect the RF signals from the hydrogen protons precessing back into alignment with the external magnetic field.*

Patient Support Table

The patient table supports the patient and allows the patient to be moved into the bore for scanning. The table must be capable of supporting at least 350 pounds. It is constructed of nonmagnetic material to avoid altering the magnetic field. The table is not used to move the patient during the scanning process as in CT scanning because the scan slice location and orientation are selected electronically using the gradient coils.

Computer

The computer is a major component in the formation of MR images. It programs the gradient coils to select different imaging planes, and it processes the RF signals from surface coils into digital data to create the MR images. The digital MR images can be transmitted, stored, and displayed just like any other digital images. Display systems allow viewing of the images on a TV monitor. A laser printer can be coupled to the computer system to produce hard copies on film.

RF SHIELDING

The MR room is surrounded by a copper screen called a **Faraday cage.** The Faraday cage prevents external RF signals from entering the room because the RF energy cannot penetrate through the copper screen. RF shielding is necessary because the RF signals from the precessing protons in the patient are very weak. In order to detect their weak signals, external RF energy must be minimized.

HAZARDS

There is no ionizing radiation associated with MR imaging, so none of the potential hazards of x-ray exposure are present during MR examinations. The strong magnetic fields and the energy from the RF signals are the major hazards in MR imaging. Ferromagnetic objects can become projectiles when they are attracted into the bore of the magnet by the fringe field. Screwdrivers and oxygen bottles are some of the more common objects that can become projectiles. Magnetic objects should not be brought into the MR room.

Patients with metallic implants, even if they are not ferromagnetic, such as metal prostheses, surgical clips and, cochlear implants, may be excluded from MR scanning because of the possible interaction between the RF energy and the metal, just as may happen if a metal fork is left in a microwave oven. Patients with pacemakers should not be near the magnet because the fringe field may interfere with the pacemaker operation.

An MRI unit uses no ionizing radiation. A Faraday cage shields the MR room from external RF energy so that the weak RF signals from the precessing protons can be detected. Magnetic objects may be violently attracted into the bore. Metal implants may be heated by the RF fields. There is also the possibility that the magnetic field will disrupt cardiac pacemakers.

SUMMARY

The protons used in MR imaging are the hydrogen nuclei in the human body. Protons in a magnetic field align in the direction of the magnetic field. Their Larmor resonance frequency depends on the magnetic field strength. Protons in stronger magnetic fields have higher Larmor frequencies. An RF excitation pulse is used to rotate the protons out of alignment with the magnetic field. As the protons precess back into alignment, they give off RF energy at their Larmor frequency. These RF signals are used to form magnetic resonance images. There are two relaxation times, T1 and T2, associated with the proton realignment. T1- and T2-weighted images of the same tissues can have different appearances. Both T1- and T2-weighted images provide excellent soft tissue contrast. The decision to obtain a T1- or T2-weighted image is based upon the structures to be imaged. The external magnetic field used to align the protons can be produced by either a permanent magnet or a superconducting magnet. Magnetic fields are measured in units of tesla or gauss. Permanent magnet units have field strengths of 0.25 to 0.5 T. MR units with superconducting magnets have field strengths of 1.0 to 1.5 T. The coils of superconducting magnets have zero electrical resistance. The coils are maintained at 23 K by liquid helium contained in a Dewar vacuum container. Gradient coils are used to select the MR imaging planes. Surface coils emit the excitation RF pulses and receive the RF signals from the protons precessing back into alignment. No ferromagnetic objects should be brought into the MR room because of the strength of the magnetic field. Metallic implants may be heated by the RF signals, causing thermal burns. A Faraday cage surrounding the room shields the MR unit from external RF signals.

QUESTIONS

1. Precession is
   a. the diameter of the bore.
   b. proton rotation around the magnetic field direction.
   c. spinning of the RF field.
   d. a unit of magnetic field strength.
2. The most abundant element in the human body is
   a. oxygen.
   b. hydrogen.
   c. carbon.
   d. nitrogen.
3. The Larmor frequency is the resonant frequency of the
   a. magnetic field.
   b. superconducting coils.
   c. protons in a magnetic field.
   d. permanent magnet.
4. Resonance is the
   a. loss of resistance at low temperatures.
   b. spinning of the hydrogen proton.
   c. absorption or emission of energy at a specific frequency.
   d. volume of a Dewar vessel.

5. The hydrogen protons are excited during MR imaging by
   a. RF pulses at the Larmor resonance frequency.
   b. RF in the fringe field.
   c. contrast material injection.
   d. RF pulses outside the bore.
6. Permanent magnets
   a. produce low fields.
   b. have a wide bore.
   c. require no external power.
   d. have/do all of the above.
7. MR images are obtained utilizing ionizing radiation.
   a. True
   b. False
8. Superconducting magnets
   a. use superconducting coils.
   b. must be maintained at a low temperature.
   c. have current flowing continuously with no electrical resistance.
   d. have/do all of the above.
9. Protons precessing back into alignment with the external magnetic field have a specific
   a. velocity.
   b. relaxation time.
   c. recombination time.
   d. orbital residence.
10. The resonance of the protons depends on
    a. their relaxation times.
    b. RF pulses.
    c. the magnetic field strength.
    d. precession.
11. Shim coils are used to
    a. select the slice to be imaged.
    b. produce and detect RF signals.
    c. prevent excess heating during scanning.
    d. improve the homogeneity of the magnetic field.
12. Gradient coils are used to
    a. select the slice to be imaged.
    b. produce and detect RF signals.
    c. prevent excess heating during scanning.
    d. improve the homogeneity of the magnetic field.
13. Liquid helium
    a. is a superconducting liquid.
    b. must be kept at temperatures above 23°C.
    c. is used in permanent magnet MR units.
    d. is used to cool superconducting coils.

14. A Dewar is
    a. liquid helium maintained at 23°C.
    b. a vacuum container.
    c. a gradient coil.
    d. a superconducting coil.
15. T1 is the time associated with the
    a. harmonic frequency bandwidth.
    b. proton's loss of phase.
    c. proton precessing back into alignment.
    d. gradient signal resonance.
16. T2 is the time associated with the
    a. harmonic frequency bandwidth.
    b. proton's loss of phase.
    c. proton precessing back into alignment.
    d. gradient signal resonance.
17. Safety concerns in MRI include
    a. effects on pacemakers.
    b. ferromagnetic projectiles.
    c. heating of metallic implants.
    d. all of the above.
18. The MR room is shielded with a
    a. superconducting coil.
    b. concrete wall.
    c. Faraday cage.
    d. lead wall.
19. Surface coils are used to
    a. select the slice to be imaged.
    b. produce and detect RF signals.
    c. prevent excess heating during scanning.
    d. improve the homogeneity of the magnetic field.
20. The MR room is shielded against
    a. ionizing radiation.
    b. RF energy leaving the room.
    c. RF energy entering the room.
    d. external magnetic fields.
21. The knocking or rapping noise during MR scanning is caused by pulsing of the
    a. magnet coil.
    b. gradient coils.
    c. signal coils.
    d. shim coils.
22. The maximum allowed table motion speed during MR scanning is
    a. 0 cm/s.
    b. 5 cm/s.
    c. 10 cm/s.
    d. 50 cm/s.

ANSWERS TO CHAPTER 19 QUESTIONS

1.	b	12.	a
2.	b	13.	d
3.	c	14.	b
4.	c	15.	c
5.	a	16.	b
6.	d	17.	d
7.	b	18.	c
8.	d	19.	b
9.	b	20.	c
10.	c	21.	b
11.	d	22.	a

20

Quality Control

OBJECTIVES

Upon completion of this chapter, the student will be able to

1. State the factors included in radiographic quality control.
2. State the factors included in processor quality control.
3. State the types and sources of film artifacts.
4. State the factors included in mammographic quality control.
5. State the factors included in fluoroscopic quality control.
6. State the factors included in computed tomography quality control.

INTRODUCTION

In the health care industry, the terms *quality assurance* and *quality control* have different meanings. Quality assurance deals primarily with personnel and their interactions with the patient and other staff. It is the term used to describe the process or program used to maintain high-quality imaging. It is a many-step process that involves identifying goals, formulating plans to achieve these goals, implementing the plans, and evaluating the success of the program. Quality assurance also includes outcomes analysis, such as how often the radiologist's report agrees with the patient's condition.

Quality control refers to the measurement and evaluation of radiographic equipment, together with the identification and correction of problems associated with the equipment. It includes periodic checks and monitoring of the operation of all equipment, initial acceptance testing of equipment, periodic testing of equipment performance, and the steps taken to correct deviations from expected performance. Quality control measurements often require specialized equipment. This chapter discusses the factors that should be moni-

tored and the frequency of monitoring. Often regularly scheduled maintenance can detect and correct potential problems before they affect image
quality. Documentation of all quality control monitoring should include the
date, the type of test, the outcome, and identification of the individual per-
forming the monitoring test.

RADIOGRAPHIC QUALITY CONTROL

Radiographic quality control consists of periodic monitoring of the x-ray tube,
the associated electric circuits, the accuracy of the exposure factors, and the
film processor. The factors that must be monitored, the test tools used, the acceptable limits, and the frequency of monitoring are presented in Table 20.1.

Measurement of the Focal Spot or System Resolution

As the tube ages, the anode surface may become rough, resulting in a larger
effective focal spot, because the rough surface leads to an increase in off-focus
radiation. Degradation of the focal spot can produce blurred structures on the
radiograph. This is known as focal spot blur. The focal spot size or spatial resolution should be measured annually. The size should be within ±50 percent of
the nominal or stated focal spot size. The **pinhole camera** and a star pattern
phantom are used to measure the focal spot size. The most accurate method is
the pinhole camera, which produces an image of the focal spot. However, the
pinhole camera is extremely difficult and time-consuming to set up and use.

Table 20-1
Radiographic Quality Control Factors

Factor	Monitoring Frequency	Limits	Test Tool
1. Focal spot size	Annual	±50%	Slit or pinhole camera
Spatial resolution	Annual	> 8 lp/mm	Bar phantom
2. Collimation	Annual	±2% SID	Film + metal markers
3. kVp	Annual	±4 kVp	Penetrometer or step wedge
4. Filtration	Annual	> 2.5 mm Al	Aluminum sheets
5. Exposure time	Annual	< 10 ms, ±20%	Exposure meter or spinning top
	Annual	> 10 ms, ±5%	
6. Exposure reproducibility	Annual	±5%	Exposure meter or ion chamber
7. Exposure linearity	Annual	±10%	Exposure meter or ion chamber
8. AEC	Annual	None	Exposure meter

The star pattern uses an image of a star to determine the focal spot size by using a formula to relate the diameter of the star image to the size of the focal spot.

The **bar phantom,** an alternating series of metal strips with different separations, gives the spatial resolution of the system directly. The advantage of the bar pattern is that it can readily detect degradation of image quality. The resolution of a film screen system should be greater than 8 line pairs per millimeter (lp/mm). Figure 20.1A and B shows photographs of the star and bar phantoms together with the star and bar pattern images used to measure the size of the focal spot or determine the resolution of the imaging system. The penny in Fig. 20.1A indicates the size of the phantoms. Today almost all annual resolution monitoring tests are performed with a resolution bar phantom.

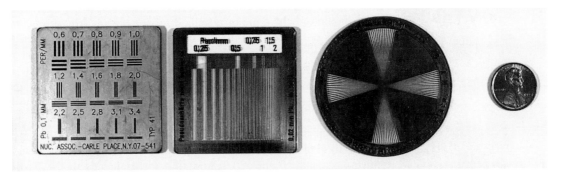

A

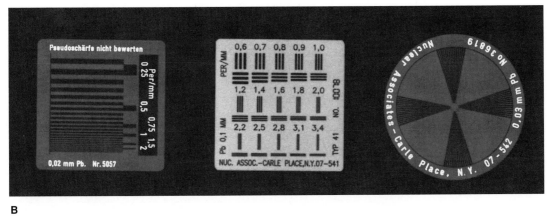

B

Figure 20.1 *A.* Star-and-bar pattern phantoms, *B.* The x-ray images used to measure spatial resolution.

Collimation

It is important that the light field and the radiation field coincide so that the x-ray field placement is correct. This is called light-radiation field congruence.

The alignment of the collimator that defines the x-ray beam and the light field must be checked annually and whenever the tube or field light is replaced. To measure the light-radiation field congruence, a film cassette is placed on the tabletop. The edges of the light field are marked on the cassette by placing metal markers such as coins or paper clips at the edge of the light field. An exposure is made, and the edges of the light and radiation fields are measured. The sum of the differences between the light and radiation field edges must be less than 2 percent of the source to image receptor distance (SID).

kVp Accuracy

If the kVp settings are incorrect, the patient dose may be increased and the image contrast compromised. The applied kVp can be measured directly using a voltage divider. This requires disconnecting the high-voltage cables from the x-ray tube and should only be done by a trained service person. Measurement of the kVp can also be made using a step wedge penetrometer. The optical density under the steps of the penetrometer is related to the kVp of the beam because higher-kVp x-rays have greater penetration. The same principle is used in modern electronic kVp meters. Electronic detectors measure the penetration of the x-ray beam through two different attenuating filters. The ratio of the readings from the two detectors is used to calculate the kVp of the x-ray beam. Electronic kVp meters are more accurate than penetrometers and are the preferred method of measuring kVp. The kVp should be within ±4 kV and should be tested annually. Figure 20.2 shows an electronic kVp meter. Electronic kVp meters are accurate to ±1 kVp and give the maximum, average, and

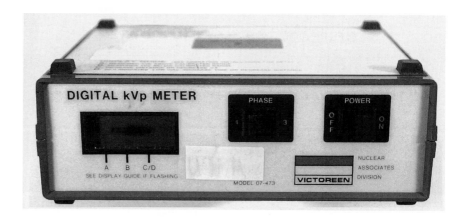

Figure 20.2 **An electronic kVp meter.**

effective kVp of the x-ray beam. kVp measurements are usually made by the service engineer or the medical physicist.

Filtration

The filtration of an x-ray beam is reported in terms of its **half-value layer (HVL),** expressed in terms of aluminum thickness. The HVL of the x-ray beam is measured annually to ensure that the penetrability of the beam has not been degraded. The HVL is measured using thin sheets of aluminum (Al). A series of output measurements is made, first with no added aluminum in the beam, then with added thicknesses of Al. The HVL is calculated from the decrease in output as the Al thickness is increased. An HVL of at least 2.5 millimeters (mm) Al equivalent is required for a tube operating at 70 kVp or higher. The tube window and light field mirror contribute about 1 mm Al to the total filtration.

Exposure Time

If the timer settings are not accurate, the mAs values may be incorrect, resulting in poor-quality images. In the past, a **spinning top** with a hole in a metal disk was used to check the timer stations. After an exposure of the spinning disk was made, the hole in the disk appeared as a series of dots on the film because the x-rays are produced only at the peak of the voltage cycle. The exposure time can be determined by counting the number of dots. For example, a 0.1-second (s) exposure would be expected to show an image with 12 dots, representing 0.1 of the 120 pulses that occur each second with a single-phase full-wave-rectified circuit. A synchronous motor was used to check the timer accuracy of three-phase units. Today all timer measurements are made electronically. A radiation detector measures the duration of the x-ray exposure. Timer accuracy should be checked annually and must be within ±5 percent for exposure times greater than 10 ms and within ±20 percent for exposure times less than 10 ms.

Exposure Reproducibility

Exposure reproducibility means that the radiation output [measured in milliroentgens (mR)] should be the same for a series of exposures in which all the technical factors are held constant. Exposure reproducibility should be measured annually using a radiation dosimeter.

    Exposure reciprocity means that each combination of mA and time that results in the same mAs should give the same radiation output (measured in milliroentgens) within ±5 percent of the average output. Table 20.2 gives examples from x-ray unit A of how different combinations of time and mA can give the same mAs value and the same radiation output.

    The differences in exposure as measured by the output in milliroentgens arise from slight differences in the calibration of the timer and mA stations.

Table 20.2
Exposure Reciprocity from Unit A

Time set	mA	mAs	Radiation Output (mR)
0.02	500	10	40
0.033	300	10	42
0.05	200	10	41
0.1	100	10	40
0.2	50	10	40
0.4	25	10	39

Unit A meets the exposure reproducibility requirements because all mAs values are within ±5 percent of the average.

Exposure Linearity

Exposure linearity is a measure of how the radiation output in milliroentgens increases with increasing mAs. The radiation output per mAs (mR/mAs) should remain the same within ±10 percent as the mAs is changed. Table 20.3 gives examples of different combinations of time and mA and different mAs from x-ray unit B.

The mR/mAs should track linearly within ±10 percent with changes in mAs. Unit B does not meet the linearity requirement because the 0.4 s, 25 mA entry differs from the average by more than 10 percent. We know that the 25 mA station rather than the 0.4 s time station is faulty because the 0.4 s, 50 mA selection gave an mR/mAs value within ±10 percent of the average value.

Table 20.3
Exposure Linearity Measurements on Unit B

Time	mA	mAs	mR	mR/mAs
0.05	100	5	19	3.8
0.025	200	5	20	4.0
0.1	50	5	21	4.1
0.1	100	10	41	4.1
0.2	50	10	38	3.8
0.4	25	10	31	2.9
0.4	50	20	79	3.9
0.2	100	20	80	4.0

Automatic Exposure Control

The automatic exposure control (**AEC**) is designed to compensate for differences in patient size by adjusting the time. The AEC measures the exit radiation and adjusts the exposure time to produce a proper-density image. The AEC circuit is tested annually to verify that the mAs increases with increasing patient thickness.

Radiographic quality control includes annual testing of focal spot size or system resolution; collimation; kVp accuracy; exposure time, reproducibility, and linearity; and AEC performance.

PROCESSOR QUALITY CONTROL

Processor quality control is necessary to ensure that the processed films produce consistently high-quality images. Processor quality control consists of daily monitoring and periodic cleaning and maintenance of the processor. All efforts expended in obtaining an excellent latent image are wasted if the latent image is not processed in a reproducible manner. Table 20.4 lists the processor quality assurance factors together with their recommended monitoring frequency.

Processor Monitoring

The overall operation of the processor is most easily monitored by preparing a sensitometric strip and processing it in the processor each morning as soon as the processor is warmed up.

The sensitometer is an instrument that exposes a test film to light through a series of filters. Using the sensitometer eliminates any variations due to x-ray

Table 20.4
Processor Quality Control Factors

Factor	Monitoring Frequency	Limits	Test Tools
Sensitometry/densitometry	Daily	Department limits	Sensitometer Densitometer
Temperature	Daily	±2°F	Digital thermometer
Crossover racks cleaning	Daily	Clean	Visual inspection
Replenishment rates	Weekly	Manufacturer's specifications	Meter or gauge
Tanks and transport roller cleaning	Depends on number of films/week	Clean	Visual inspection

output variations. The output of the sensitometer is a film with a series of densities extending from base plus fog level to completely black in discrete steps. For this reason, this process is also called a step wedge exposure. Figure 20.3 shows a sensitometer and a densitometer.

A densitometer is used to measure the optical density (OD) of each step. The background density (which is the base plus fog density), average speed, and contrast in the middensity range are calculated from the measured optical density values. These values are then recorded and compared with previous measured values. The optical density values from the daily sensitometric strip must be within acceptable limits, which are set by the department. The base plus fog value must be less than 0.05 OD. If the readings are outside the acceptable limits, the processor cannot be used clinically until the problem is corrected. Figure 20.4 shows a sensitometer strip image.

The temperatures of the processor solutions should be checked with a digital thermometer and recorded daily. Mercury thermometers should never be used to measure processor temperatures because mercury contamination of a processor is almost impossible to eliminate. Slight changes in the temperature of the developer solution will produce significant density changes in the final radiograph. The developer temperature should be maintained within ±2°F of the set value. The developer and fixer replenishment rates should be monitored weekly and maintained within the supplier's tolerances.

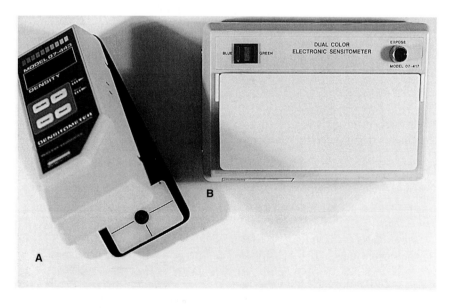

Figure 20.3 A densitometer (A) and a sensitometer (B).

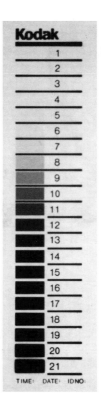

Figure 20.4 **Sensitometer strip.**

IMAGE ARTIFACTS

An **artifact** is an unwanted density or image on the radiograph. Film artifacts can be divided into three categories based on their source. The major sources of artifacts are exposure artifacts, handling artifacts, and processor artifacts.

Exposure Artifacts

Exposure artifacts occur during the exposure of the patient rather than after the exposure has been made. They can be present with both film and digital image receptors. Exposure artifacts are caused by improper positioning, technical factors, or patient motion. Grid cutoff due to improper alignment of the grid also can produce artifacts; these appear as lighter areas on one or both sides of the image.

Lack of patient preparation can also be a significant source of exposure artifacts. Failure to remove eyeglasses, jewelry, rings, watches, and hair clips will produce exposure artifacts. Hair, especially if braided or wet, can cause exposure artifacts. Figure 20.5 presents an example of an exposure artifact due to a necklace.

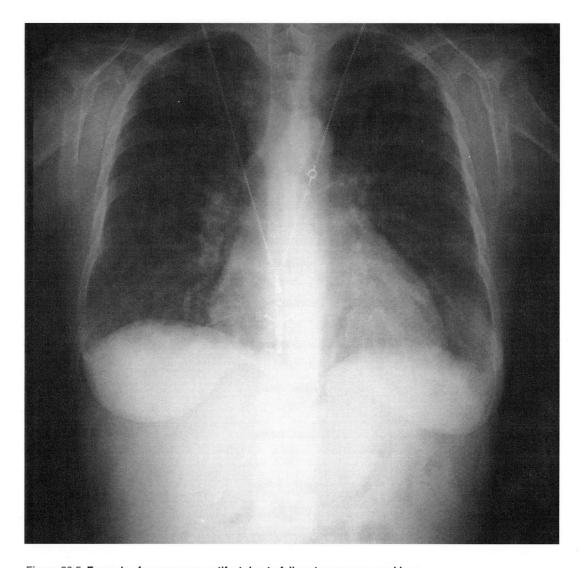

Figure 20.5 Example of an exposure artifact due to faliure to remove a necklace.

Exposure artifacts can be reduced or eliminated by careful attention to detail before taking the exposure.

Handling and Storage Artifacts

Handling artifacts occur because of improper handling and storage of the film. Handling artifacts include light leaks, static, crease marks, and fingerprints. The source of handling artifacts is usually easy to identify because the cassettes must be light-tight; any physical damage or rough handling may destroy the light-tight integrity. Light leaks appear as **positive-density areas,** darker areas on the image. Screens should be cleaned monthly with a special cleaning fluid and lint-free wipes to prevent static buildup. Static artifacts are caused by electrical discharges and appear as positive dark lines on the image. They are most common in winter, when the air is dry and relative humidity is low. The three types of static artifacts are tree, which appear with branches; crown, which have many lines radiating from a common area; and smudge, which appear as slightly positive areas on the image. Film should be stored under conditions where the relative humidity is between 40 and 60 percent and the temperature is below 72°F.

Rough handling of the undeveloped film can produce crease or kink marks, sometimes called fingernail marks because they resemble fingernail clippings. These positive-density marks result from bending or creasing of the film during loading, unloading, or processing. Handling the film with sweaty, greasy, or oily hands can result in **negative-density** areas, or lighter areas, in the form of fingerprint marks on the film.

Figure 20.6 presents examples of handling artifacts.

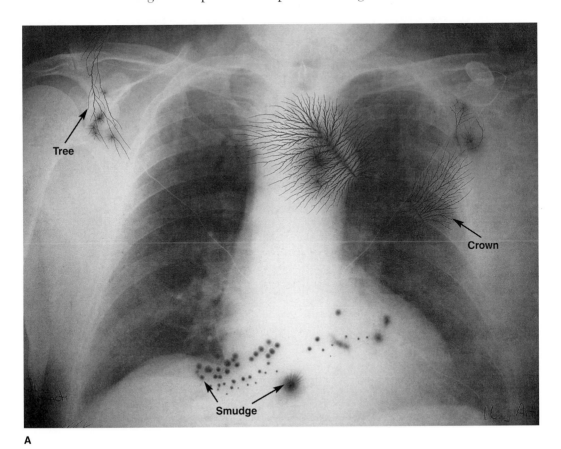

A

Figure 20.6 **Examples of handling artifacts: A, static, tree, smudge, and crown.**

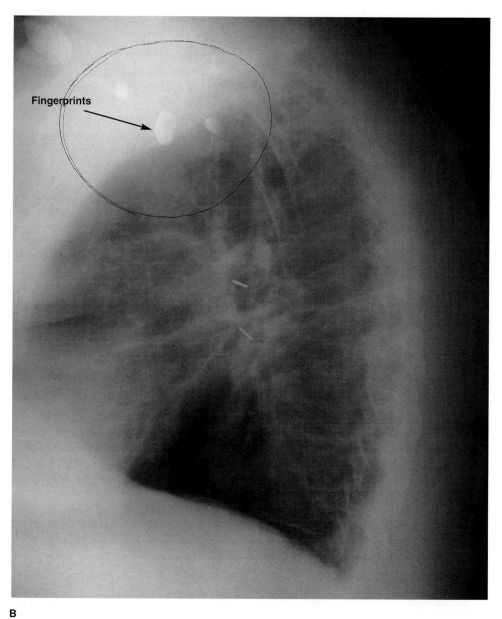

B

Figure 20.6 *(continued)* B, Fingerprint artifacts.

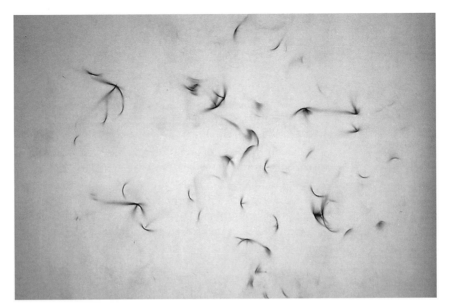

C

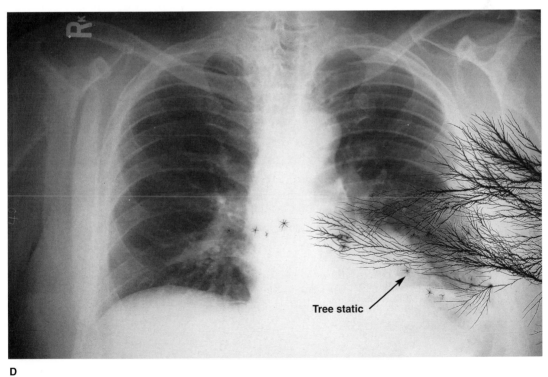

Tree static

D

Figure 20.6 *(continued)*   C, Crease marks (fingernails). D, Tree static.

Processor Artifacts

Processor artifacts occur as a result of improper processor quality control. Processor artifacts include pi marks, guide-shoe marks, and chemical stains.

A deposit of dirt or chemicals on a portion of a roller will make a dark or positive mark on the film on each revolution. These **pi mark** artifacts are perpendicular to the direction of film travel through the processor and are spaced pi, or 3.14, times the roller diameter apart. Typical transport rollers are 1 inch (in.) in diameter, so pi marks are usually 3.14 in. apart.

Regularly scheduled processor cleaning will eliminate pi marks and many other processor artifacts. It is essential to clean the crossover racks daily.

Guide-shoe marks are caused by the guide shoes, which are used to reverse the direction of the film. Guide-shoe marks indicate that the guide shoes are misaligned and are scratching the film emulsion. These marks appear as light lines or negative densities parallel to the film direction. Realignment of the guide shoes will eliminate guide-shoe marks. Figure 20.7 shows guide-shoe marks.

Exposure artifacts result from improper positioning, improper technical factors, and faulty patient preparation. Film storage and handling are critical to avoiding artifacts. Film should be stored at temperatures below 72°F and relative humidity between 40 and 60 percent. Base fog should be less than 0.05. Processor artifacts include pi marks, guide-shoe marks, and chemical stains. Regularly scheduled processor maintenance and cleaning will eliminate most processor artifacts.

COMPUTED RADIOGRAPHY QUALITY CONTROL

Artifacts in computed radiography (CR) systems are usually produced by sudden failure of internal components. Such artifacts are easy to detect because they occupy all or a significant portion of the image and take the form of streaks or lines.

As part of a computed radiography quality assurance program, it is important to monitor the sensitivity and dynamic range of the system annually to ensure that there has been no degradation of the detector plates' efficiency. The dynamic range is the difference between the lowest and highest signals the system can process.

FLUOROSCOPY QUALITY CONTROL

There are two types of fluoroscopic units, stationary and mobile. Stationary fluoroscopic units must be installed with a source to skin distance (SSD) of at

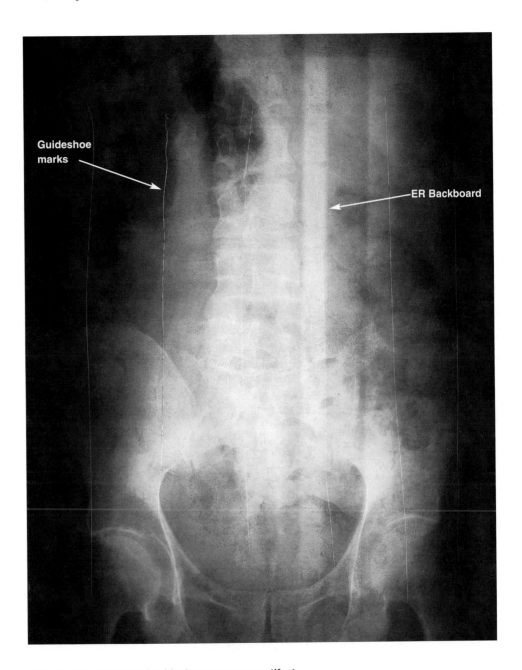

Figure 20.7 **Example of guideshoe processor artifact.**

least 38 centimeters (cm) (15 in.) at tabletop. Mobile C-arm fluoroscopy units must have an SSD of at least 30 cm (12 in.). Quality control of fluoroscopic systems consists of monitoring the radiation output exposure rate, the spatial and contrast resolution, and the operation of the automatic brightness control (ABC) of the system.

Radiation Output or Exposure Rate

The exposure rate must be checked with an attenuation phantom placed in the beam to ensure that the measurements are made under conditions similar to those in clinical practice. Typical entrance skin exposure rates **(ESE)** are about 3 rad per minute (min) [3 milligray (mGy)/min]. Under normal conditions, the ESE should be less than 5 rad/min (50 mGy/min), and it must always be less than 10 rad/min (100 mGy/min). Because the ESE is higher with higher magnification modes, it must be measured at all magnification modes. The ESE of a fluoroscopic system must be measured annually. A general rule of thumb is that the ESE is about 2 rad/min per mA.

EXAMPLE 1:

What is the ESE if a 3-min examination uses a tube current of 1.3 mA?

ANSWER:

$$ESE = 2 \text{ rad/min} \cdot (mA \times 3 \text{ min} \times 1.3 \text{ mA}$$
$$ESE = 7.8 \text{ rad}$$

Resolution

The spatial resolution of a fluoroscopic system is checked by placing a resolution phantom in the beam and observing the system resolution. The resolution phantom consists of a series of lead bars of differing separation labeled in line pairs per millimeter. The higher the number of line pairs per millimeter visible, the better the resolution of the system. Modern fluoroscopic systems have resolutions between 1.2 and 2.5 lp/mm. The resolution must be checked annually at all magnification modes. Figure 20.8 shows an example of an image obtained with a fluoroscopic resolution phantom.

Automatic Brightness Control

Automatic brightness control circuits are designed to maintain a constant image brightness regardless of the thickness of the patient. The operation of an

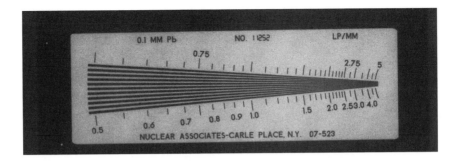

Figure 20.8 X-ray image obtained with a fluoroscopic resolution phantom.

ABC circuit is measured by placing attenuators of different thicknesses in the beam. The mAs should increase with increasing attenuator thickness. The operation of the backup timer in the radiographic mode can be verified by placing a lead sheet in the beam. The beam should be terminated at the backup timer setting, usually about 500 mAs or 5 s. ABC circuits should be tested annually. Some fluoroscopic quality control tests and their limits are shown in Table 20.5.

PROTECTIVE APPAREL QUALITY CONTROL

Protective aprons and other radiation shields must be checked for tears, gaps, holes, and voids at least annually. All protective apparel should be visually inspected and also tested radiographically. This inspection may be performed fluoroscopically or by taking radiographs of the apparel. Figure 20.9A shows a photograph of a normal-appearing lead glove. Figure 20.9B shows a radiograph of the same glove that shows a gap in the protection because the internal lead shielding is torn and shifted.

Table 20.5
Fluoroscopic Quality Control Tests

Factor	Frequency	Limits	Tools
Exposure rate	Annual	<10 rad/min	Exposure meter
Resolution	Annual	None	Resolution phantom
Automatic brightness control	Annual	None	Exposure meter
Protective apparel	Annual	No cracks or gaps	Fluoroscope or film

COMPUTED TOMOGRAPHY QUALITY CONTROL

Computed tomographic quality control includes annual tests of system noise and uniformity, linearity, spatial resolution, contrast resolution, slice thickness, patient exposure, and support table increment accuracy.

The test for noise and uniformity is performed daily. A water phantom is scanned and the computer adjusts the system so that the CT number of water equals zero. The uniformity should be such that there is variation of less than ±10 CT units across the image.

CT linearity is measured using a special phantom with plastic rods of different calibrated densities. The unit is initially calibrated so that water has a CT number of 0 and air has a CT number of −1000. Other quality control tests of a CT unit are similar to those performed on a conventional radiographic or fluoroscopic unit. These include tests of the spatial resolution, contrast resolu-

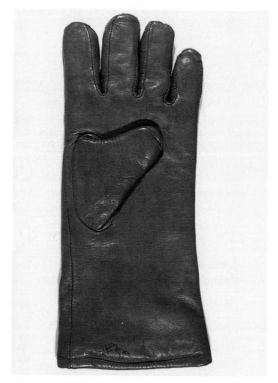

A

Figure 20.9 **A, Photograph of lead glove.**

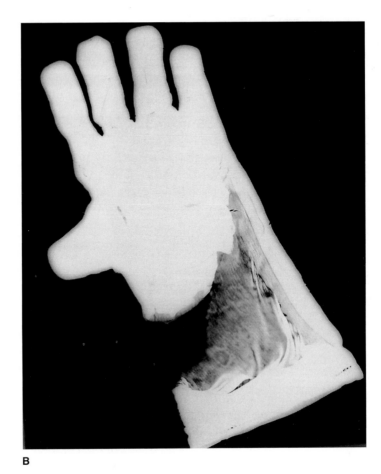

Figure 20.9 *(continued)* B, X-ray of a lead glove showing a gap in protection.

tion, and patient exposure. Tests unique to the CT unit include support table increment accuracy and slice thickness. Table 20.6 lists the quality control tests for a CT scanner.

MAMMOGRAPHIC QUALITY CONTROL

A facility must be accredited by a recognized agency to perform mammographic examinations. The federal Mammography Standards Quality Act (MQSA) sets out the standards that accredited facilities must meet. The mam-

Table 20.6
CT Quality Control Tests

Factor	Frequency	Limits
Noise	Daily	±10 HU
Uniformity	Daily	±0.04%
Spatial resolution	Annual	±20%
Contrast resolution	Annual	±0.5%
Slice thicknesses < 5 mm	Annual	0.5 mm
Slice thicknesses > 5 mm	Annual	1 mm
Support table indexing	Annual	±1 mm

mography technologist is responsible for a series of daily, weekly, monthly, quarterly, semiannual, and annual monitoring tests. These tests must be documented, and records must be available for the annual inspection.

The tests, their limits, and their required frequency are shown in Table 20.7.

Computed radiography quality control includes annual monitoring of the sensitivity and dynamic range of the system. Fluoroscopic quality control includes monitoring the output rate and resolution at all magnification modes. The output rate is limited to no more than 10 rad/min. Protective apparel must be inspected for gaps, voids, and tears at least annually. The required quality control tests for mammography are spelled out in the Mammography Quality Standards Act. The results of each of these monitoring tests must be

Table 20.7
Mammography Quality Control Tests

Test	Frequency
Darkroom cleanliness	Daily
Processor quality control	Daily
Screen cleaning	Weekly
View box cleaning	Weekly
Phantom image quality	Weekly
Visual inspection of equipment	Monthly
Repeat analysis	Quarterly
Fixer retention	Quarterly
Film/screen contact	Semiannually
Compression device	Semiannually
Darkroom fog	Semiannually

documented, and the records must be available for review during the annual inspection.

SUMMARY

Quality assurance deals with personnel and the performance of the team required to produce high-quality radiographs. Quality control deals with equipment performance. Radiographic quality control includes monitoring the components that affect radiologic image quality. These include focal spot size, kVp, the timer, exposure linearity, and processor performance, including monitoring of processor temperature and replenishment rate. The focal spot size or system resolution should be measured at least annually to detect gradual degradation of image resolution. The focal spot must be within ±50 percent of the nominal focal spot size. Spatial resolution should be greater than ±8 lp/mm. Regular processor quality control tests are necessary to ensure that the processed films are of high quality. An exposure made with a sensitometer and measured with a densitometer gives a good measure of processor operation. Artifacts are unwanted densities or images on a radiograph. Pi marks are positive-density artifacts perpendicular to the direction of film travel through the processor and separated by 3.14 in. Guide-shoe marks are negative-density straight-line artifacts parallel to the direction of film travel through the processor. CT quality assurance tests include daily scanning of a water phantom to monitor CT number and field uniformity. Fluoroscopy quality control involves monitoring the exposure rate and spatial resolution. The tabletop dose rate must be less than 0.01 Gy/min (10 rad/min). Mammographic quality control tests are specified by the federal Mammographic Quality Standards Act.

QUESTIONS

1. The sum of the differences between the light and the x-ray field edges must be within _____ of the SID.
   a. 1 percent
   b. 2 percent
   c. 5 percent
   d. 10 percent
2. The _____ measures the system resolution directly.
   a. pinhole camera
   b. optical densitometer
   c. spinning top
   d. bar phantom

3. The _____ measures the size of the focal spot.
   a. pinhole camera
   b. optical densitometer
   c. spinning top
   d. bar phantom
4. The kVp of the beam should be within ±_____ kVp of the kVp setting.
   a. 2
   b. 4
   c. 5
   d. 10
5. The penetrability or filtration of an x-ray beam is reported in terms of its
   a. EMF.
   b. RTV.
   c. HVL.
   d. MAQ.
6. An x-ray tube operating above 70 kVp must have an HVL of at least
   _____ mm Al.
   a. 1.5
   b. 2.5
   c. 3.5
   d. 5
7. The same mAs value achieved with several different mA and time settings
   must produce the same radiation output within _____ percent of the
   average.
   a. ±2
   b. ±5
   c. ±10
   d. ±20
8. The mR/mAs _____ increase with increases in mAs.
   a. should
   b. should not
9. During the exposure linearity test, the mR/mAs should vary by no more
   than ±_____ percent from the average.
   a. 2
   b. 5
   c. 7
   d. 10
10. The developer temperature should be maintained within _____°F of the
    set value.
    a. ±2
    b. ±4
    c. ±5
    d. ±8

11. The _____ can be used to measure timer accuracy.
    a. pinhole camera
    b. optical densitometer
    c. spinning top
    d. bar phantom
12. Mammographic quality control requirements are specified in the
    a. RSNA.
    b. LSMFT.
    c. DDT.
    d. MQSA.
13. During the daily CT quality control procedure, the CT number of water is set to
    a. −1000.
    b. 0.
    c. +500.
    d. +1000.
14. A 4-min fluoroscopic examination with a 1.5-mA tube current results in a patient dose of _____ rad.
    a. 4
    b. 8
    c. 12
    d. 16
15. In this series of four different exposures, which mAs station does not meet the exposure linearity criteria?
    a. 5 mAs, 3.2 mR/mAs
    b. 100 mAs, 5.8 mR/mAs
    c. 200 mAs, 6.0 mR/mAs
    d. 400 mAs, 6.2 mR/mAs
16. Which combination of temperature and humidity should be used for film storage?
    a. 68 percent relative humidity, 10°F
    b. 10 percent relative humidity, 10°F
    c. 98 percent relative humidity, 68°F
    d. 50 percent relative humidity, 68°F
17. The base fog density should be less than _____ OD.
    a. 0.02
    b. 0.05
    c. 0.2
    d. 0.5

ANSWERS TO CHAPTER 20 QUESTIONS

1. b
2. d
3. a
4. b
5. c
6. b
7. b
8. b
9. d

10. a
11. c
12. d
13. b
14. c
15. a
16. d
17. b

Unit V

Radiation Protection

21

Biologic Effects of Radiation

OBJECTIVES

Upon completion of this chapter, the student will be able to

1. Describe the reproductive cycle of the human cell.
2. Identify the relative radiation sensitivity of human cells, tissues, and organs.
3. Describe the linear nonthreshold dose response model.
4. Identify the stages of acute radiation effects.

HUMAN BIOLOGY

About 80 percent of the human body is water. The remainder of the body consists of 15 percent proteins, 2 percent lipids, 1 percent carbohydrates, 1 percent nucleic acid, and 1 percent other materials. These constituents are combined into cells. The human body is made up of many different types of cells. The cells of a specific type combine to form tissues, and tissues combine to form organs. The functions of cells can differ greatly, but all cells in the body have many common features. They absorb nutrients, produce energy, and synthesize molecular compounds. These activities are called metabolism. There are two types of cells in the body, genetic and somatic. **Genetic cells** are cells of the reproductive organs. **Somatic cells** are all the other cells in the human body (skin, nerve, muscle, etc.).

The central nucleus of a human cell contains the genetic code, which is held in large macromolecules of deoxyribonucleic acid **(DNA).** The cell's genetic information is transferred by **chromosomes,** which are clusters of DNA

361

molecules. The cell nucleus is surrounded by the cytoplasm. This cytoplasm contains organelles that produce energy, synthesize proteins, and eliminate waste and toxins. The entire cell contents are contained within the cell membrane. Figure 21.1 illustrates the structure of a human cell.

The genetic information about a cell's form and function is contained in the DNA molecule. This molecule is shaped in the form of a double helix. The two helices of the DNA molecule are connected by base pairs attached to the side chains like the rungs of a ladder. The rungs are made up of four different base pairs: adenine, guanine, thymine, and cytosine. The sequence of these bases and how they are connected to the side chains encodes the information in the DNA molecule. Figure 21.2 shows a schematic diagram of a DNA molecule.

Ribonucleic acid (**RNA**) molecules, which are contained in both the cell nucleus and the cytoplasm, are similar to DNA molecules, but they have only a single strand of nucleic acid, whereas the DNA molecules have two strands. The RNA molecules serve as templates for the replication of DNA molecules.

The human body is composed of 80 percent water and 15 percent proteins, with the remainder made up of lipids, carbohydrates, nucleic acid, and other materials. Human cells have a nucleus containing DNA molecules and surrounding cytoplasm containing organelles. There are two types of human cells, genetic cells and somatic cells. Genetic cells are cells of the reproductive organs; somatic cells are all other cells in the human body.

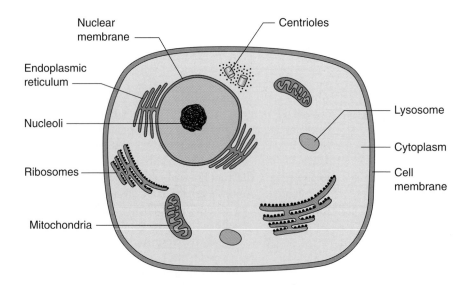

Figure 21.1 A typical cell contains a nucleus surrounded by cytoplasm contained within a cell membrane.

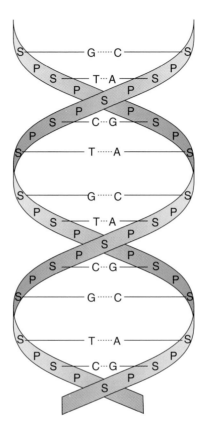

Figure 21.2 **Schematic representation of a DNA molecule.**

CELL DIVISION

Cells go through a sequence or cycle during division. The end result of the cycle is the division of a single cell into two cells. The division of somatic cells is called **mitosis,** and the division of genetic cells is called **meiosis.** Both mitosis and meiosis occur during one phase of a well-defined cell cycle. Table 21.1 lists the phases of the cell cycle.

Cell division occurs during the M phase of the cell cycle. At the beginning of the M phase the DNA molecules clump together to form visible chromosomes. Cell division results in two cells. After cell division, each new cell passes through a growth phase, G_1, in which it prepares for DNA synthesis. During the S phase, each DNA molecule is duplicated to form two identical daughter DNA molecules. These DNA molecules will combine to form duplicate chromosomes during the S phase. After synthesis is completed, the cell enters into

Table 21.1
Phases of the Cell Cycle

Phase of Cell Cycle	Description
M	Mitosis or meiosis
G_1	Pre-DNA synthesis, cell growth
S	DNA synthesis
G_2	Cell growth following DNA synthesis

the post-DNA synthesis, or G_2, phase, during which the cell continues to mature. At the end of the G_2 phase, the cell again enters the M phase, where mitosis or meiosis occurs. Different cell types have different cell cycle times. For example, some blood cells progress through their cell cycle in a few days, while other cells require many months to progress through their cell cycle.

Mitosis

Mitosis describes the division of somatic cells. The cell division, or M, phase of the cell cycle is divided into four subphases, which are listed in Table 21.2. Before cell division begins, the cell has 46 chromosomes arranged in 23 pairs. During prophase, the nucleus begins to swell and the chromosomes become visible under a microscope. During metaphase, the chromosomes align themselves on fibers along the center of the nucleus. During anaphase, the chromosomes begin to divide, forming two sets of chromosomes. During telophase, the two sets of chromosomes divide into two separate nuclei, forming the two daughter cells. Each daughter cell nucleus contains 46 chromosomes. The newly formed daughter cells are immature or young somatic cells and are called **stem cells.** They remain stem cells until they grow, develop, and mature.

Meiosis

Immature genetic cells, called **germ cells,** begin with the same number of chromosomes as somatic cells have. However, genetic cell division during meiosis differs from somatic cell division during mitosis. During meiosis, the

Table 21.2
Subphases of Mitosis or Meiosis

First	Prophase
Second	Metaphase
Third	Anaphase
Fourth	Telophase

number of chromosomes is reduced to half of the normal 46, so that each germ cell contains only 23 chromosomes. Following conception, each of the two germ cells contributes half of the chromosomes when they combine to form a daughter cell containing the standard number of 46 chromosomes. Genetic cells progress through the same phases in meiosis as somatic cells do in mitosis.

The process of cells dividing into two daughter cells is called cell division or replication. During cell division, the cell progresses through a series of phases. Somatic cell division is called mitosis; genetic cell division is called meiosis. Meiosis results in daughter cells that have only 23 chromosomes, rather than the 46 chromosomes arranged in 23 pairs in daughter cells resulting from mitosis.

TISSUES AND ORGANS

Cells in the body combine to form specific tissues. These tissues combine to form organs. Organ systems perform specific functions. Different types of tissues and organs have cells with different structures and functions. Examples of major organ systems include the nervous, respiratory, digestive, endocrine, circulatory, and reproductive systems.

THE LAW OF BERGONNE AND TRIBONDEAU

Two French scientists, Bergonne and Tribondeau, studied the effect of radiation on cells, tissues, and organs. Their observations relate to the sensitivity of cells, tissues, and organs to ionizing radiation. Important points of the Bergonne and Tribondeau law are as follows:

1. Younger or immature cells are more radiosensitive.
2. Rapidly dividing cells are more radiosensitive.
3. Mature cells are less radiosensitive.
4. Rapidly growing cells are more radiosensitive.

These points are important in diagnostic radiology because the fetus, which contains younger or immature cells, and cells that are rapidly dividing, is more sensitive to radiation than adult cells. Cells are most sensitive to radiation exposure during the M phase of the cell cycle. They are most resistant to radiation exposure in the late S phase. Germ and stem cells are more radiosensitive than mature cells of the same type. Stem cells of a particular type are identified with the suffix -*blast*. For example, immature red blood cells are known as erythroblasts, and bone stem cells are known as osteoblasts. Blastic

Table 21.3
Radiation Sensitivity of Some Cells, Tissues, and Organs

Most sensitive	Lymphocytes
	Gonads
	Spermatogonia
	Oogonia
	Hemopoietic tissues/erythroblasts
Intermediate	Intestine/intestinal crypt cells
	Bone/osteoblasts
	Skin/epithelial cells
	Lens of eye/cornea
	Thyroid
Least sensitive	Muscle cells
	Nerve cells
	Spinal cord
	Brain

cells are more radiosensitive than mature cells of the same type. Cells that are less sensitive to radiation are called radioresistant. Radioresistant cells show fewer biologic effects of radiation than do radiosensitive cells. In keeping with the law of Bergonne and Tribondeau, nerve cells of the brain and spinal cord are most radioresistant because once they are developed, these nerve cells do not undergo further cell division. Lymphocytes and gonadal cells are the most radiosensitive because they undergo rapid cell division and are constantly developing.

Table 21.3 lists several cells, tissues, and organs in radiation sensitivity categories.

The law of Bergonne and Tribondeau states that immature, rapidly dividing, or rapidly growing cells are the most radiosensitive. Mature, slowly growing cells are the most radioresistant.

LINEAR ENERGY TRANSFER

The characteristics of particulate and electromagnetic radiation can affect the amount of biologic damage. The radiation characteristic that is most important in determining cell damage is the rate at which the radiation deposits its energy.

The term linear energy transfer (**LET**) describes how the ionizing radiation energy is deposited along a tract or path in tissue. LET has units of kiloelectron volts per micrometer (keV/μm). As the radiation passes through tissue, it produces ionization. Different types of ionizing radiation have different LET values. As high-LET radiation passes through tissue, it deposits large amounts of energy in a short distance. Accordingly, high-LET radiation has a greater biologic effect but very little penetrating ability because it loses all its energy in a short distance.

Low-LET radiation is very penetrating because it spreads its energy over large distances. There is little chance that a low-LET radiation will deposit more than one ionization in any one cell. Current theories suggest that two or three ionizations in a cell nucleus are required to produce biologic effects. Because the ionizations from low-LET radiation are spread over many cells, this radiation does not usually cause significant damage in any one cell. Figure 21.3 compares the ionization along the tracks of a high- and a low-LET radiation.

Alpha and beta particles and protons are types of high-LET radiation, with alpha particles having the highest LET. High-LET radiation has values from 10 to 200 keV/μm with ranges of a few millimeters in tissue. X-rays and gamma rays are types of low-LET radiation, with values from 0.2 to 3 keV/μm and ranges of many centimeters in tissue.

The biologic effects of radiations with different LET values are compared by comparing their relative biologic effectiveness (**RBE**) values. RBE is the ratio of doses of a standard radiation to a test radiation required to produce the same biologic effect. Diagnostic x-rays and gamma rays have a RBE value close to 1. High-LET radiations have higher RBE values because they produce the same effect at lower doses.

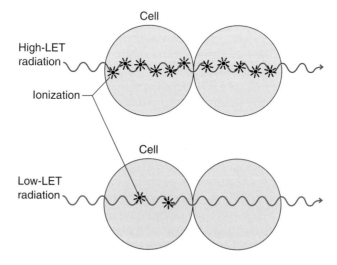

Figure 21.3 Comparison of high-LET and low-LET ionization tracks.

TYPES OF CELL DAMAGE

Several things can happen when ionization occurs within a cell. The cell can die and form scar tissue. The cell can repair itself from the damage. Repaired cells can continue to function normally after repair. Alternatively, the cell can be transformed into an abnormal cell. Transformed cells may begin the process of becoming cancer cells.

If a large number of ionizations occur in a cell over a short period of time, the cell's repair mechanisms may be overwhelmed, and it may not be able to repair the damage. Biologic effects of low dose rate exposures are less than those from high dose rate exposures. Long-term exposures over months or years show about half the effect as those caused by short-term exposures involving the same dose.

DIRECT AND INDIRECT EFFECTS

The amount of cell damage depends on both the quantity of radiation and how the radiation is deposited in the cell. If the radiation directly damages the cell nucleus, the damage is called a direct effect. If the radiation deposits its energy outside the nucleus, the damage is called an indirect effect.

Direct effects result from ionizing radiation depositing its energy within the cell nucleus and breaking the DNA molecular bonds. The target for direct effects is the DNA molecule. High-LET radiation primarily produces direct effects. High-LET ionizations are deposited inside the cell nucleus and damage so many DNA molecules that the cell is unable to repair all the damage. High-LET radiation usually results in cell death.

Indirect effects result from ionizing radiation depositing its energy within the cytoplasm outside of the cell nucleus. Low-LET radiation primarily produces indirect effects.

Low-LET radiation can damage the cell by producing an intermediate, toxic product in the cytoplasm that then interacts with the DNA in the nucleus. The most common toxic product is produced by the radiolysis of water. In radiolysis of water, the water molecule is broken into two uncharged particles, H° and OH°, which are free radicals. Although free radicals are uncharged, they have an unpaired electron and are very chemically reactive. Free radicals can easily break DNA bonds. Free radicals, which are produced primarily in the cytoplasm, have a short life, but they exist long enough to reach the nucleus and damage the DNA molecules. Free radicals produced from the radiolysis of water can also combine to form hydrogen peroxide, H_2O_2, which is toxic to cells. Most damage from low-LET radiation is caused by indirect effects because the low-LET ionizations are separated by distances much larger than a cell. Figure 21.4 shows the formation of a free radical pair by radiolysis of water.

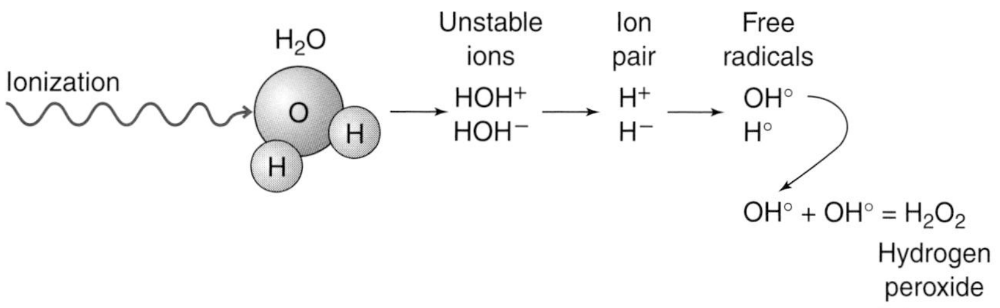

Figure 21.4 Radiolysis of water to form the free radicals H° and OH°.

Free radicals are produced more readily when there is an abundance of oxygen present. The cytoplasm, which consists primarily of H_2O, is an abundant reservoir of oxygen. The effect of oxygen is measured by the oxygen enhancement ratio **(OER),** which is the ratio of the radiation doses necessary to produce the same effect without and with oxygen present. OER values for high-LET radiations are close to 1 because the high-LET radiations are so effective in producing damage that the presence or absence of oxygen does not matter. Low-LET radiations typically have OER values of 2 to 3, meaning that oxygen enhances the effects of radiation.

More indirect effects occur if there is more oxygen present, because free radicals are readily produced by ionizations in the presence of oxygen. Oxygen is a radiosensitizer because cells in the presence of oxygen are more sensitive to radiation. Cells in tissues with a poor blood supply are more resistant to radiation damage because they have a diminished oxygen supply. Many tumors are radioresistant because they are avascular, that is, they lack an adequate blood supply.

Different radiations have different characteristics, which are characterized by their LET values. High-LET radiation produces cell damage primarily by direct effects. Low-LET radiation produces cell damage primarily through indirect effects. Radiolysis of water produces free radicals and is a indirect effect. Direct effects produce damage to the DNA in the cell nucleus, Indirect effects produce their effects through production of toxins in the cytoplasm. X-rays and gamma radiation have low LET values. Most of the radiation damage to the cell is produced by indirect effects.

CELL SURVIVAL CURVE

The number of cells that survive after being exposed to radiation depends on the radiation dose. A cell survival curve is a plot of the fraction of cells surviving as a function of radiation dose. It is obtained through a series of experiments in which groups of cells are exposed to different doses of radiation. Figure 21.5 shows the fraction of surviving cells plotted against the radiation dose.

The cell survival curve can be divided into two parts, the S, or shoulder, region and the L, or linear, region. The shoulder of the curve in the S region indicates the amount of cell repair or recovery. At very low doses, almost 100 percent of the cells survive. As the dose is increased, some of the cells are killed, but most recover from the radiation damage and survive. The dose at which an extrapolation of the straight-line portion of the survival curve intersects the 100 percent survival line is known as D_Q, the threshold dose. D_Q is a measure of the amount of cellular repair or sublethal damage. Cells with greater repair or recovery capability have a larger shoulder region and a larger D_Q value. High-LET radiations produce cell survival curves with almost no shoulder region and very small D_Q values. High-LET radiations overwhelm the cell's repair mechanism.

The linear region occurs at higher doses, where the survival curve becomes a straight line when cell survival is plotted on a logarithmic scale. In the L region, cell survival is inversely proportional to dose. An increase in dose produces a decrease in cell survival. The dose required to reduce the population of surviving cells to 37 percent of the original value is D_0, the mean lethal dose.

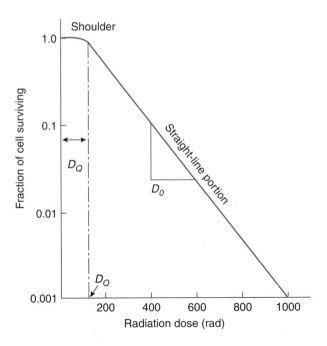

Figure 21.5 **Cell survival curve.**

Different cell and tissue types have different D_0 and D_Q values. Radioresistant cells have large D_0 values because they require a large radiation dose to reduce the number of surviving cells to 37 percent of the original population. Radiosensitive cells have small D_0 values because they require a smaller radiation dose to reduce the number of surviving cells to this degree.

LINEAR AND NONLINEAR DOSE-RESPONSE MODELS

A dose-response curve shows the relationship between the radiation dose and the resulting biologic effects. Biologic data on humans are available only at doses greater than about 1 gray (Gy) (100 rad). No biologic effects have been observed at doses of a few milligray. These are the dose levels usually encountered in diagnostic radiology.

Data obtained at higher doses can be extrapolated to lower doses to estimate biologic effects at the lower dose levels. These extrapolations are done using dose-response models. There are two types of dose-response models, the linear and nonlinear models. A linear model predicts a doubling of the effect if the dose is doubled. A nonlinear model predicts some other relation between the dose and its effect. Each of these models may or may not have a threshold. A **threshold dose** is defined as the minimum dose at which biologic effects become evident. A linear model can have either a threshold or a nonthreshold response. A linear curve that passes through the origin is a nonthreshold curve. A linear curve that rises at some dose greater than zero is a threshold response. The dose at which the curve rises above zero is also a threshold dose response.

The linear model extrapolates by using a straight line to connect the data for high doses to the 0,0 point, the origin of the graph. The linear model predicts that biologic effects are directly proportional to the radiation dose. The nonlinear model, which is also called the linear quadratic model, predicts small effects at low doses. The magnitude of the effects gradually increases with increasing radiation dose until the two models predict the same biologic effects at high doses, where human data are available.

Figure 21.6 shows the linear dose-response model with and without a threshold.

Figure 21.7 shows the curves obtained from the nonlinear model with and without a threshold. In practice, almost all nonlinear curves have a threshold below which there are no observed biologic effects.

The **linear nonthreshold (LNT) dose-response model** is used to estimate radiation effects in the diagnostic energy range. Diagnostic x-rays are assumed to follow a linear nonthreshold dose-response.

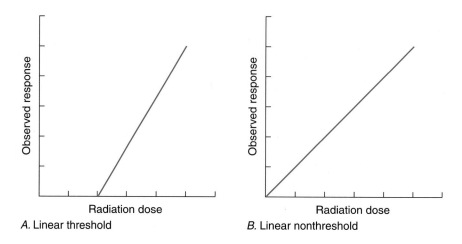

Figure 21.6 **Dose-response curves for (*A*) linear threshold model and (*B*) linear nonthreshold model.**

The cell survival curve plots the percentage of surviving cells as a function of radiation dose. The linear nonthreshold dose-response model is used to estimate the radiation damage in humans in the low-dose diagnostic energy range.

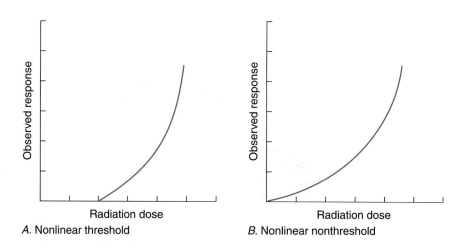

Figure 21.7 **Dose-response curves for (*A*) non-linear threshold model and (*B*) nonlinear nonthreshold models.**

HIGH-DOSE RADIATION EFFECTS

Acute radiation effects result from high radiation doses delivered to the whole body in a few hours or less. The clinical signs and symptoms of radiation exposure present themselves in four stages:

1. The prodromal stage
2. The latent period
3. The acute stage
4. The final stage, resulting in recovery or death

The duration of each stage and the severity of each stage depend on the radiation dose.

Prodromal Stage

The first stage of radiation response following an exposure is the **prodromal stage.** The early effects of radiation exposure are manifest in the prodromal stage. The prodromal stage shows the clinical signs and symptoms resulting from radiation exposure to the whole body. Individuals who are exposed to radiation levels greater than 1 Gy (100 rad) usually show prodromal symptoms, which include varying degrees of nausea, vomiting, and diarrhea. The prodromal stage can begin within a few minutes to hours following exposure and last for a few hours to a few days. The time between the exposure and the onset of prodromal symptoms is an indication of the magnitude of the exposure. Higher exposure levels result in shorter times to the onset of the prodromal symptoms. The onset of prodromal symptoms shortly after exposure indicates a major radiation exposure to the whole body.

Latent Period

The second stage of high-dose effects is the **latent period.** During the latent period the exposed individual has no clinical symptoms or illness from the radiation exposure and appears to have recovered with no ill effects. However, even though there are no symptoms, there may be ongoing cell damage. The latent period can extend from a few hours to several days, depending on the dose. Higher doses result in shorter latent periods.

Acute Stage

During the **acute stage** of radiation response, the full clinical effects are evident. The three syndromes that become manifest during the acute stage are the **hematologic syndrome,** the **gastrointestinal (GI) syndrome,** and **central nervous system (CNS) syndrome.**

The whole-body dose determines the effects an individual will display during the acute stage. At higher dose levels, the acute effects observed may include more than one **syndrome.** Thus, an individual exposed to 3.5 Gy (350 rad) will display the symptoms of both the hematologic and the gastrointestinal syndromes.

The three acute-phase syndromes resulting from high-dose whole-body exposures are dose-related. The first syndrome to appear is the hematologic syndrome; then, if the whole-body dose is high, the gastrointestinal syndrome will appear. At very high doses, the central nervous system syndrome becomes evident.

Hematologic Syndrome

The major hematologic effect of radiation exposure is a decrease in leukocytes, erythrocytes, thrombocytes, and lymphocytes. This means that the body's defenses against infection are reduced or eliminated. Individuals exposed to whole-body dose levels above about 1 Gy (100 rad) experience nausea and vomiting during the prodromal stage. Hematologic effects follow a latent period of a few weeks. During the latent period, there are no apparent symptoms, but blood cell damage is still being expressed. Death at these exposure levels is due to infection. The body's defense mechanisms begin to recover about 30 days after exposure. When these defense mechanisms against infection are fully active, complete recovery can be expected. Individuals exposed to doses as high as 6 Gy (600 rad) can recover if they are given medical care to prevent infection.

Gastrointestinal Syndrome

Gastrointestinal symptoms appear at whole-body doses of 3 Gy (300 rad) or higher. Whole-body doses above 6 Gy (600 rad) kill most of the stem cells in the gastrointestinal tract. Following the prodromal stage, there is a latent period of about 10 days. After the latent period, the individual experiences another bout of diarrhea and infection as the intestines break down, allowing a loss of body fluids and an invasion of bacteria. This occurs just as the body's defenses are beginning to fail because of the hematologic effects. Death usually occurs about 2 weeks after exposure.

Central Nervous System Syndrome

At doses greater than 50 Gy (5000 rad), the radiation damages the nerve cells, and so the body's regulatory mechanisms fail within a few days. The latent period may be as short as a few hours with very high doses. Higher doses result in shorter latent periods. After the latent period, the exposed individual loses consciousness and stops breathing. Exposures at these dose levels always result in death.

Table 21.4 presents the high-dose acute stages, the dose levels at which they begin to appear, and their latent periods following whole-body exposure.

Table 21.4
Dose Levels at which Biologic Effects Appear

Dose Level at which Effects Appear		Biologic Effect	Latent Period
Gy	rad		
<1	<100	No observable effect	
1	100	Hematologic	2–4 weeks
3	300	Gastrointestinal	10–14 days
>50	>5000	Central nervous system	A few hours

Final Stage: Recovery or Death

The survival of an individual depends on many complex factors, including the amount and distribution of the radiation, the individual's general health, the individual's sensitivity to radiation, and the medical treatment obtained. No individuals have survived whole-body exposures of 10 Gy (1000 rad) or greater. Human data on exposures at these levels are sparse, but it appears that survival from doses of 6 to 7 Gy (600 to 700 rad) is possible with vigorous medical treatment that includes large doses of antibiotics and maintenance of body fluids and electrolyte balance. The mean survival time is the average time of survival and is dose-related; higher doses have shorter mean survival times. Although there are no absolute values, the mean survival time for the hematologic syndrome is 45 days, that for the gastrointestinal syndrome is 8 days, and that for the CNS syndrome is 2 days.

LD$_{50/30}$

The **LD**$_{50/30}$ is used to express the lethal dose of radiation to humans. LD$_{50/30}$ is a threshold response: It is the radiation dose to the whole body that will produce death in 50 percent of the exposed population within 30 days. The LD$_{50/30}$ is about 3 Gy (300 rad) for individuals without medical treatment, and somewhat higher for individuals with proper medical care.

The effects of high-dose whole-body radiation appear in four stages. The initial appearance of damage is in the prodromal stage, which includes symptoms of nausea, vomiting, and diarrhea. The prodromal stage is followed by a latent period, during which the victim appears to return to good health. The latent period may last from hours to weeks, depending on the dose. The acute stage follows the latent period. During the acute stage, the victim may demonstrate hematologic, gastrointestinal, or even central nervous system symptoms, depending

*on the whole-body dose received. The final stage is recovery or death.
Doses in diagnostic radiology are not high enough to produce these
high-dose acute effects. The LD$_{50/30}$ is the whole-body dose that will
produce death in 50 percent of the exposed population within 30 days.
The LD$_{50/30}$ for exposed individuals without medical care is about 3 Gy
(300 rad).*

Effects of Partial Body Irradiations

Exposure of localized portions of the body to radiation produces different effects from exposure of the whole body. Localized exposures show striking, but
nonlethal effects, including erythema, epilation, and cataracts. Radiation exposures to limited portions of the body can also induce cancer and leukemia.

Localized exposure to the skin will produce **erythema,** or skin reddening,
at dose levels near 6 Gy (600 rad). The skin erythema dose for 50 percent of
the population (SED$_{50}$) is 6 Gy (600 rad). The radiation causes local damage to
the skin stem cells, producing reddening of the skin within a few days. The latent period for skin erythema is a few days.

Epilation, or temporary hair loss, occurs at doses above a threshold of 3
Gy (300 rad) with a latent period of a few weeks. Regrowth of the hair begins
in about 2 months and is complete in about 6 months.

Cataracts, or cloudiness or opacity, of the eye are produced by a single
acute dose of 2 Gy (200 rad) to the lens of the eye. Exposures occurring over a
period of months or years demonstrate a threshold dose of 10 Gy (1000 rad).
The latent period for cataract development is several years.

Cancer and Leukemia Induction

Cancer is the second leading cause of death in the United States, exceeded
only by cardiovascular disease. More than one in five individuals will die from
cancer. Ionizing radiation can cause cancer and leukemia; it is a **carcinogen.**
Leukemia is a cancer of the blood. There are many other carcinogens, including smoking, diet, and environmental factors. It is difficult to determine the
exact cause of any particular cancer because cancers induced by radiation have
latent periods of from 10 to 25 years. In a unexposed population of one million, there will be over 200,000 cancer deaths. The current best estimate of
the risk of dying from a radiation-induced cancer is 5 percent per gray (0.05%
percent per rad). In other words, if one million individuals were exposed to 10
mGy (1 rad), an extra 500 deaths due to radiation-induced cancers would be
predicted. Deaths due to cancer would rise from 200,000 to 200,500 in the exposed population. These estimates are based on the linear nonthreshold dose-
response model.

*Effects of localized radiation exposure follow a threshold dose response.
The SED$_{50,}$ which is the skin erythema dose, is 6 Gy (600 rad).*

> *Cataract induction has a threshold of about 10 Gy (1000 rad). Cancer induction is assumed to follow the linear nonthreshold dose-response model. Radiation is a carcinogen, with an estimate of cancer induction of 500 extra cancer deaths per million persons exposed to 10 mGy.*

RADIATION AND PREGNANCY

The fetus is very sensitive to radiation because it is made up of rapidly dividing cells. The fetus is most sensitive to radiation during the first trimester of pregnancy. The effects on the fetus depend on the stage of fetal development at which the radiation exposure occurs. There appears to be a threshold of about 0.1 Gy (10 rad) for fetal damage. Routine diagnostic procedures never reach this level. There is no reason to recommend an elective abortion if the dose to the fetus is less than 0.1 Gy (10 rad). At fetal doses above 0.25 Gy (25 rad), serious discussion with the parents is advisable. The overlying tissue and amniotic fluid provide significant shielding to the fetus. The dose to the fetus is usually about 25 percent of the entrance skin dose. All institutions should have a policy regarding x-ray examinations of potentially pregnant patients to ensure that all patients are treated the same way. Medically necessary examinations should never be delayed because of pregnancy because an examination that can be postponed until the birth of the baby is not a necessary examination. The technologist should give special attention to proper positioning and should seek to minimize the number of exposures. Shielding the abdomen of a pregnant patient is not advisable. If the pelvis is being examined, shielding will compromise the examination. If the pelvis is not in the collimated direct beam, only internal scattered radiation will reach the fetus. External shielding will not attenuate the internal scattered radiation. However, providing a pregnant patient with an abdominal shield demonstrates commendable concern for the safety of her baby.

GENETIC EFFECTS

There are 110,000 abnormalities per million live births in an unirradiated population. Many experiments have been conducted to evaluate the effect of radiation damage on future generations. Germ cells are radiosensitive because they are immature genetic cells. The extrapolated estimate of genetic damage is that an additional 100 abnormalities per million live births would be expected if the reproductive organs of the parents were irradiated to 10 mGy (1 rad). That is, if the parents of 1 million babies were exposed to 10 mGy, the number of abnormalities would rise from 110,000 to 110,100. This is less than a 1 percent increase.

Genetically Significant Dose

The genetically significant dose **(GSD)** measures the effect on the genetic pool of radiation exposure to the gonads. The GSD is defined as that dose which, if delivered to every member of the population, would produce the same genetic effect as is produced by the actual doses to the individual members of the population. Medical exposures contribute about 200 µGy (20 mrad) to the GSD in the United States.

Doubling Dose

The **doubling dose** is defined as that radiation dose that produces twice the genetic mutation rate in a population as is seen in the population without the radiation dose. The doubling dose is estimated to be between 0.5 and 1 Gy (50 and 100 rad).

> *Fetal doses from diagnostic x-ray examinations rarely are as high as 10 rad. There is no reason to contemplate an abortion if the fetal dose is 10 rad or less. The genetically significant dose provides an estimate of the genetic effects of radiation. The contribution to the GSD from medical radiation is about 200 µGy. The doubling dose is about 0.5 Gy.*

SUMMARY

Cell division consists of four phases, M, G_1, S, and G_2. The M phase consists of mitosis or meiosis. Somatic cell division is called mitosis, and the division of genetic cells is called meiosis. Cells are most sensitive to radiation exposure during the M phase and most radioresistant in the late S phase. Immature somatic cells are called stem cells, and immature genetic cells are called germ cells. Germ and stem cells are more radiosensitive than mature cells. The law of Bergonne and Tribondeau states that younger, immature, and rapidly dividing cells are more radiosensitive. Direct effects result from ionization and breaking of DNA molecule bonds in the cell nucleus. Indirect effects are produced when radiation interacts with the cytoplasm to produce free radicals that damage the cell. The effect of oxygen on tissue radiosensitivity is measured by the oxygen enhancement ratio. Well-vascularized tissues are more radiosensitive than tissues with smaller blood supplies and less oxygen. Linear energy transfer describes how energy is deposited along the radiation path in tissue. High-LET radiation produces direct biological effects; low-LET radiation produces biologic effects through indirect effects. The effects of radiations with different LET values can be evaluated by comparing their relative biological effectiveness values. X-rays and gamma radiations are forms of low-LET radiations. Alpha and beta particles are high-LET radiations. A cell survival curve plots the percentage of surviving cells against the radiation dose. A radiation dose-response curve plots the relationship between the radiation dose and the biologic effects produced. Different dose-response models use linear and nonlinear, threshold and nonthreshold curves. The effects of diagnostic radiation are assumed to follow the linear nonthreshold dose-response model. Acute effects from high-dose whole-body radiation include the hematologic effect, which appears at doses of about 1 Gy (100 rad); the gastrointestinal effect, which appears at about 3 Gy (300 rad); and the CNS effect, which appears at doses of about 50 Gy (5000 rad). Dose levels in diagnostic radiology are not high enough to produce acute effects. Local effects and their threshold dose levels include epilation [3 Gy (300 rad)], erythema [6 Gy (600 rad)], and cataract formation [10 Gy (1000 rad)]. The increase in cancer due to radiation is estimated to be 5 percent per gray. No ill effects on the fetus have been observed at doses less than 100 mGy (10 rad). Genetic effects are described by the genetically significant dose. The doubling dose is about 0.5 Gy.

QUESTIONS

1. The most radiosensitive part of the cell cycle is the _____ phase.
   a. S
   b. G_1
   c. M
   d. G_2
2. The least radiosensitive part of the cell cycle is the _____ phase.
   a. S
   b. G_1
   c. M
   d. G_2
3. The most radiosensitive tissues and organs are
   1. muscle.
   2. nerve.
   3. gonads.
   4. intestine.
   a. 1 and 3.
   b. 1 and 2.
   c. 1 and 4.
   d. 3 and 4.
4. The most radioresistant tissues are
   1. muscle.
   2. nerve.
   3. gonads.
   4. intestine.
   a. 1 and 3.
   b. 1 and 2.
   c. 1 and 4.
   d. 3 and 4.

5. The law of Bergonne and Tribondeau states that
   1. younger cells are more radiosensitive.
   2. rapidly dividing cells are more radiosensitive.
   3. mature cells are less radiosensitive.
   4. rapidly growing cells are more radiosensitive.
   a. 1 and 2
   b. 1, 2, and 4
   c. 1, 3, and 4
   d. 1, 2, 3, and 4
6. The least radioresistant cells in the human body are
   a. epithelial cells.
   b. nerve cells.
   c. osteocytes.
   d. lymphocytes.
7. The technical term for cell division of genetic cells is
   a. mitosis.
   b. meiosis.
   c. growth.
   d. other.
8. The stage of high-dose radiation effects in which the individual appears to
   have recovered but may still exhibit symptoms at a later date is called the
   a. prodromal stage.
   b. latent period.
   c. acute stage.
   d. recovery stage.
9. The high-dose effect occurring at doses from 1 to 2.5 Gy (100 to 250 rad)
   is the
   a. prodromal syndrome.
   b. hematologic syndrome.
   c. gastrointestinal syndrome.
   d. central nervous system syndrome.
10. The high-dose effect occurring at doses from 3 to 5 Gy (300 to 600 rad) is
    the
    a. prodromal syndrome.
    b. hematologic syndrome.
    c. gastrointestinal syndrome.
    d. central nervous system syndrome.
11. A direct effect of radiation exposure to the cell involves the
    a. DNA bond.
    b. cell membrane.
    c. cytoplasm.
    d. organelles.

12. An indirect effect of radiation exposure to the cell involves the
    a. DNA bond.
    b. cell membrane.
    c. cytoplasm.
    d. organelles.
13. The D_0 in a cell survival curve describes the
    a. cell repair or recovery.
    b. organelle damage.
    c. DNA damage.
    d. dose that will kill 63 percent of the cells and leave 37 percent of the cells surviving.
14. The D_Q in a cell survival curve describes the
    a. cell repair or recovery.
    b. organelle damage.
    c. DNA damage.
    d. dose that will kill 63 percent of the cells.
15. It is assumed that biologic effects from diagnostic radiology exposures follow the _____ dose-response model.
    a. linear threshold
    b. linear nonthreshold
    c. nonlinear threshold
    d. nonlinear nonthreshold
16. Higher doses result in _____ latent periods.
    a. shorter
    b. longer
    c. unchanged
    d. none of the above
17. Ionizing radiation is a
    a. carcinogen.
    b. cytoplasmicogen.
    c. nucleonogen.
    d. orangelistigen.
18. The fetus is most sensitive to radiation during the _____ trimester of pregnancy.
    a. first
    b. second
    c. third
    d. fourth
19. The doubling dose for genetic effects is about _____ rad.
    a. 10
    b. 50
    c. 200
    d. 500

20. Which of the following types of radiation has the highest LET?
    a. Gamma rays
    b. Bremsstrahlung
    c. Alpha particles
    d. X-rays
21. Immature somatic cells are called
    a. germ cells.
    b. stem cells.
    c. genetic cells.
    d. oogonia.
22. The $LD_{50/30}$ represents a radiation dose that will kill
    a. 30 people in 50 days.
    b. 30 percent of the cells in 50 days.
    c. 50 percent of the people in 30 days.
    d. 50 percent of the cells in 30 days.
23. The skin erythema dose (the SED_{50}) is approximately _____ rad.
    a. 50
    b. 100
    c. 300
    d. 600
24. The dose to produce epilation is approximately _____ rad.
    a. 50
    b. 100
    c. 300
    d. 600
25. The $LD_{50/30}$ dose with no medical support is approximately _____ rad.
    a. 50
    b. 100
    c. 300
    d. 1600
26. The term *epilation* is used to refer to
    a. loss of hair.
    b. loss of white blood cells.
    c. metabolism.
    d. cataract formation.
27. The most radiosensitive cells are
    a. nerve cells.
    b. lymphocytes.
    c. muscle cells.
    d. brain cells.
28. Genetic effects of radiation are associated with
    a. RBE.
    b. OER.
    c. LET.
    d. GSD.

29. The first stage of radiation response following an exposure is the _____ stage.
    a. prodromal
    b. latent
    c. acute
    d. final

30. The target molecule for direct radiation effects is
    a. H_2O.
    b. RBE.
    c. LET.
    d. DNA.

ANSWERS TO CHAPTER 21 QUESTIONS

1.	c	16.	a
2.	a	17.	a
3.	d	18.	a
4.	b	19.	b
5.	d	20.	c
6.	d	21.	b
7.	b	22.	c
8.	b	23.	d
9.	b	24.	c
10.	c	25.	c
11.	a	26.	a
12.	c	27.	b
13.	d	28.	d
14.	a	29.	a
15.	b	30.	d

22

Radiation Protection

OBJECTIVES

Upon completion of this chapter, the student will be able to

1. Describe the methods of reducing radiation exposure.
2. State the exposure limits for radiation workers and for the general public.
3. State the requirements for personnel monitoring.
4. Describe ALARA.
5. State the three components of natural background radiation.

INTRODUCTION

The purpose of radiation protection is to reduce the radiation exposure to staff, patients, and public as much as possible while still maintaining image quality. This reduction is accomplished by both reducing the amount of radiation to the patient and reducing the amount of scattered radiation. Exposure is the number of x-rays, measured in milliroentgens (mR), and dose is the energy deposited, measured in milligray (mGy) or millirads (mrad). When dealing with diagnostic x-rays, the relation 1 mR = 1 mrad = 1 mrem is approximately correct. Radiation exposures occur only when the x-ray beam is "on." The patient does not become radioactive and is not a source of radiation after a diagnostic exposure is completed. X-rays dissipate after the exposure, just as light disappears when a lamp is switched off.

REDUCTION OF RADIATION EXPOSURE
OF THE STAFF

The three methods of reducing the radiation exposure of the staff are to

1. Reduce time.
2. Increase distance.
3. Increase shielding.

The radiation exposure of the technologist and radiologist can be reduced by reducing the time the individual is exposed to radiation, increasing the individual's distance from the radiation source, and increasing the amount of shielding between the radiation source and the individual. The major source of radiation to the radiologist and technologist is scatter from the patient. The diagnostic x-ray beam should always be collimated to the smallest field size applicable for each examination. Smaller field sizes produce less scatter because less tissue is irradiated. The technologist should never be in the direct beam or in the room during a diagnostic radiographic exposure. The technologist should never hold a patient during the exposure.

Time

Patient exposure during fluoroscopy is determined by the length of time the patient is in the x-ray beam. Shorter fluoroscopic exposure times result in lower doses to patients and staff. Regulations require that fluoroscopic units be equipped with a timer to indicate the total fluoroscopic beam on time. This timer must provide an audible reminder to indicate when 5 minutes (min) of beam on time has elapsed. Most fluoroscopic procedures require less than 5 min, although the timer can be reset when necessary.

Distance

During fluoroscopy, when the technologist must be in the room while the beam is on, the patient is the source of scattered radiation. The intensity of scattered radiation is less than that of the primary beam by a factor of 1000. That is, the intensity of the scattered radiation 1 meter (m) from the patient is 1/1000 of the primary beam intensity. Increasing the distance from the patient decreases the scattered radiation reaching the staff. According to the inverse square law, doubling the distance from the source reduces the radiation intensity to one-fourth its original value. Moving one step away from the edge of the fluoroscopic table reduces the radiation exposure significantly. Figure 22.1 presents typical exposure levels at various distances from a fluoroscopic table.

The patient is also the source of scatter during portable examinations. Increasing the distance from the patient during portable examinations de-

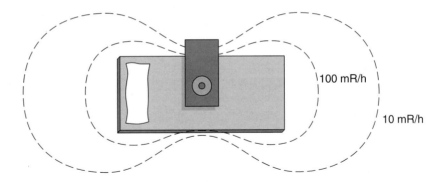

Figure 22.1 **Exposure levels around a fluoroscopic table.**

creases scattered radiation to the technologist. Portable units are equipped with an exposure switch on the end of a 180-centimeter (cm) [(6-foot (ft)] cord to allow the technologist to move away from the patient before making the exposure.

Shielding

Protective Apparel

Protective aprons have equivalent lead thicknesses of 0.25, 0.5, or 1.0 millimeter (mm) lead. The protection is equivalent to that of pure lead of the thickness indicated. Drapes hanging from the image intensifier, protective aprons, gloves, Bucky slot covers, and fold-up shields are designed to intercept the scattered radiation and reduce the radiation exposure of the staff. The Bucky tray should be moved to the foot of the table when possible to ensure that the Bucky slot cover is in place. Lead glasses and thyroid shields can also be used to protect specific areas of the body. Table 22.1 presents the types of protective shielding, their equivalent lead thickness, and the approximate attenuation of scattered radiation.

Table 22.1
Protective Apparel Thickness in Millimeters Lead Equivalent and Attenuation Values

Apparel	Thickness, mm	Attenuation, %
Apron	0.50	99.9
Gloves	0.25	99
Thyroid shield	0.25	99
Glasses	0.25	99
Fluoroscopic drape	0.25	99

Lead aprons are worn to protect vital organs. They are made of a vinyl-lead mixture covered with a smooth vinyl surface to aid in cleaning. The interior vinyl-lead composition is flexible but will crack if it is bent too far or bent repeatedly in the same location. Lead aprons must never be tossed in a heap or folded over for storage. They must be stored properly on reinforced hanging racks or laid flat on a table. Because they are so susceptible to cracking when stored improperly, lead aprons and other protective apparel should be inspected annually, both visually and under fluoroscopy or by taking radiographs. This inspection must be documented. If a defect in a protective apron, glove, or shield is detected, the item must immediately be removed from service. Figure 22.2 shows a photograph of a protective apron and a glove. A protective apron should be assigned to every portable unit.

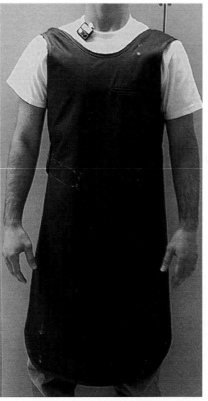

A

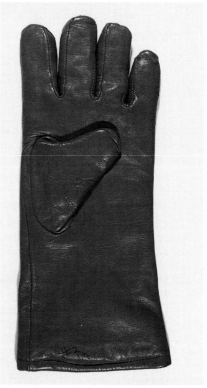

B

Figure 22.2 **Lead apron (*A*) and glove (*B*).**

Room Shielding

Room shielding is designed to prevent the transmission of radiation through the room walls. Almost all diagnostic and fluoroscopic rooms have shielding in at least some of the walls. The radiation shielding required is specified in terms of thickness of lead or concrete. The thickness of the protective barrier depends on the distance from the radiation source, the workload, the use of the space on the other side of the wall, and the amount of time the beam is pointed at the wall. The workload is a combination of the number of patients and the technical exposure factors used. Typical shielding in diagnostic room walls is 1.6 mm [1/16 inch (in.)] of lead. The floors and ceilings of diagnostic x-ray rooms do not require additional shielding if they are made of concrete because the thickness of concrete required to support the floor also provides adequate shielding against scattered radiation.

Room shielding must protect against both primary and secondary radiation. **Primary radiation** is the direct, collimated, useful x-ray beam. **Secondary radiation** is made up of scattered and leakage radiation. Primary barriers protect against the primary beam, which is directed against them. Secondary barriers protect against secondary radiation. Secondary radiation has lower energy than the primary beam, and so less shielding thickness is required. Usually only a few walls of a room are primary barriers. The wall on which the vertical Bucky is mounted is always a primary barrier. The floor of a radiographic room is usually a primary barrier. The wall of the control booth and its window are always a secondary barrier because the beam is never directed at the control booth. The primary beam is never directed at a secondary barrier.

Secondary radiation includes scatter from the patient and leakage radiation escaping through the tube housing in all directions. Regulations require that leakage radiation be less than 100 mR per hour (h) at 1 m. Leakage radiation is not a problem with modern x-ray tubes because they are manufactured with adequate shielding in their housing.

Half-Value Layer

The half-value layer (**HVL**) is that amount of shielding required to reduce the radiation intensity to half the original value. The tenth-value layer (**TVL**) is the amount of shielding required to reduce the radiation to one-tenth its original value. The TVL is used in determining the amount of shielding required for primary and secondary barriers.

The three methods of reducing radiation exposure are reducing time, increasing distance, and increasing shielding. Reducing the time reduces radiation exposure. The patient is the source of most scattered radiation. Increasing the distance from the patient reduces the scattered radiation to the staff. Increased shielding reduces the exposure of the staff. Lead aprons protect vital organs. Primary radiation is the direct x-ray beam;

secondary radiation is scattered or leakage radiation. Leakage radiation must be less than 100 mR/h at a distance of 1 m from the tube housing. Scattered radiation is lower in intensity and energy than the primary beam. The HVL is the amount of shielding required to reduce the intensity to one-half its original value; the TVL is the amount of shielding required to reduce the intensity to one-tenth its original value.

REDUCTION OF RADIATION DOSE TO THE PATIENT

The radiation dose to the patient can be reduced by careful selection of exposure techniques and adherence to good radiographic procedures. Selection of higher-kVp, lower-mAs techniques reduces the patient dose.

The single most important factor in reducing the patient dose is limiting or eliminating retakes. A retake doubles the patient dose to obtain information that should have been obtained with the initial exposure. Retakes can be reduced by careful patient positioning, selection of correct exposure techniques, and good communication so that the patient knows what is expected of her or him. Reducing the exposure time, by choosing a higher-mA station with a corresponding shorter time or by selecting a faster film/screen combination when one is available, will reduce retakes due to patient motion. Shielding of the patient's gonads when it does not compromise the diagnostic content of the image will reduce the gonadal dose.

EFFECTIVE DOSE

The **effective dose** of an examination is that dose to the whole body that would cause the same harm as a partial or localized dose for a particular x-ray examination. Effective dose is introduced to account for the irradiation of different parts of the body. The hazardous effects of whole-body radiation have been extensively studied. Irradiating a portion of the body does not produce the same ill effects as a whole-body exposure to the same dose. A whole-body exposure of 7 Gy (700 rad) is a lethal dose, but if the radiation dose is delivered to a localized portion of the body, the effects are less severe. Radiation therapy patients routinely receive 70 Gy (7,000 rad) to portions of their body during cancer treatment and survive for many years.

The effective dose relates the actual dose to a portion of the body to the dose that would produce the same harm if delivered to the whole body. The effective dose is obtained by multiplying the dose to a particular organ by a weighting factor. Table 22.2 gives the organs and the weighting factors that are used in calculating the effective dose.

Table 22.2
Organs and Weighting Factors Used in Calculating Effective Dose

Organ	Weighting Factor
Gonads	0.20
Active bone marrow	0.12
Colon	0.12
Lungs	0.12
Stomach	0.12
Bladder	0.05
Breasts	0.05
Esophagus	0.05
Liver	0.05
Thyroid	0.05
Bone surfaces	0.01
Skin	0.01
Remainder	0.05
Total	1.00

The effective dose from a posteroanterior chest examination is about 0.1 millisievert (mSv) [10 millirem (mrem)] although the entrance dose is about 0.70 mSv (70 mrem). The difference between the entrance dose and the effective dose occurs because many of the organs used to calculate the effective dose are not exposed to the primary beam during the examination.

REGULATIONS

Federal and state regulations have been established to limit occupational exposures. An occupational exposure is a radiation exposure received during normal work duties. There are limits on the whole-body dose, the dose to the lens of the eye, and the dose to any other organ of the body. Table 22.3 presents a summary of the limits on annual doses to occupational workers, the public, and the fetuses of declared pregnant radiation workers. The employer must ensure that no worker's annual dose exceeds these limits.

The limit on the whole-body dose for a radiation worker is 50 mSv (5 rem or 5000 mrem) per year. The dose limit per quarter is 12.5 mSv (1.25 rem or 1250 mrem). There is also a limit on the total dose that can be accumulated in a lifetime, which is called the cumulative limit. The cumulative limit is the age in years times 10 mSv (or the age in years times 1 rem). For example, the cumulative limit for a 32-year-old technologist is 320 mSv (32 rem). The annual

Table 22.3

Regulations on the Annual Exposures of Workers, the Fetus, and the Public to Radiation

Classification	Effective Dose Limit
Radiation workers	50 mSv (5000 rem)
Lens of the eye	150 mSv (15,000 mrem)
Extremities or any other organ	500 mSv (50,000 mrem)
Cumulative dose to worker	Age in years × 10 mSv (Age × 1 rem)
General public	1 mSv (100 mrem)
Fetus	5 mSv (500 mrem)

limit for nonradiation workers and the general public is 1 mSv (100 millirem). The fetus of a pregnant radiologic technologist must be limited to a dose of less than 5 mSv (500 millirem) for the entire pregnancy, and it is recommended that the dose be spread out so that the fetal dose is less than 0.5 mSv (50 millirem) per month.

Although most x-ray technologists never receive even a small fraction of the annual dose limit, they are still issued personnel radiation monitors. The regulations require issuing a personnel dose monitor to any staff member who might be exposed to more than 10 percent of the limits listed in Table 22.3. Most radiology departments change the personnel monitors monthly, but the monitoring interval can be as long as 3 months. A pregnant technologist must be furnished with a second personnel monitor to be worn under the protective apparel at the abdominal level (the "belly badge") to provide an estimate of the monthly fetal dose. The personnel monitoring reports should be available for review by all monitored individuals.

To reduce the dose to patients, the technologist should use increased kVp, lower mAs, and faster film/screen combinations. Decreased exposure time will reduce patient motion artifacts. Careful positioning and good communication with the patient will reduce retakes. The effective dose relates the actual dose given to a portion of the body to the dose that would produce the same harm if delivered to the entire body. The dose to a radiation worker is limited to 50 mSv (5 rem or 5000 mrem) per year to the whole body, 150 mSv (15 rem or 15,000 mrad) per year to the eye, and 500 mSv (50 rem or 50,000 mrem) per year to the extremities. The cumulative dose cannot exceed 10 × N mSv (N rem), where N is the worker's age in years. The fetus of a pregnant technologist cannot receive more than 5 mSv (0.5 rem or 500 mrem) throughout the entire pregnancy. Pregnant technologists must be issued a second "belly badge" to be worn at the abdominal level under the apron to estimate the dose to the fetus. Personnel radiation monitors must be issued to staff members who might receive 10 percent or more of the annual limits.

EQUIPMENT REGULATIONS

There are also federal and state regulations on radiation-producing equipment.

Fluoroscopic and radiographic tubes operating at 70 kVp must have a half-value layer of at least 2.5 mm aluminum equivalent. The leakage radiation from the housing of the x-ray tube must be less than 1 mSv/h (100 mR/h) at a distance of 1 m. There must be a timer that sounds an audible alarm after 5 min of fluoroscopy beam on time.

Fluoroscopy units must have dose rates of less than 100 mSv/min (10 R/min) at the tabletop, unless there is an audible alarm that sounds during the high-dose-rate mode. Fixed fluoroscopic units must have at least 38 cm (15 in.) distance between the focal spot and the tabletop. C-arm and portable fluoroscopic units must have 30 cm (12 in.) distance between the focal spot and the patient entrance surface.

RADIATION DETECTORS

Gas-Filled Detectors

Ion chambers and **Geiger counters** are gas-filled detectors that collect the ions produced by radiation. The ions are collected and amplified to produce the output signal.

Gas-filled detectors are sensitive to low levels of radiation. They are used in survey instruments to detect radioactive contamination, as detectors in CT scanners, and as calibration instruments for the calibration of x-ray tubes and nuclear medicine dose calibrators. Figure 22.3 shows portable Geiger counters and ion chambers used for radiation surveys.

Scintillation Detectors

Scintillators are crystals that give off light when struck by radiation. The amount of light depends on the radiation energy deposited in the crystal. Higher radiation energy deposited results in greater light emission. The light emitted by the crystal is detected by a photomultiplier tube, which converts the light output into an electrical output signal. Scintillators are used as detectors in CT scanners and nuclear medicine cameras.

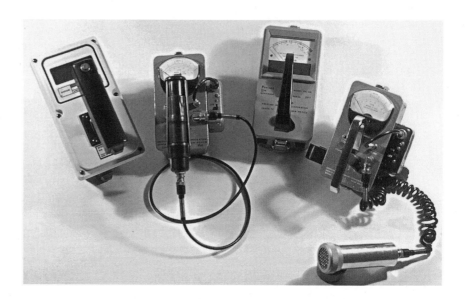

Figure 22.3 Portable survey meters.

Personnel Monitors

There are two types of personnel monitors: film badges and TLD monitors. Film badges contain a small piece of film that will have a specific optical density after exposure to radiation and development. The higher the exposure, the greater the optical density. Personnel monitors using film as a detector have copper and aluminum filters to estimate the energy of the radiation. An energy correction, obtained from the optical densities under the filters, is applied to calculate the radiation dose from the unfiltered optical density. TLD monitors do not require a set of filters because their energy response is effectively the same as that of tissue. Figure 22.4 shows a variety of personnel monitors.

Film

Film is used as a radiation detector in personnel monitor dosimeters. These are often referred to as **film badges.** The optical density of the film is measured after exposure to radiation and converted into a radiation dose in tissue. The silver halide in the film emulsion makes the film response very sensitive to x-ray energy. Radiation energies near the K-edge of silver are preferentially absorbed and produce correspondingly higher optical densities. Filters must be included in the personnel monitor to determine the radiation energy so that appropriate corrections can be applied to obtain the correct dose to tissue. Film is sensitive to heat, light, and moisture as well as radiation. Personnel monitor dosimeters that use film must be kept dry and cool. Storing them in a hot car during the summer or passing them through a washing machine will render them useless.

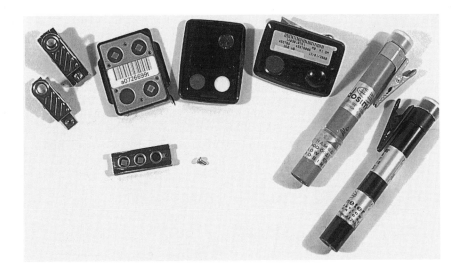

Figure 22.4 Personnel radiation monitors.

Thermoluminescent Dosimeters

A thermoluminescent dosimeter (**TLD**) uses a lithium fluoride crystal as the radiation detector. When it is exposed to x-rays, the lithium fluoride crystal traps the radiation energy. This trapped energy can be released as light by heating the crystals to over 100°C. The light is detected by a photomultiplier tube and converted into an electrical output signal. These dosimeters are called thermoluminescent dosimeters because they give off light after heating. The amount of light is proportional to the radiation dose absorbed in the crystal. Lithium fluoride has almost exactly the same energy response to radiation as human tissue.

Monitoring Period

The monitoring period for personnel dosimeters is usually 1 month. After the monitoring period is over, the film badge or TLD monitor is returned to the supplier for reading. The film is developed, and the optical density is converted to a radiation dose in tissue. The lithium fluoride crystal from the TLD monitor is heated to over 100°C, and the amount of light released is converted to a radiation dose in tissue. Both types of personnel monitors can detect radiation levels below about 20 mrad. The personnel monitor must be worn on the collar or sleeve outside the protective apparel. The clip on the monitor should be closest to the body, with the face of the monitor directed outward away from the body. Radiation received as a patient is not included in the occupational exposure. An individual's personnel monitoring badge must not be worn during an x-ray examination as a patient.

ALARA

All radiation protection programs must operate under the principle of keeping the radiation exposure to staff, patients, and public as low as reasonably achievable (**ALARA**). This means that steps must be taken to reduce radiation exposure below regulatory limits. Technical factors such as kVp, mA, distance, shielding, filtration, collimation, SID, beam area, and type of image receptor all influence the radiation levels to the staff and public.

NATURAL BACKGROUND RADIATION

Natural background radiation arises from three sources: cosmic rays from outer space, terrestrial radiation from radioactive dirt and rocks, and internal radiation. Table 22.4 compares the natural background radiation levels of cities at sea level, such as Chicago, and cities at higher altitudes in the west, such as Denver, Salt Lake City, or Albuquerque. Both the terrestrial radiation from the earth and the cosmic radiation are higher for cities at higher altitudes. Internal radiation is primarily from ^{40}K, which is naturally present in potassium-rich foods such as nuts and bananas. Internal radiation does not change with geographic location. The values in Table 22.4 do not include contributions from radon gas, which may contribute an additional 2 mSv (200 mrem) per year but varies greatly from location to location. Table 22.5 lists some representative radiographic examinations and their effective doses for comparison with natural background radiation.

Both film and thermoluminescent dosimeters are used as personnel monitors. Annual exposures must be limited to less than 50 mSv (5000 mrem) to the whole body, 500 mSv (50,000 mrem) to other organs, and 150 mSv (15,000 mrem) to the eye. Personnel monitors must be worn at collar level outside protective apparel. Radiation protection programs must follow the principles of ALARA and keep exposures as low as reasonably achievable. Workers must be monitored if they might

Table 22.4
Annual Natural Background Radiation

	Denver	Chicago
Internal	0.40 mSv (40 mrem)	0.40 mSv (40 mrem)
Cosmic	0.80 mSv (80 mrem)	0.30 mSv (30 mrem)
Terrestrial	0.80 mSv (80 mrem)	0.35 mSv (30 mrem)
Total	2 mSv (200 mrem)	1 mSv (100 mrem)

Table 22.5
Examples of Effective Doses from Representative Diagnostic Examinations

Examination	Effective Dose
Head (AP and LAT)	51 µSv (5.1 mrem)
Chest (AP and LAT)	82 µSv (8.2 mrem)
Abdomen (AP)	490 µSv (49 mrem)
Lumbar spine (AP and LAT)	700 µSv (70 mrem)
Pelvis (AP)	500 µSv (50 mrem)
Barium enema	
(6 spot films and 1 min fluoroscopy)	3700 µSv (370 mrem)
Fluoroscopy	720 µSv/min (72 mrem/min)
CT	
Head	2000 µSv (200 mrem)
Body	13,500 µSv (1350 mrem)

AP = anteroposterior; CT = computed tomography; LAT = lateral.

receive 10 percent or more of the annual limits. Natural background radiation contributes from 1 to 3 mSv (100 to 300 mrem) annually. Natural background radiation is made up of cosmic, terrestrial, and internal radiation.

SUMMARY

The three methods for reducing radiation exposure are reduction of time, increase in distance, and increase in shielding. Primary barriers protect against primary radiation; secondary barriers protect against secondary radiation, which includes scatter and leakage radiation. The effective dose is the whole-body dose that would produce the same harm as a partial-body dose. It is obtained by adding up the doses from a selected group of organs. The maximum allowed annual effective dose to the whole body of a radiation worker is 50 mSv (5000 mrem). The maximum allowed annual effective dose to the eyes of a radiation worker is 150 mSv (15,000 mrem). The maximum allowed annual effective dose to other organs of the body is 500 mSv (50,000 mrem). The public is limited to no more than 1 mSv (100 mrem) per year. Radiation workers who might receive more than 10 percent of the maximum annual effective dose must be monitored. The personnel monitor should be worn on the outside of the protective apparel near the collar. Gas-filled detectors are used to calibrate x-ray units. TLDs are used in personnel monitors and must be heated to obtain a reading. ALARA means that steps must be taken to reduce radiation levels to the staff and public to as low as reasonably achievable. Natural background radiation arises from cosmic radiation from outer space, terrestrial radiation from the earth, and internal radiation. The natural background in locations about 1 mile high, such as Denver, Salt Lake City, or Albuquerque, is 2 mSv per year, whereas locations at sea level have background radiation of about 1 mSv per year.

QUESTIONS

1. The natural background radiation at sea level is about _____ mSv per year.
   a. 0.5
   b. 1.0
   c. 2.0
   d. 3.0
2. The natural background radiation in Denver or some other mile-high city is _____ mSv per year.
   a. 0.5
   b. 1.0
   c. 2.0
   d. 3.0
3. The maximum allowed effective dose to a radiation worker is _____ mSv per year.
   a. 15
   b. 50
   c. 500
   d. 1500
4. The maximum allowed effective dose to the eyes of a radiation worker is _____ mSv per year.
   a. 50
   b. 150
   c. 500
   d. 1500
5. The maximum allowed effective dose to other organs of the body of a radiation worker is _____ mSv per year.
   a. 15
   b. 50
   c. 500
   d. 1500
6. The personnel monitor should be worn
   a. under the protective apparel near the waist.
   b. outside the protective apparel near the collar.
   c. under the protective apparel near the collar.
   d. outside the protective apparel near the waist.

7. The detector that requires heating to obtain a dose reading is the
   a. gas-filled detector.
   b. scintillator.
   c. TLD.
   d. GM counter.
8. The detector that is used to calibrate x-ray units is the
   a. gas-filled detector.
   b. scintillator.
   c. TLD.
   d. GM counter.
9. Methods to reduce radiation exposure are to the staff include
   1. Reduce time.
   2. Increase distance.
   3. Reduce shielding.
   4. Reduce field size.
   a. 1, 2, 3, and 4.
   b. 1, 2, and 4.
   c. 2, 3, and 4.
   d. 1 and 2.
10. ALARA means
    a. as low as readily achievable.
    b. always low and readily accessible.
    c. always low and really achievable.
    d. as low as reasonably achievable.
11. Radiation workers must be badged if they may receive more than _____ percent of the maximum allowed annual dose.
    a. 5
    b. 10
    c. 20
    d. 25
12. The components of natural background are
    1. cosmic radiation
    2. medical radiation
    3. terrestrial radiation
    4. internal radiation
    a. 1, 2, 3, and 4.
    b. 1, 2, and 3.
    c. 2, 3, and 4.
    d. 1, 3, and 4.
13. The maximum allowed effective dose to the general public is _____ mSv per year.
    a. 1
    b. 5
    c. 50
    d. 150

14. Primary barriers protect against _____ radiation.
    a. direct
    b. leakage and scatter
15. Secondary barriers protect against _____ radiation.
    a. direct
    b. leakage and scatter
16. Lead aprons and other protective apparel should be inspected for hidden cracks at least
    a. daily.
    b. weekly.
    c. monthly.
    d. annually.
17. The HVL is the amount of shielding required to reduce the transmitted intensity to _____ the original intensity.
    a. 0.1
    b. 0.25
    c. 0.5
    d. 1.5
18. Secondary radiation is made up of _____ radiation.
    a. leakage and scattered
    b. primary, leakage and scattered
    c. scattered and secondary
    d. leakage and primary
19. The major source of radiation exposure to radiology personnel is the
    a. primary beam.
    b. Bucky.
    c. image intensifier.
    d. patient.
20. The technologist is allowed to hold a patient during an exposure
    a. when the patient is in danger of falling.
    b. when the patient is a baby.
    c. when the patient is in pain.
    d. never.
21. A protective apron should be assigned to _____ portable units.
    a. all
    b. most
    c. many
    d. no
22. The typical lead shielding thickness in diagnostic x-ray room walls is _____ mm.
    a. 0.25
    b. 0.50
    c. 1.6
    d. 2.5

23. Which of the following is a primary barrier?
    1. Wall with vertical Bucky cassette holder
    2. Wall of the control booth
    3. Floor
    a. 1
    b. 1 and 3
    c. 2 and 3
    d. 1, 2, 3, and 4
24. The x-ray tube housing must limit leakage radiation to less than ____ mR/h at 1 m.
    a. 50
    b. 100
    c. 250
    d. 500
25. Which of the following is *not* an occupational exposure?
    a. Scattered radiation received from an orthopedic C-arm fluoroscopic unit
    b. Scattered radiation received from a portable examination
    c. Scattered radiation received from a fluoroscopy unit
    d. Radiation received as a patient

ANSWERS TO CHAPTER 22 QUESTIONS

1.	b	14.	a
2.	c	15.	b
3.	b	16.	d
4.	b	17.	c
5.	c	18.	a
6.	b	19.	d
7.	c	20.	d
8.	a	21.	a
9.	b	22.	c
10.	d	23.	b
11.	b	24.	b
12.	d	25.	d
13.	a		

Glossary

A

ABC. Automatic brightness control of a fluoroscope.

absorption. Complete transfer of the x-ray's energy to an atom.

ADC. Analog-to-digital converter.

AEC. Automatic exposure control.

air gap. A technique that uses increased OID to reduce scatter radiation reaching the image receptor.

ALARA. As low as reasonably achievable.

alternating current. Current that flows in a positive direction for half of the cycle and then in a negative direction for the other half of the cycle.

ammonium thiosulfate. The clearing agent in the fixer solution. It removes the undeveloped silver halide crystals from the emulsion.

ampere. The unit of electric current; it is the number of electrons flowing in a conductor.

AMU. Atomic mass unit. One AMU equals 1.6×10^{-27} kilogram, the mass of the proton or neutron.

anode. The positive electrode of an x-ray tube which contains the target that is struck by the projectile electrons.

anode angle. The angle between the anode surface and the central ray of the x-ray beam.

artifact. An unwanted density or image on the radiograph.

Atomic mass. The number of nucleons (neutrons plus protons) in the nucleus.

Atomic number. The number of protons in the nucleus.

Atomic weight. The average of the atomic masses of the isotopes of an element weighted by their natural occurrence.

attenuation. The removal of x-rays from the beam by either absorption or scattering.

automatic brightness control. A circuit that maintains the fluoroscopic image at a constant brightness.

autotransformer. Transformer with a single winding used to change the input voltage to a step-up or step-down transformer.

B

bar phantom. An alternating series of radiopaque and radiolucent strips of different separations used to directly measure the imaging system resolution.

beam quality. The penetrating characteristics of the x-ray beam.

beam quantity. The amount or intensity of the x-ray beam.

BMD. Bone mineral densitometry.

bore. The opening in an MRI magnet.

bremsstrahlung. X-rays produced when projectile electrons are stopped or slowed in the anode.

Bucky factor. The ratio of the mAs required with a grid to the mAs required without a grid to produce the same optical density. The amount of mAs increase required when a grid is added.

Bucky grid. A moving grid designed to blur out the grid lines and absorb scatter radiation.

C

capacitor An electrical device used to temporarily store electrical charge.

carcinogen. A material agent which causes cancer. Ionionizing radiation is a carcinogen.

cassette. A light-tight container with intensifying screens used to hold the x-ray film.

cataract. A cloudiness or opacity of the lens of the eye.

cathode. The negative electrode of an x-ray tube which contains the filament that emits electrons for x-ray production.

characteristic curve. A graph of optical density and relative exposure which is characteristic of a particular type of x-ray film.

characteristic x-ray production. X-ray production that occurs when an orbital electron fills a vacancy in the shell of the anode.

chromosomes. Clusters of genes made up of DNA molecules.

cine. Cinefluorography is associated with rapid (30 frames per second or more) sequence filming.

CNS syndrome. Central nervous system syndrome following high-dose, whole-body radiation exposure.

coherent scattering. Low-energy scattering involving no loss of photon energy, only a change in photon direction.

conduction. Transfer of heat through solid materials.

conductor. A material in which electrons can move freely.

contrast agent. Material added to the body to increase the subject contrast. Contrast media have densities and atomic numbers very different from body tissues.

convection. Transfer of heat through motion of air or a liquid.

conversion efficiency. A measure of a screen's efficiency in converting x-ray energy into light energy.

coulomb. The unit of electric charge.

Coulomb's law. The law describing the force between two electric charges.

CR. Computed radiography.

crossover racks. Part of the automatic film processor system designed to transport the film from one solution to the next solution.

CT. Computed tomography.

D

DAC. Digital-to-analog converter.

densitometer. A device used to measure the amount of light transmitted through the film and giving the numerical value of its optical density.

detail. The degree of geometric sharpness or resolution of an object recorded as an image.

detail screens. Intensifying screens used for higher resolution imaging such as extremity examinations.

developer. The chemical solution in the x-ray processor that converts exposed silver halide grains into metallic silver.

dewar. An insulated vacuum container.

direct current. Current that flows in only one direction.

DNA. Deoxyribonucleic acid. The genetic material in each cell. DNA molecules have two strands of nucleic acid.

D_O. The mean lethal dose as obtained from a cell survival curve.

domains. Small groups of iron molecules in magnets.

doubling dose. The radiation dose which would double the genetic mutation rate.

D_Q. The threshold dose in a cell survival curve.

DR. Direct radiography.

E

effective dose. The dose to the whole body which would cause the same harm as the actual dose received from the examination.

electric current. The movement of electrons in a material such as a conductor or semiconductor.

electrical generator. A device that converts mechanical energy to electrical energy.

electromagnetic induction. Production of a current in a conductor by a changing magnetic field near the conductor.

E_{max}. The maximum energy of the x-ray beam.

EMF. Electromotive force; electrical potential which is measured in volts (V) or kilovolts (kV).

emulsion. The gelatin layer containing the silver halide grains coated on the film base.

epilation. Loss of hair.

erythema. Skin reddening.

ESE. Entrance skin exposure.

exit radiation. The combination of transmitted and scattered radiation that passes through the patient.

exposure linearity. Measures the change in radiation output as the mAs are increased. The mR/mAs should remain constant with changes in mAs.

exposure reproducibility. A series of exposures with the same mAs, but different values of mA and time should produce the same radiation output.

F

Faraday cage. A screen surrounding an MRI room to prevent external RF energy from entering the room.

ferromagnetic. Material that is strongly attracted to a magnet and can be magnetized.

FFD. Focus film distance. The distance between the focal spot and the film. This term has been replaced by SID.

fifteen percent rule. To maintain the same optical density, a 15% change in kVp requires a factor of 2 compensating change in mAs.

filament. The source of electrons in the cathode.

film badge. A personal dose monitor which uses film as the radiation detector.

film cassette. A light-tight container with intensifying screens used to hold the x-ray film.

film contrast. The difference in optical density between a region of interest and its surroundings.

film speed. A measure of film sensitivity; faster films require less exposure.

fixer. The chemical solution in the x-ray processor that stops the reducing action of the developer and removes the unexposed silver halide crystals from the plastic film base.

fluorescence. The production of light in the intensifying screen phosphor by x-rays.

fluoroscopy. Dynamic x-ray technique for viewing moving structures.

focal spot. The area on the anode where the projectile electrons strike, the source of x-rays.

focused grid. A grid whose radiopaque lead strips are tilted to align, at a predetermined SID, with the divergent x-ray beam.

FOV. Field of view.

frequency. The number of cycles per second of a wave, usually expressed in hertz (Hz).

fringe field. The magnetic field extending outside the bore of an MRI magnet.

G

gas-filled ionization chamber. A radiation detector based on measurement of the ionization of a gas. Used for calibration of x-ray units.

gauss (G). A unit of magnetism.

GBX filter. A safelight filter which produces a deep red light, which is safe for green sensitive orthochromatic films.

Geiger counter. A gas-filled radiation detector used to survey for leakage radiation and detect areas of radioactive contamination.

genetic cells. Cells of the reproductive organs.

germ cells. Immature genetic cells.

GI syndrome. The gastrointestinal syndrome following a high dose, whole-body radiation exposure.

glutaraldehyde. A chemical in the developing solution which retards film emulsion swelling and hardens the emulsion during drying.

gradient coils. Coils used to select the imaging plane in MRI.

grid. Scatter reduction device consisting of alternating strips of radiopaque and radiolucent material.

grid cutoff. The interception of transmitted x-rays by the radiopaque strips of a grid, resulting in lighter density at one or both edges of the field.

grid frequency. The number of lead strips per cm or per inch.

grid ratio. The ratio of the height of the lead strips to the distance between the lead strips in a grid.

GSD. Genetically significant dose.

guide shoe marks. Negative density line artifacts parallel to the direction of film travel through the processor. Caused by scratches in the film emulsion by improperly aligned guide shoes.

guide shoes. Part of the automatic processor film transport system which changes the direction of the film in the developer, fixer, or wash solutions.

Gurney Mott theory. A theory of how the silver halide grains are exposed to form a latent image and developed to form a visible radiographic image.

H

Heel effect. Decreased intensity from the cathode side of the x-ray beam to the anode side. The lightest part of an image is at the anode side of the image.

hematologic syndrome. The depression of blood cells and the body's infection fighting ability following whole-body radiation exposure.

high-speed screens. Intensifying screens used for examinations that require short exposure times. The use of high-speed screens results in lower patient dose.

high-voltage transformer. A high-voltage transformer converts low voltage to high voltage.

HVL. Half-value layer. A measure of the penetration of an x-ray beam. The thickness required to reduce the x-ray intensity to half its original value.

hydroquinone. A reducing agent in the developing solution that changes the silver halide crystals into metallic silver.

I

image intensifier. Converts x-rays into a brighter visible image.

indexing. Movement of the patient support table by a specified amount.

insulator. A material in which electrons are fixed and cannot move freely.

intensification factor. The ratio of mAs values required to produce the same optical density without and with an intensifying screen.

intensifying screen. Increases the efficiency of x-ray absorption and decreases the dose to the patient by converting x-ray energy into visible light energy.

inverse square law. The inverse square law states that the intensity is inversely proportional to the square of the distance.

ion chamber. A gas-filled radiation detector used to calibrate x-ray tube output.

ion pair. A positive and a negative ion is termed an ion pair.

isotopes. Isotopes are atoms of the same element whose nuclei contain the same number of protons but a different number of neutrons.

K

keV. Kiloelectron volts. A measure of the energy of an x-ray photon or an electron.

kVp. Kilovoltage potential. A measure of the voltage applied to the x-ray tube.

L

Larmor frequency. The resonant frequency of a hydrogen proton in a magnetic field.

latent image. The undeveloped distribution of exposed silver halide grains in the film emulsion.

latent period. During the latent period the exposed individual has no clinical symptoms or illness from the radiation and appears to have recovered with no ill effects.

$LD_{50/30}$. The whole body dose, which will produce death in 50% of the exposed population within 30 days.

leakage radiation. Radiation outside the primary x-ray beam emitted through the tube housing.

LET. A description of how ionization energy is deposited along the radiation path in tissue.

level control. The electronic control that sets the density value to displayed as the center of the density range.

linear nonthreshold dose response model. The dose response model, with no threshold, based on a linear response to radiation exposure.

liquid helium. Helium gas cooled below 23°K to produce a liquid.

LNT. Linear nonthreshold dose-response model.

long-scale contrast image. An image with many densities between black and white. A low-contrast image.

M

mA. Milliamperes, 1/1000 ampere.

magnification. An increase in the image size of an object.

main magnet coil. The superconducting coil, which produces the external magnetic field in an MRI system.

mammography. The radiographic examination of the breast used to detect breast cancer.

mAs. Milliampere-seconds; milliamperes multiplied by the exposure time.

matrix. A group of numbers arranged in rows and columns.

medium-speed screens. Intensifying screens used for routine imaging.

meiosis. Division of genetic cells.

mitosis. Division of somatic cells.

molybdenum. A metal element used in mammographic filters and anodes.

motor. An electrical device used to convert electrical energy into mechanical energy.

MQSA. Mammographic Quality Standards Act. The federal standard for mammographic imaging.

MR. Magnetic resonance.

MRI. Magnetic resonance imaging.

N

natural background radiation. Radiation from natural sources.

negative density area. An area of lighter density on the film.

NM. Nuclear medicine.

nucleons. Nuclear particles, either neutrons or protons.

O

OER. Oxygen enhancement ratio. A measure of how much the radiosensitivity of a cell type is increased by the presence of oxygen.

ohm. The unit of electrical resistance (Ω)

Ohm's law. The relation between voltage, current, and resistance.

OID. Object to image receptor distance..

optical densitometer. A device to measure the blackness or optical desnity of a film.

optical density. A measure of the degree of blackness of the film expressed on a logarithmic scale.

orthochromatic film. Film sensitive to light from green-light-emitting screens.

output taps. The output connections of an autotransformer.

P

panchromatic film. Film sensitive to all wavelengths of visible light.

parallel grid. A grid that has parallel lead strips.

paramagnetic materials. Materials that react weakly to magnetic fields.

PBL. Positive beam limitation device. An automatic collimator that adjusts the field size to match the cassette size in the Bucky tray.

permanent magnet. An MRI magnet made of ferromagnetic material which utilizes an electric current to produce the magnetic field.

phenidone. A reducing agent in the developing solution that changes the silver halide crystals into metallic silver.

phosphor. Material which converts x-rays into visible light.

phosphorescence. The continuation of light emission from intensifying screens after the stimulation from the x-rays ceases (afterglow).

photocathode. Converts x-rays into electrons in the image intensifier.

photoelectric interaction. Complete absorption of the incident photon by the atom.

photoelectron. An electron ejected from an atom following a photoelectric interaction.

photomultiplier. A tube which converts light into an electrical signal.

photomultiplier tube. An electrical device that converts a light signal into an electrical signal.

photon. Electromagnetic radiation acting as a particle.

pi marks. Positive density artifacts on a film perpendicular to film travel through the processor separated by 3.14 inches.

pinhole camera. A device used to produce an image of the x-ray tube focal spot.

pixel. A picture element of a matrix which contains information on its location and intensity.

PMT. Photomultiplier tube.

positive density area. Darker area on the film.

power. The amount of energy used per second. Electric power is the current multiplied by the voltage and is measured in watts.

precession. The rotation of a spinning hydrogen proton around the external magnetic field.

primary beam. The useful x-ray beam emitted from the x-ray tube.

primary radiation. The direct, collimated, useful x-ray beam.

primary winding. The input winding of a transformer.

prodromal stage. The first stage of radiation response following an exposure, in which signs and symptoms are demonstrated.

Q

quality. The penetrating characteristics or energy of the x-ray beam.

quality control. The measurement and evaluation of radiologic equipment.

quantity. The intensity or amount of x-rays.

quantum mottle. The random speckled appearance of an image, similar to the "snow" seen with poor TV reception. Quantum mottle is greater when high-speed screens and low-mAs techniques are used, because there are fewer interacting x-rays.

R

radiation heat transfer. Transfer of heat by infrared radiation.

radioactive decay. The transformation of radioactive nuclei into a different element followed by the emission of particulate or electromagnetic radiation.

radiographic contrast. A combination of film and subject contrast.

radiographic noise. Also termed *quantum mottle*. The random speckled appearance of an image caused by too few interacting x-rays. Often seen in images produced with high-speed screens and low-mAs techniques.

radioisotope. An unstable isotope which spontaneously transforms into more stable isotopes with the emission of radiation.

radiolucent. Low-attenuating material.

radiopaque. Highly attenuating material.

rare-earth screens. Rare-earth phosphors employed in intensifying screens such as gadolinium, lanthanum, and yttrium.

RBE. Relative biologic effectiveness. A measure of biologic damage from radiation.

reciprocity law. The same mAs, regardless of the values of mA and seconds, should give the same image density.

rectifier. An electrical device that allows current to flow only in one direction. Rectifiers are used to convert AC into DC.

resistance. The opposition to current flow.

resonance. The absorption or emission of energy only at a certain specific frequency.

RF. Radio frequency.

RF pulse. A short burst of RF energy at a specific frequency; used in MRI.

rhodium. A metal element used in mammographic anodes and filters.

ripple. The variation between the maximum voltage and minimum voltage.

RNA. Ribonucleic acid. RNA molecules are similar to DNA molecules but have only a single strand of nucleic acid whereas the DNA molecules have two strands.

rotor. The central rotating component of an electric motor, used to rotate the anode.

S

safelight. A light in the darkroom, usually red filtered, designed to provide low-level, low-energy illumination without exposing the film.

scattering. The photon interaction with an atom resulting in a change of direction and loss of energy.

scintillation detectors. A radiation detector that, when irradiated, emits a burst of light.

scintillator. A crystal which gives off light when struck by radiation.

secondary radiation. A combination of scattered and leakage radiation.

semiconductor. A material which can act as conductor or insulator, depending on how it is made and its environment.

sensitometer. A device that uses light to produce a stepwedge image for processor quality assurance.

shim coils. Coils used to improve the uniformity of the main magnetic field in an MRI unit.

short-contrast-scale image. An image with few density differences between black and white. A high-contrast image.

SID. Source to image receptor distance. The distance from the radiation source to the image receptor.

SOD. Source to object distance. The distance from the radiation source to the object under examination.

sodium sulfite. Chemical added to both the developer and fixer solutions to remove oxidizing agents and maintain chemical balance.

solid-state detector. A radiation detector based on measurement of ionization in a solid.

somatic cells. All cells in the human body that are not genetic cells.

spatial resolution. The minimum separation at which two objects can be recognized as two separate objects.

spectral matching. Matching the wavelength or color of the light from the intensifying screen to the film sensitivity.

spinning top. A quality control test tool formerly used to measure timer accuracy.

SSD. Source to skin distance.

stator. The fixed windings of an electric motor.

stem cells. Young or immature somatic cells.

step-down transformer. A transformer that has more turns in the primary winding than in the secondary winding, which decreases the voltage.

step-up transformer. A transformer that has more turns in the secondary winding than in the primary winding, which increases the voltage.

subject contrast. The difference in x-ray transmission between different areas of the body. The primary controlling factor is kVp.

superconducting magnet. A magnet whose coils are made of a superconducting material and which produce the external magnetic field in an MRI unit.

superconductor. A material in which electrons can flow freely with no resistance when the material is cooled to an extremely low temperature.

surface coils. Coils which detect the weak RF signals from the precessing protons that produce the MR image.

syndrome. A group of signs or symptoms associated with a specific condition, such as acute radiation exposure.

T

T1 relaxation time. The time it takes a proton to relax back into alignment with the external magnetic field.

T2 relaxation time. The time it takes the protons to lose their phase after being moved out of alignment by an RF pulse.

tesla. A unit of magnetism.

thermionic emission. The emission of electrons by heating of the filament in the cathode.

thermostat. Electrical device to control the developer solution temperature.

threshold dose. The radiation dose at which biologic effects become evident.

TLD. Thermoluminescent dosimeter. A radiation detector which, when heated, gives off an amount of light proportional to the radiation exposure.

transformer. An electrical device to change voltage from low to high or vice versa.

tube current. The current of projectile electrons that passes inside the x-ray tube from cathode to anode. Measured in mA.

turns ratio. The ratio of the number of turns of coils in the secondary windings to the number of turns in the primary windings of a transformer.

TVL. Tenth-value layer. The amount of shielding material required to reduce the radiation intensity to one-tenth its original value.

U

US. Ultrasound.

V

VCR. Video cassette recorder.

voltage. A measure of electrical force or pressure.

voxel. A volume element in a CT or MR examination.

W

wavelength. The distance between adjacent peaks or adjacent valleys of a wave.

window control. For digital images, the electronic control that sets the number of density differences between black and white that are displayed.

Index

Note: Page numbers in italics indicate figures; those followed by t indicate tables.

NOTES

NOTES

NOTES

NOTES

NOTES

NOTES

NOTES